Your Blueprint for Strong Immunity

This book is dedicated to anyone who has ever suffered with poor health alone, without compassion.

Your Blueprint for Strong Immunity

Personalise your diet and lifestyle for better health

Dr Jenna Macciochi

yellow kite

The information in this book is not intended to constitute medical advice, nor is it intended to replace or conflict with the advice given to you by your doctor or other health professional. Before implementing any recommendations on diet, supplements and exercise set out in this book, you should discuss them with your doctor, especially if you have any medical condition or if you are taking any medication. The author and publisher disclaim any liability directly or indirectly from the use of the material in this book by any person.

First published in Great Britain in 2022 by Yellow Kite
An Imprint of Hodder & Stoughton
An Hachette UK company

5

The image on page 308 is from Shutterstock
All other images are by Dr Jenna Macciochi

A CIP catalogue record for this title is available from the British Library

Trade Paperback ISBN 978 1 529 36360 9
eBook ISBN 978 1 529 36361 6

Typeset in Freight Text Pro by Palimpsest Book Production Ltd, Falkirk, Stirlingshire

Printed and bound in Great Britain by Clays Ltd, Elcograf S.p.A.

Yellow Kite
Hodder & Stoughton Ltd
Carmelite House
50 Victoria Embankment
London EC4Y 0DZ

www.yellowkitebooks.co.uk

Contents

Introduction 1

PART 1:
Getting Started – What You Need to Know **11**

1 Meet Your Immune System 15
2 Forget Boosting – It's All About Balance 21
3 Write Your Own Immunobiography 32
4 How Long Does it Take to Build Strong Immunity? 54

PART 2:
Building Your Foundations **71**

5 You and Food 74
6 Metabolic Health – and Why it Matters 86
7 Immune-Nourishing Nutrition 103
Recipes 151
8 The Immune–Brain Romance 192
9 Sustainable Movement 215
10 Sleep and the Science of Rest 236
11 Outside-In Immune Support – Curating a Healthy Environment 245

PART 3:
Supporting Specific Conditions **269**

12 The Battle Against Infection 273
13 Supporting Immunity When You Suffer From Allergies 294
14 Thriving with an Autoimmune Disease 325

Final Word 357
Acknowledgements 359
References 361
Index 389

A Brief Note

Your immune system is really an all-embracing and all-encompassing wellness system. It's as indispensable as your heart or lungs. But before we journey into the mysterious system that keeps us well, this is a brief note for readers and the obligatory disclaimer.

Infection, illness or any kind of disease can be scary and unsettling. But by understanding more about your immune system, my hope is that this book will provide not only a new appreciation for disease and illness, but some comfort that will allow you to nurture your health with less fear and alleviate some of the anxiety that illness brings.

The highly complex nature of the immune system means that it is subject to endless speculations and opinions. By reading this book, you will also be less susceptible to snake oil and 'immune boosting' quick fixes and learn to cast a critical eye on pervasive immunity-marketing claims. I want to leave you understanding more about this amazing system that keeps you well and feel confident in how to support your immune system both now and for the future.

This book is intended for the general population, not healthcare professionals or research scientists. The information contained within this book is not intended to constitute medical advice nor to replace or conflict with the advice given to you by your doctor or other health professional. Please view this book as a broadening of the lens to consider all the inputs into your health across your whole life and offer up some gentle practices and supplements to support you in your own health journey. Before you implement any recommendations on diet, supplement, exercise and other lifestyle changes set out in this book, you should discuss them with your doctor, especially if you have any medical condition or are taking any medication. The author and publisher disclaim any liability directly or indirectly from the use of the material in this book by any person.

Although it is not written for healthcare professionals or research scientists, you are of course very welcome to read it (and I'd be delighted if you did!). But just be aware that won't find the level of detail that this vast and complex subject area demands as I tried to keep it compassionate and clear for the general reader without a background in this field.

Introduction

Your immune system is your greatest health asset. It is nothing short of amazing.

The immune system's role in protecting you from infection is the main feature in conversations around immunity. But the immune system is not only for infection protection; it matters for so much more. As such, it should really be called your wellness system. Every inch of your mental and physical health runs through your immune system. It is a collection of incredible immune cells, cell subtypes, organs and molecules scattered throughout your body, all of which want to unleash their superpowers and keep you healthy and vital. For that to occur, you need to give your immune cells the proper resources and environment. Care for your immunity well and it will repay you in a health span rendering you less susceptible to both infection and chronic inflammatory disease.

PRIORITISE YOUR IMMUNE SYSTEM EACH DAY

You and your immune system – you're on a longevity journey together. And here's an important point to consider about longevity: you don't just want extra years tacked onto your life; you want healthy years. You want better health, and you want it for longer. Just as you care for your mind so that you can be productive and focused when needed, you care for your immune system so that you can do the things you enjoy. Prioritising your immune health is for life, not just for fighting illness.

In today's society, more and more people are living with lifestyle-related poor health. One in three adults globally suffers from multiple chronic conditions. Fifty per cent of GP appointments are with people with long-term conditions. Seventy-five per cent of the NHS budget is spent on chronic disease.[1] The reality is that our wellbeing deteriorates so insidiously over time that by the time of disease diagnosis the only option is to manage symptoms rather than address the root cause.

The issues facing us today are extremely complex. Solving them is far from a simple, quick fix and requires both a holistic view and a consistent approach.

WHY YOU NEED THIS BOOK

In the big picture of health, there are few things that can be resolved or transformed quickly. Before we can start to improve our immune systems, we need to understand its complexities – to appreciate that there are a lot of factors involved. But the overall thrust of wellness culture can make it feel like a very ambitious task to take on alone. Who to follow? What supplements to take? Is this even applicable to your personal health situation? Enthusiasm at the beginning of your health journey can quickly descend into feelings of overwhelm, confusion and self-blame if you don't achieve what you set out to do. Fear, guilt and shame as motivators for transforming your health are neither sustainable nor health-promoting in themselves.

And that's where this book comes in. It will help you to create your unique health recipe, with the 'right ingredients' used in the 'right way' for you. It is your personalised blueprint, not a one-size-fits all.

In Part 1, you will meet the bits and pieces that make up the beautiful biology of your immune system. You will get acquainted with what is considered to be one of the most complex systems in the body and the breadth of vital roles it plays. I will outline why we want a *balanced* not boosted immunity, and set the record straight on inflammation – the immune system's way of responding to things that cause harm and injury. There will be a little bit of technical language (no way to avoid that), but ultimately, you will acquire the knowledge and tools to embark upon creating your own immune-support blueprint.

I will help you to conduct an honest appraisal of your immune system, looking upstream – to identify root causes of any issues – and figuring out any areas where you are not showing up for your immune system and where balance is missing in your life. A self-assessment on pp. 41–53 allows you to consider your relationship with each of the pillars of immune health and will orientate you towards the 'lifestyle lever' you need to pull the hardest; it highlights your own Achilles heel – the part of your everyday life that is stealing your health the most. You will identify weak spots and personal imbalances in immune function that enable you to develop a truly personalised blueprint for a long lifetime of wellness. I will be helping you to learn about your individual needs for your own unique health journey, providing the knowledge and tools to make the decisions that improve it. It's about being strategic with your health by setting out clear and measurable goals, addressing negative self-talk and being tactical with your knowledge – knowing which tools to employ and when.

In Part 2, we dive into the practical steps to take across each of the five core elements of the blueprint; these are the lifestyle levers that are deeply entwined with and connected to our immunological health:

1. Inside-out immune support – what (and how) you eat
2. Mental health – navigating your immune–brain romance
3. Sustainable movement – gaining mobility, muscle and momentum
4. Sleep – and the science of rest to improve your energy and the quality of your sleep
5. Outside-in immune support – how to curate healthy surroundings

Think of it as a pie, comprised of several pieces, but the portion that needs the most focus will be different for each of us. And the journey to health and healing will look different for everyone, too. The knowledge shared in each chapter provides the framework upon which you can personalise your approach as you learn the facts, the science-backed tools and recommendations to jumpstart your lifestyle transformation on the trajectory to strong immunity. It's about exploration of you and becoming the expert in your own health by constructing your blueprint around each of the pillars of immune health.

Living well happens through the small things we do each day – every morning, afternoon and evening. No one magical supplement, superfood, diet plan or exercise routine can ensure you'll stay healthy. In these pages, however, you'll find a 360-degree approach. It's about making changes that stick – checking in on all the parts of your life that you have control over to support yourself, physically, mentally and immunologically. That way, you will be well prepared from the inside out, no matter what the future brings. When it comes to your immune system, the strongest evidence shows that simple daily actions across each of the lifestyle levers listed on p. 4 add up to a meaningful difference. I'll guide you on how to start taking effective steps in the right direction, embrace the small victories and make them count towards your wellbeing, for long-term shifts and consistent results. There's nothing wrong with starting small. That's where the greatest progress often begins.

Finally, in Part 3, we'll take a look at immunity both in crisis and in recovery. I will help you to make sense of the science and commit to the right evidence-based actions to help and heal. Although we do our best to circumvent illness, sometimes it's unavoidable. So I will address specific immune imbalances with an empowering guide to combating common, yet debilitating health challenges, such as infections, allergies and autoimmune diseases. When our circumstances put us in a situation that feels out of our control health-wise, we can seize the reins by making the right lifestyle choices. These can play a huge role in how we feel, cope and recover through different health challenges.

Your immune system is for life, not just for when you feel ill. It is as much about taking positive and preventative measures as it is about dealing with the consequences of an immunity crisis once it has engulfed you.

Immunity is not only biological but societal. COVID-19 has painfully demonstrated our vulnerabilities, reminding us that no matter how robust we might believe we are, disease can loom just around the corner reminding us that many other aspects of modern life are contagious, too: obesity, loneliness and a plethora of negative psychosocial and socioeconomic issues that have collectively been silently eroding our health. Pandemics, like any health crisis, often call for extreme temporary measures but there is opportunity in every crisis, nudging us to change our health habits for the better. Though there is no diminishing the difficulties that a jolt to your health can have.

Remember, your health is your responsibility, so when applying the tools in this book, please filter it through that lens: talk to a healthcare professional if you are going to explore any new practices and, finally, be self-compassionate in your pursuit of wellbeing.

IT'S NOT ABOUT BEING HEALTHY; IT'S ABOUT BEING HEALTH*IER*

Health is not an endpoint, nor is it a passive status quo. It's a process, a mindset, an exploration. It is ongoing across our lives. And it is highly individual.

Many of you will be familiar with the term pathogenesis. We use it quite often in the biomedical sciences to refer to the processes by which a disease develops, including the factors that contribute to its progression. The word comes from the Greek *pathos* ('suffering', 'disease') and *genesis* ('origin'). The lesser-known term 'salutogenesis' comes from the Latin *salus* ('health') and, again, the Greek *genesis*, and poses the question: how can we move towards greater health? Pathogenesis and salutogenesis are two sides of the same coin. Sadly, much of our modern-day medicine is focused on the pathogenic model: emphasis on all the scary illnesses and diseases that can await us if we don't take good care of ourselves (and sometimes even if we do). It is easier to conceptualise a disease state than a healthy state of an individual. We know that disease is caused by the presence of an insult that can be genetic, environmental or caused by a decline in normal physiological function, such as during ageing. Health, on the other hand, seems to be more metaphysical – a so-called state of 'wellbeing'.[2] As an absence of disease, health becomes somewhat passive.

Let's flip this to a different orientation – one where you are an active participant, where you are taking on particular behaviours and adopting a particular stance towards your diet, lifestyle and environment in order to promote your wellbeing above and beyond where it would otherwise be. For example, it is powerful to engage in exercise to 'burn off' those junk foods you just ate, to avoid undesirable changes in body composition or to help you move away from a family risk of heart disease. Salutogenesis involves a mindset and an orientation towards engaging in physical movement to feel good and enhance your wellbeing. It's not only moving away from sickness (pathogenesis), but towards wellness (salutogenesis). A salutogenic point of view means that rather than asking, 'How should we treat disease?' we might instead ask, 'How can we promote and maintain health?' It is proactive rather than reactive – because ultimately it is easier to stay well than it is to overcome sickness.

Attaining a healthy lifestyle is never going to be effortless because our modern-day environment just isn't conducive to it. In fact, there is almost no example in healthcare where the same thing helps everybody.

While there are undeniable benefits to the ever-increasing number of health 'experts', plans, programmes, books, resources . . . the sheer volume of information can invoke a feeling of understandable overwhelm about where to start. But with the knowledge shared in this book, we can remove some of the obstacles and make the path a little easier to navigate.

HOW TO BUILD YOUR HEALTH FROM THE BOTTOM UP

Our health is our most precious asset, and we must protect and nourish it. But defining what health actually is means different things to different people and depends very much on your starting point.

For me, health is a dynamic state of wellbeing in which our internal and external environments, mental and physical wellness collectively fulfil the demands of our lives. Your immune system – aka your wellness system – is constantly interpreting signals from the outside (and your inside) world, and your body's ability to process all that information efficiently and accurately equates to health.

On your journey to be healthier it is key to remind yourself that your journey will look different from someone else's. However, there are certain fundamentals within your control that offer universal benefit, regardless of your starting point or life circumstances, including habitual diet and exercise, sleep quality and mental wellbeing and the environments you frequent. If you practise working with these fundamentals consistently, you will be on the right path towards your own personal best health. And the most exciting part? They don't generally require fancy equipment, a financial investment or even hours of time.

The information discussed in this book should be viewed and interpreted in the context of your immunobiography (which we will go into in Chapter 3) and your individual and current health, while each chapter in Part 2 will help you to identify what taxes your immune system the most, as we explore each of the five big foundational pillars or levers of a strong and well-functioning immune system, as mentioned previously (nutrition, mental wellbeing, movement, sleep and environment). But having knowledge and appreciating the science behind it is just part of the process. The rest is about taking action. For example, I know that I feel better and more energised when I go to bed at a consistent time and ensure that I get enough quality sleep. But I don't always do that. Sometimes I find excuses to stay up late, or sometimes life just gets in the way. So I want to share more than just knowledge here. I want to help you take action to get your health back on track, maintain consistency in your actions and live more healthily and for longer.

This book will make sure you have all the tools to nail the best foundations; and, of course, I'll throw in some of my non-essential but nice-to-have extras for elevating your health from just ok to absolutely optimal.

PART 1

Getting Started – What You Need to Know

To start you on the right path, you first need a blueprint to shape that path in the direction you want it to take. Every part of your immune system functions better when protected from environmental assaults and bolstered by healthy living.

Here, in Part 1, you will get better acquainted with your immune system and the many team players that defend and protect you to keep your body working to its fullest potential. I'll tackle the million-dollar question – 'Can you build healthy immunity?' – and disentangle some of the fad from the facts.

You will learn of the myriad inputs that shape this system, and how true optimum health means being able to constantly calibrate the internal environment of your own body with your external one.

Of course, improving your health requires both practical tools and consistent application, and it can be challenging to know where to start. I will guide you upstream, exploring how your 'immunobiography' has shaped your current health to date and helping you to become an expert in your own immune system.

We have somehow reached a strange phase of human existence whereby we inadvertently sacrifice our wellbeing because life gets in the way. Acquiring the deep knowledge that I'm about to share with you will also set you up for Part 2, where I lay out the practical stepping stones to help you implement your new-found knowledge (even if you think you don't have time) by focusing on realistic goals and developing the habits that will help you achieve them.

CHAPTER 1:

Meet Your Immune System

Research has convincingly shown that the immune system plays a major role in every single aspect of our mental and physical health, from metabolism to mood, brain function, cancer surveillance, healing and repair and even pregnancy.

The immune system consists of an intricate network of cells, molecules and organs that have evolved over millions of years, shaped by the environments in which we live. Like a collection of scattered listening posts, it sits as a crossroads of our physical and mental health.

A STRONG IMMUNITY TEAM

When it's working properly, the immune system will reduce your susceptibility to infection and disease, support proper immune function, better prepare your body to fight off infection, improve your ability to recover if you do get sick, and stave off unwanted inflammation, age-related immune decline and chronic disease.

There is a lot more to the immune system than meets the eye. It is made up of synergistic segments, which are constantly responding to our internal and external environments. Included in our definition of the immune system are:

- physical barriers: saliva, tears, the respiratory tract, the gastrointestinal tract
- microbiological barriers: the collections of microbes that live on and in us
- innate immunity: a diverse collection of white blood cells and molecules that form our first line of defence (for example, the inflammation, tissue damage and acute pain we experience immediately when we hurt ourselves)
- adaptive immunity: the highly specific T cells and B cells and the chemicals and antibodies they produce; this is the immune response with memory – we become immune to certain germs via previous exposure or a vaccine
- cytokines: messenger proteins that communicate between immune cells and our bodies.

The innate and adaptive arms of the immune system act both independently and co-operatively, interlacing their cells and molecules to keep us well. When the first line of defence (innate immunity) hasn't been able to fix the problem, the adaptive system is activated to support it. Innate immune cells called phagocytes display antigens, which the adaptive system recognises, rallying the appropriate T cells to kickstart a further immune response. Genetics play quite an important role here. Innate cells 'show' bits of a germ (called antigens) to our adaptive immune cells in order to switch on the right 'flavour' of immunity for that particular germ. Antigens sit on molecules called HLA – human leukocyte antigens. Our HLA immunity genes are the ones that vary the most between us.[1] This means that although we might differ genetically in the obvious things, such as eye and skin colour, we are actually much more genetically different from each other in our immune systems. The HLA system is highly complex, and it's incredibly important to be aware of this because it explains why we all respond differently to the same germ. For example, your immune system might effectively detect and mount an immune response to a germ such as SARS-CoV-2. But how effectively your T and B cells do this will depend, in part, on your personal HLA molecules. These molecules determine how easily we switch on our adaptive immune response.[2] It is a kind of Russian roulette, whereby your innate immune cells chop the virus up into tiny pieces but only some of these will fit onto your unique HLA molecules. These 'bits' of virus will then be presented to T cells, but your HLA molecules might inadvertently send your T cells off to battle the least effective target on the virus. This results in a poorer immune response compared to another person who has a different set of HLA molecules. There is no hierarchy in the HLA system – it's partly genetic lucky dip. So you might be very good at fighting bacteria but suck at fighting viruses. And while we cannot control this aspect of our immune defences, there are lots of things we *can* do to shape our immune system.

We have many different types of immune cells and, like players in a football team, they each have unique (though sometimes overlapping) roles. If the team is poorly configured or has imbalances, then it won't function effectively or at the level required. The cascade of effects results in a variety of negative health outcomes, only some of which – such as infection, autoimmunity and allergy, for example – are commonly recognised as 'immune' problems. But an unbalanced immune system can be counterproductive to your health in many more subtle ways by impacting unwanted inflammation, energy levels and ageing. This is where the T regulatory cells come in – it's their job to shut down the immune reaction at the end of a response, bringing your body back into homeostasis (a self-regulating process geared towards stability) once the other immune cells have done their job. So keeping these guys happy is particularly important.

CAN YOU BUILD HEALTHY IMMUNITY?

This isn't a trick question, I promise. But it's also not an easy one to answer.

Like an athlete, the immune system needs to balance training and practice with adequate rest and repair to become strong and adept. And despite the commonly used metaphor in which the immune system is compared to a defence army, protecting us against a threatening, germy world, what is becoming clear is that it is, in fact, also partly a peacekeeping force.

The internet is awash with new ways to restore immune health. Most, however, are superficial attempts at remedying a deeper problem because there's a faulty assumption that the only thing separating us from a healthy immune system is a massive dose of a specific vitamin or mineral. We also tend to cast all germs as the villains because a tiny minority of them cause disease. But it's important to realise that health is complex, and the immune system more complex still. We can't expect to address such complexity with an overly simplistic solution.

A better way to think about it is that our immune health is a reflection of things we can control and things we can't. It's the interface between our genes (epigenetics), diet, lifestyle and our environment. Immunity is how our bodies learn to protect our insides from the world outside. It's a sensing-and-reacting system, so by its very definition it is a shared experience that cannot be separated from social, cultural and environmental contexts. For example, did you know that soil has an immune system? As do the sea, the sky and all living things on this planet. The health of your immune system depends on the health of the planetary immune system. Through diet, lifestyle and environment, we can provide the right set of inputs not only to support proper

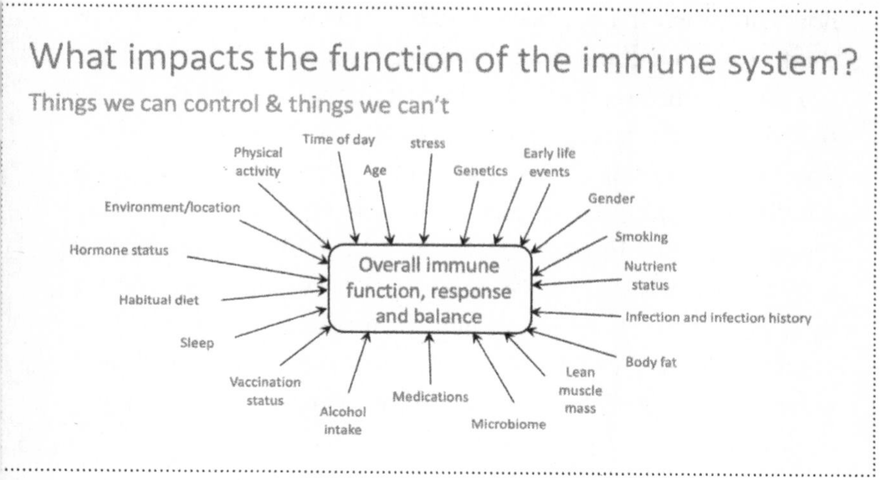

Figure 1 The immune system is shaped by things we can control and things we can't

day-to-day immune function, but to keep it rejuvenated, reducing our risk of (or symptoms of) inflammatory disease.

'The best doctor gives the least medicine.' So said Benjamin Franklin. I love this quote, but I don't mean to denigrate medicine at all. However, so many people are not feeling their best, not because of a medical diagnosis but because of a messy combination of diet, lifestyle and environment which in many cases cannot be easily fixed by medicine. No matter where you are on your health journey, there are almost always small things within your reach that can be used to help you thrive and embrace a salutogenic approach to health. As someone who grew up on a farm, I always find myself trying (and sometimes failing) to grow things – from house plants or tiny city-balcony gardens to, more recently, my sustainable kitchen garden. Along my growing journey I've had to learn a lot to keep these plants alive. The ecological term 'permaculture' (an approach based on an understanding of how nature works) has been a useful framework and one I now think of when it comes to maintaining immunity. Let me explain.

Permaculture serves to design sustainable habitats for things to grow and thrive, regardless of climate, environment or scale. Specifically, it means that by creating the right harmonious conditions, minimal interference is required. Australian researcher Bill Morrison developed the permaculture theory stated: 'The only ethical decision is to take responsibility for our own existence.' Taking this idea from permaculture, we can curate the right diet, lifestyle and environment (both inside and outside our bodies) to thrive with little need for intervention.

CHAPTER 2:

Forget Boosting – It's All About Balance

The benefits of quick fixes and 'immune-boosting' supplements have been touted for decades, but as an immunologist, I find that most conversations around building a strong immune system are woefully inadequate, superficial attempts at remedying a deeper problem. This is one reason why 'immune boosting' is a phrase that I really can't get along with.

Of course, it's always a good idea to do everything we can to have the immune system firing away at full speed. But if we can't boost it, what can we do? Well, first, we need to deepen our understanding of the delicate balance of this complex system.

BALANCING INFLAMMATION

Inflammation is your immune system's response to germs, damage or disease. It's your body's way of responding to things that cause harm, such as injury or infection.[1] It's a sophisticated and highly orchestrated process involving many cells and molecules. You will know when your body is responding with inflammation when you spot the following cardinal signs of acute inflammation:

- Heat or fever
- Pain

- Loss of function
- Erythema (Greek for redness, but this is misleading. Redness is easier to see in people with less pigmented skin, but can be a subtle darkening of existing skin colour in more deeply pigmented skin)
- Swelling

We used to assume that any damage done when we have an infection was caused by the infecting organism. Slowly, however, it became clear that many of the symptoms we suffer when we're ill – fever, weight loss, tissue damage, even fatigue and depression – are triggered not by pathogens but by inflammation from our own immune system. Whether it's a paper cut, grazed knee, infection or broken bone, your immune system responds to damage, danger or infection with inflammation, which works hard to keep us well, stopping minor issues from escalating, actively resolving them and repairing tissue. Inflammation is a normal and essential part of the body's defence mechanism; it's integral to our wellbeing – we really couldn't survive without it.

Although the cardinal signs of inflammation are often local to the immediate area affected, it has broad-ranging physiological impacts throughout the body, acting on the cardiovascular and circulatory systems, brain, muscles, bones and breathing, as well as the pancreas and liver.

With such far-reaching effects, too much inflammation can be harmful. As can its frequency, lack of regulation and failure to resolve.[2] It might seem hard to grasp, but this system that keeps us healthy and protects us from harm, paradoxically becomes the very thing that threatens the foundations upon which a healthy immune system is built. Contained and short-lived, it is useful, designed to damage the germs and other threats once they enter our bodies. When it is not contained, however, and continues over a prolonged period, inflammation becomes problematic, and now scientific evidence supports the fact that this chronic unwanted inflammation can make it challenging for the body to manage infections such as influenza and even COVID.[3] Unwanted inflammation is the key risk factor for a multitude of chronic diseases, including certain cancers, heart disease, metabolic conditions, such as type-2 diabetes, neurodegenerative disease and many other conditions that are now overtaking infections as the leading cause of poor health and death worldwide. Not only that, but it can also subtly impact quality of life through things such as fatigue, headaches, fertility issues, ageing or just feeling that we can't lean effectively into the life we desire because things are not quite working as they should. It's also the common thread in allergy and autoimmunity, as we will explore later. We can't say that inflammation is causal to disease or a specific state of ill health, but it is a contributing factor.

INFLAMMATION AT WORK

Our planet is a wise, self-regulating system with carefully crafted flows and feedback loops, but when things get out of balance, global warming starts to harm the delicate ecosystems that call it home. I see inflammation as being much the same. The immune system has mechanisms in place to self-regulate inflammation, but when conditions become unbalanced, it transforms into a damaging, low-grade version of itself, in the form of 'chronic' inflammation.

Chronic inflammation creates a vicious cycle with molecular damage that is not always obvious but slowly accumulates over time (see figure 2[4]).

Recognising that inflammation isn't always a temporary protective response but can sometimes morph into chronic inflammation

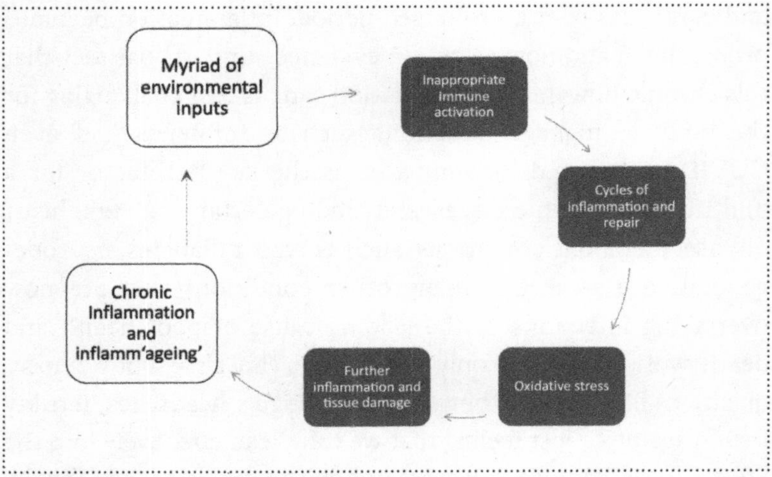

Figure 2 Inflammation vicious cycle

has redefined how we understand our wellbeing. Chronic inflammation is now considered a path to poor health. It can increase infection risk, susceptibility to certain cancers and the likelihood that we will become prone to a chronic disease. Chronic inflammation can also give rise to symptoms such as fatigue, lack of mental clarity, skin irritations and pain, and limit your ability to recover. It can even negatively influence how well you respond to medical treatments.[5] Chronic inflammation and a raised inflammatory baseline plague modern life; the body's way of expressing an internal immune imbalance can also result in reduced ability to fight infection. It can also mean that the usual checks and balances that close the loop on an acute inflammatory response to an infection can be overridden. This is something we have seen in severe cases of COVID-19 infection, whereby a 'runaway' inflammatory response to the virus ends up damaging the person it is meant to protect.[6] But the good news is that by identifying the root causes of chronic inflammation, there are many ways to quench it, as we will explore in the following chapters.

IMMUNE RESILIENCE

If your immune system was represented by a set of scales, perfectly balanced weights would symbolise optimum health. On one side of the scales is the high-tech, highly advanced special-ops team, comprising the co-ordinated actions of innate and adaptive immune cells that react and cause inflammation to beat infection. How do we make sure this highly trained team is prepared and ready to go? We not only need to furnish our special-ops team with everything it needs and the right environment to deal with the unexpected, but we need to support the proper functioning of the much-underappreciated regulatory arm of the immune system that ensures proper regulation of the special ops, preventing them from fighting with each other and ensuring they are targeting only the bad guys. Essentially, one half of your immune system is designed to turn the other half off. By lowering the body's unwanted inflammation, it gives you more bandwidth to fight an infection if it comes along.

There is no general rule regarding which type of immune response may be considered 'good' or 'bad'. A strong pro-inflammatory response, for example, may provide faster or more effective clearance of germs, but it also comes with a greater risk of collateral damage. When chronic inflammation is in the mix, it can be a tale of an immunological Goldilocks: for some people, chronic inflammation leads to a too-'boosted' immune system driving uncomfortable symptoms and signs of poor health, while in another person, it leads to a too-weak system that isn't able to deal with infections adequately. If you suffer from chronic inflammation, these two scenarios are not mutually exclusive. The aim, as I said earlier, isn't to boost, rather to balance – to achieve an immune system that is 'just right'. Immune resilience is a term used to define an optimal and balanced immune response that attacks and eliminates the microbe without hurting your own body cells or causing excessive inflammation. Therefore, the best immune reaction is the most regulated, balanced and economic one – the one that provides the best cost–benefit ratio to you as an individual, according to whatever challenges you face. If you pile more weight onto one side of the scales, the delicate balance is interrupted, potentially tipping your immune system into chaos and threatening your immune resilience.

Oxidative stress

Oxidation is a normal and necessary process that takes place in your body. Free radicals are oxygen-containing molecules with an uneven number of electrons. The uneven number allows them to react easily with other molecules, and because they react so easily, they can cause large chain chemical reactions in the body. These reactions are called oxidation. We generate oxidants normally every day as part of our metabolism. Our immune systems use free radicals to help fight off germs.

As free radicals can be damaging to our own tissues, they are normally neutralised by antioxidants. Antioxidants come either from within our bodies, produced by our own cells, or they can be consumed in the form of antioxidant-rich foods. Oxidative stress occurs when there is an imbalance between free radicals and antioxidants. This results in biological damage to our DNA and the proteins that make up our bodies. This, in turn, can accelerate ageing and lead to or worsen a vast number of inflammatory health conditions over time.

During an immune response, inflammation can increase the production of free radicals, resulting in oxidative stress. This is a necessary and important part of our immune defences. You can't completely avoid exposure to these free radicals, but you can reduce unwanted inflammation and the negative health impacts of oxidative stress through the right diet and lifestyle choices which help keep your body in balance and prevent free-radical damage and disease. While you can't completely avoid exposure to free radicals, I will show you how the right diet and lifestyle choices can help keep your body in balance and prevent damage and disease.

IMMUNOLOGICAL AGEING

Some degree of chronic inflammation is attributed to genetics, of course, but much of it is a consequence of the cumulative effects of our lifestyle, life load and everything we are exposed to. It's becoming clear, particularly since COVID-19 came on the scene, that we have to pay more attention to the immune system with age, given that almost every age-related malady – from infectious-disease susceptibility to cancer or heart disease – has inflammation as part of its process. In fact, if you are chronically inflamed, it can now be used as a predictor for your immunological age, as well as other hallmarks of age-related decline.[7]

During COVID-19 we have learned that a healthy immunological age is one of the most vital things we can aspire to in order to avoid infectious complications and co-morbidities. The rate of immunological ageing can vary considerably between people. Differences are already apparent among people in their twenties.[8] Just because you are a certain age does not mean your body and immune system will act in a corresponding way. So even if you are still fairly young, mitigating your immunological ageing is something you need to be considering.

Accumulating damage and a decline in how well immune cells function over time (known as immune senescence) contribute, to a large degree, to how well the immune system ages. This is also linked to levels of chronic inflammation in the body.

Individual immune cells face three major fates: to survive, to 'senesce' or to commit suicide. The balance between these processes ensures that the total number of immune cells in our bodies – called our immunological space – is essentially in equilibrium. Senescent immune cells lose their ability to behave in an orderly fashion. Instead, they secrete a pro-inflammatory cocktail of cytokines (a condition known as senescence-associated secretory phenotype – SASP) and cause oxidative stress, which further contributes to the vicious cycle of inflammation known as inflamm-ageing. This is part of an age-related immune change that leads to a decline in immune reliability.

Accumulating senescent immune cells will, over time, reduce the 'space' available for fresh, new, well-functioning immune cells. Their inflamm-ageing and oxidative stress signals prevail, causing ageing-related deterioration to delicate organs and tissues. When this happens, chances are that not only will you not you feel your best, you will also be fast-tracking a vicious cycle to further immune senescence, increasing your risk of serious illness from infections like COVID-19 and countless others, reducing your ability to heal and elevating your risk of chronic inflammatory and degenerative conditions, such as heart disease, metabolic dysfunction, neurological deterioration and even certain cancers through the common denominator of unwanted inflammation.[9, 10, 11]

Key examples of things that can accelerate immunological ageing include long-term or recurrent infections, a calorie-rich diet deficient in essential nutrients and antioxidants, lifestyle factors – such as being sedentary or smoking – and exposure to environmental toxins or stress. Each of these can add more weight to the same side of your immunological scales.[12]

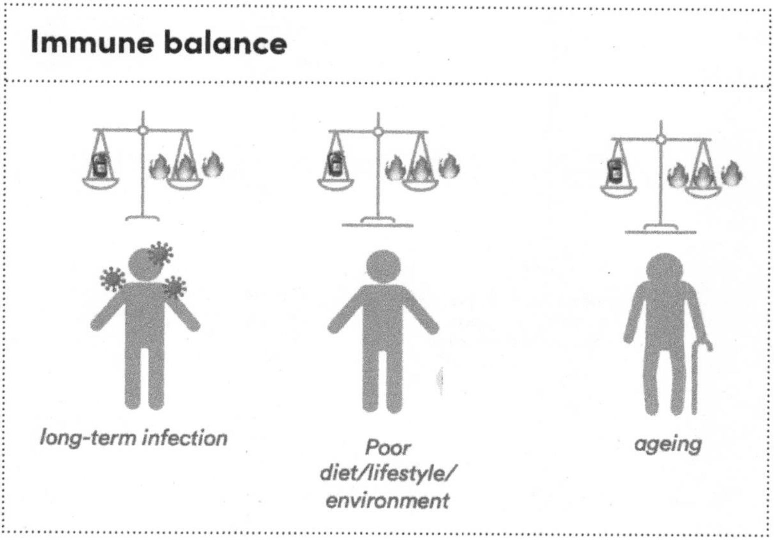

Figure 3 The pro- and anti-inflammatory immune balance

REJUVENATING IMMUNE FITNESS

A well-functioning immune system – or a state of immune fitness, as I like to call it – is where an individual's immune system is both balanced *and* resilient. This doesn't mean never getting sick, but it's about the capacity to respond and adapt to challenges effectively, followed by a return to a baseline healthy state of wellbeing.

True optimum health is being able to constantly calibrate the internal environment of our own bodies with our external environment and the challenges it brings. We differ less in our vulnerability to challenge and more in our resilience to cope with a hit – from fighting off those seasonal colds and flu in a timely manner to minimising flares of chronic conditions and recovering easily from injury or toxic exposures.

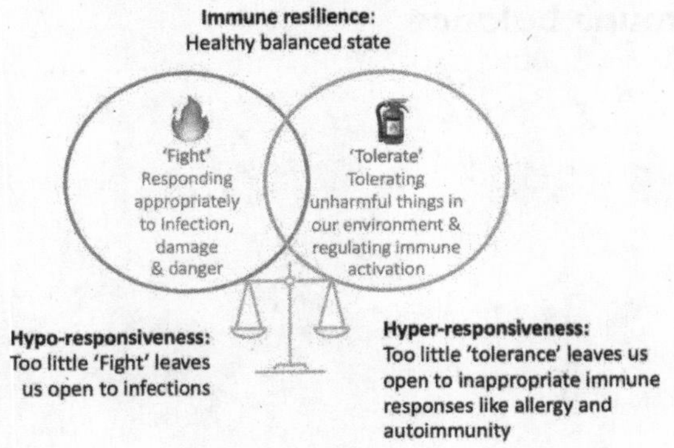

Figure 4

As we've seen, a fit, resilient and rejuvenated immune system needs both the production of fresh, new cells and the removal of old, tired and ineffective ones.

Many people don't realise that the entire immune system turns itself over rapidly, with millions of new white blood cells being produced in the bone marrow every second, and a complete turnover every 100 days. This means you have the opportunity to change the cycle with the decisions you make about the variables that are within your control – i.e. the pillars or lifestyle levers of this book. New bone-marrow-derived immune cells start their lives as blank canvases, called hematopoietic stem cells (HSC). They are naive cells, which means they don't have a personality yet. You want these to be better than the ones they are replacing because when they emerge from the bone marrow into the body, they will convert themselves into specific subpopulations of immune cells based upon 'the many inputs that shape our health. But many aspects of modern life can create small insults to these bone-marrow stem cells: poor diet, radiation, environmental toxins.[13, 14, 15] So if you are already not nourishing your body, this will be imprinted onto your fresh, new immune cells and they will be less resilient from the outset, carrying forward injuries to their DNA and less favourable epigenetic changes, making them more likely to malfunction and cause unwanted inflammation. This can now be measured and we know that damaged immune cells emerging from the bone marrow are directly linked to the age of your immune system. The effects won't show up straight away but accrue over the years.

On the other side are immune cells floating around in our bodies which have already been imprinted with our immunobiography. Some of these might not be in such good shape. These are more likely to malfunction, become immunosenescent (see p. 28) and cause an inappropriate inflammatory response. Higher levels of these aged immune cells are seen in certain chronic diseases, such as autoimmunity.[16]

This means, just like physical fitness, the immune system needs a certain level of work to stay vital and balanced – namely, all the right inputs from diet and lifestyle – so it can continually remove the old to make space for the new.

Although we can't completely stop unwanted inflammation and age-related immune decline, it is modifiable to some degree. For example, we know that an epigenetic process called methylation is fundamental to mitigating elements of immunological ageing and operates in many behind-the-scenes activities of a healthy balanced immune system.[17] This and other processes and practices to tidy up unwanted inflammation, rejuvenate the immune system and work towards reversing the ageing process will be explored in the following chapters.

CHAPTER 3:

Write Your Own Immunobiography

Each of us is unique when it comes to our immune system. This is because the immune system is designed to be highly adaptive. 'Immuno-plasticity' refers to the ability of the immune system to undergo changes in both characteristics and functions, in response to the world around us and the lives we lead. A small part of this, of course, is somewhat predetermined by genetics, which are with us from birth, and cannot be changed (though it can be modulated via epigenetics – see box opposite). But in reality, everyone's health is the sum total of their life factors cumulatively working together in synergistic and antagonistic relationships to bring them where they are today.[1] These factors, or antecedents – genetic or acquired – weave into how predisposed we may be to illness and poor health today. They can include our parents' health, our birth, childhood events, past infection, medications, even our relationships with the people who have come and gone in our lives, past traumatic events that keep cropping up, a chaotic home life or unhealthy lifestyle habits, as we will discuss. All of these can shape and sculpt the immune system.

Life brings continuous exposure to a large variety of threatening and potentially damaging agents, both internal and external. As I often say, the immune system is made, not born. Our allostatic load is 'the wear and tear on the body' which accumulates over time. For each of us, this will be unique. I liken it to a rubber band that can stretch in response to challenge; but every band will have a breaking point. The end result? We become sick.

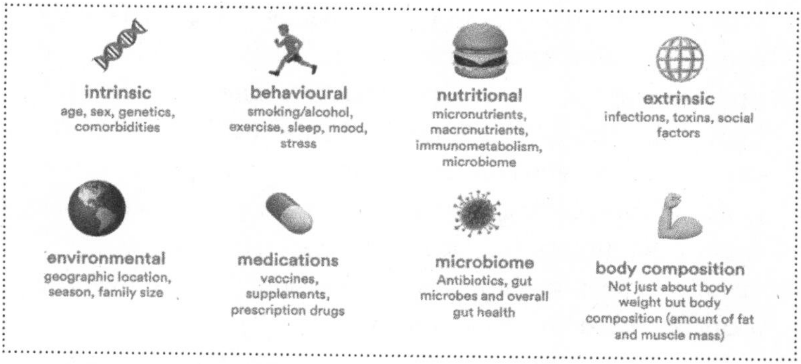

Figure 5 Factors that shape your immunobiography

Nature nurture: does it even matter?

Far from being independent or at odds, nature and nurture engage in a complex dance. Conventional wisdom has long held that our health is majority heredity: a product of our DNA and a small proportion everything else. So for sure, our inherited DNA has a lot to say in our immune systems. But for humans to thrive, we rely on adaptability. This means we need more than genetics. Our genes have evolved mechanisms to be switched on and off based on the information our bodies receive throughout our lives. This happens via a molecular tagging process known as epigenetics, meaning above genetics.

Genetic hardware and software

Epigenetics refers to modifications that attach to our DNA and regulate how our genes work. Both our genetic hardware and our epigenetic software shape who we are. Mutations in our genes are rare but our epigenetics change constantly over time, influenced by how we live, just as regular software updates over the course of our lives. Why have we evolved to have such a cool and complex mechanism? Life has constant ups and downs, and epigenetic changes – in response to tangible lifestyle factors, such as diet, smoking and alcohol, as well as the intangibles, such as stress, trauma, exposure to chemicals, relationships, habits and thoughts – allow us to adapt and become better prepared for all of these.

Why am I telling you this? Well, your immune system is the primary translator of information from the outside world – whether that's a germ or a signal through lifestyle. This means that challenges to your health, no matter what they are, can scar the epigenome of your immune cells and your health can suffer as a consequence.

But through epigenetics, we know that this doesn't necessarily mean being hardwired for poor health. As individuals, we can do so much within our circle of epigenetic influence to steer ourselves towards better health, irrespective of what genetic cards we were dealt. We can intervene through lifestyle to reduce and possibly reverse the impact of any scratches in our epigenome (and also those of future generations, as epigenetic changes are multigenerational and can be passed down from parent to child). We will look at a key epigenetic mechanism known as methylation later on in relation to practical ways that we can support our immunity.

TELLING YOUR 'STORY'

Before we come to assessing your current health, it's important to cast a wide net with regard to your individual history. Welcome to your 'immunobiography'. Think of it as your personal pattern of immune function that results from your lifetime of exposures and the various challenges that came up until this moment. In essence, this means your 'immune-biography' is unique to you, and the product of this is called your exposome. Your health, therefore, is dependent on consideration of the sum of all these factors. This can provide hints to the underlying causes of any present issues or challenges.

I'd like you to start by writing your own immunobiographical history. A form of 'narrative' medicine, this means basically telling your own story to help you to recognise the complex events that have shaped where your health stands today.[2]

The factors that affect your health are more extensive than most people realise. Scientifically, the most well-studied example is 'adverse childhood experiences',[3] but there are many more subtle influences of the journey to our current health, as you will see.

A number of questions may help guide you in starting this process. Using a form of chronological storytelling is often a useful approach, considering the characters (people in your life, including a family history of disease) and plot points (major and minor life events, any stresses and anxieties or antecedents) that stand out as you collect comprehensive information from your entire life. As you examine your history in this way, watch carefully for clues as you chart your own health, linking symptoms, exposures and life events to reveal emergent patterns. This will not only lead to 'a-ha' moments, but you will also begin to see how your health has potential. Acknowledging and accepting all the events that have led to your current starting point is a powerful tool when it comes to informing your own personalised approach on p. 41.

Perhaps your doctor has done this for you to some extent on the journey to a specific diagnosis. But as you live inside your body, you can review your own situation and history in a way that no one else can. You know it better than anyone. Sketch out a timeline that is divided into stages, beginning with pre-conception and ending with your current age. Identify and mark on the timeline all events and health issues you have experienced. You may need to consult with family members for early childhood reminders. Note down points in the following categories in a way that makes sense to you:

Predisposing antecedents

These can be in your genetic inheritance or acquired through things such as past illnesses, exposure to environmental toxins or adverse events that predispose you to poor health.

- What health issues run in your family?
- How was your mother's health before and during pregnancy?
- Note down any previous medications, including the number of courses of antibiotics.
- Note down any previous diagnoses, surgeries and medical interventions.
- Note down any periods of drug and alcohol abuse.
- Have you ever been exposed to environmental toxins (more about these in Chapter 11)?

Triggers

A trigger is anything that initiates an acute illness or the emergence of symptoms. Are there any acute events that may have pushed you over the edge or caused the sudden activation of an unwanted immune response resulting in symptoms such as allergy? Were there any life events that occurred just before or around the onset of an illness or symptom? These might include:

- An acute infection, such as pneumonia or gastroenteritis, that seemed to leave you 'not quite right'
- Any physical or emotional traumas, adverse events or periods of stress and anxiety (perhaps something like a car crash or a psychological stressor)
- Periods of inadequate social or emotional support.

Mediators

What is keeping the fire going and perpetuating poor health?

- Hormones or psychosocial issues
- Ongoing poor diet, lack of exercise, chronic stress or even living or working in a poor environment
- Habitual beliefs about your health, social reinforcement or social conditioning

The above are just examples of the kind of things to look at. It's possible that some may fall into several categories. Simply use them as a guide as you complete your timeline. For some people the optimal goal is maintaining good health and prevention, while I'd encourage others with active health issues to consider:

- What do you think led to your poor health?
- What was your health like before this problem?

I'd also encourage you to write all this down, if you feel comfortable doing so. Writing is different from talking or thinking; it can fulfil a far deeper reflective and educative function, enabling the writer to express and clarify experiences, thoughts and ideas that are problematic, troublesome, hard to grasp or hard to share with another. Writing also allows you to discover and explore issues, memories, feelings and thoughts you might not previously have acknowledged. Sometimes it's more helpful to start with your recent past and then work back. This process reveals the how and why of how you are feeling today. You can explore the particularities of your health: what conditions you have experienced, when they began, periods of your life you associate with better or worse health. Understanding all this helps to craft effective solutions and build the foundation of your personalised health plan for attending to your current and future wellbeing.

To best help yourself, you must understand the breadth and depth of what you are facing, and how it came to be. Everyone alive has suffered. It is the wisdom gained from our wounds and from our own experiences of suffering that makes us able to heal. To tell a story is perhaps what makes humans different from other living beings. Creating this narrative connects us with our own humanity.

Your immunobiography is all about you, the individual, and what makes you unique. It is about identifying the path that got you to where you are today so that you can change your trajectory to one of health, vitality and resilience. It is personalised, and it is participatory. It is the aspect of human knowledge that is not accounted for in a short appointment with your GP. And, as such, it will help to ground you in your own body, experiences and subjectivities in a way that cannot be matched by the one-size-fits-all wellness protocols that fill the internet.

Once you have an idea of your immunobiography, the extent of your allostatic load (that wear and tear we discussed) will be clear, and you can start to gain a deeper understanding of your immune system. I'm here to tell you that it's possible to take back control of your health and put the brakes on that allostatic load. You can start to build resilience and improve fitness, just as you build muscle and improve your ability to exercise in the gym. Think of yourself as the coach, and the immune cells as your team. Every team has its strengths and weaknesses, and every team can respond to good coaching. The better the training, the better the response.

MAKE YOUR IMMUNOBIOGRAPHY YOUR OWN

Neglecting your immune system is like building a house that isn't earthquake-proof in the middle of an earthquake zone. But instead of waiting and hoping for the best, you can start working on a solid foundation upon which you build an appropriate structure that can withstand assaults from earthquakes. If you personalise your foundation, i.e. your immune system, it will protect your structure and gear you up to the specific challenges you face.

I've developed a quiz to help you consider your overall quality of life and what you can do to improve it. The first step is to examine your personal relationship with each of the five foundational elements of a strong immune system:

1. How's your diet and your relationship with food?
2. How's your immune–brain romance?
3. How active are you?

4. How's your sleep and rest?
5. How healthy are your surroundings?

I will then help you to improve in each of these areas, creating personalised blueprints to focus on where you need the most help. We will also look at setting new goals and working towards small, manageable actions that will form your health investments for the long term. Finally, we will focus on consistency because this is the key to getting the results you want.

But before setting goals and implementing changes, you first need to take stock of your current health. How often do you stop and ask yourself 'How am I really doing, healthwise?' Poor health can bring down everything, but sometimes it's insidious. Most of the time, we are involved in a juggling act between work and life. Maybe you're overwhelmed by daily demands. Maybe you don't feel like you have enough time and energy. Or maybe you are running on empty, so the slightest hitch knocks you for six.

No matter how far along your health journey you have travelled, no matter how dialled-in you think you are with your body, there is always more you can learn or relearn, refine or tweak. So are you ready and willing for change? Let's start.

What are you struggling with most?

This is the question everyone should ask themselves. Making any change is challenging and requires adaptability. The first step is to take stock of your current health. Knowing where you stand in terms of your general health today is the key to levelling up to where you want your health to be tomorrow. If you are feeling lost, I hear you. It's now time for you to turn detective and spot unhelpful patterns.

Immunity and inflammation assessment

Although there are many things at play when it comes to how well your immune system is working, including things that are out of our control (see p. 19), thinking about certain signs and symptoms over the past year can be a good way to gauge whether you need to make improvements or keep up the good work.

Mark answers from 0 to 3.

1. How do you feel physically? Consider this over the past six months.

- O 0 = I feel great.
- O 1 = I feel pretty good.
- O 2 = I'm ok-ish.
- O 3 = I'm not really feeling great.

2. Does your doctor have concerns about your current health or symptoms you have been experiencing over the past year?

- O 0 = No concerns.
- O 1 = Maybe.
- O 2 = Yes, they are somewhat concerned.
- O 3 = Yes, they are very concerned.

3. How often do you pick up mild infections? (Mild indicates that the infection was short term and responded well to rest, home remedies or short courses of treatments, such as antibiotics from your doctor.) Examples include coughs, colds, ear, eye or sinus infections. Consider this over the last year and remember it's quite normal to experience up to six mild infections each year.

   - O 0 = Never.
   - O 1 = Occasionally.
   - O 2 = Often.
   - O 3 = Yes, all the time.

4. Do you suffer from poor wound healing? This is about the course of the last year.

   - O 0 = Not at all.
   - O 1 = I suffer mildly.
   - O 2 = I suffer a lot.
   - O 3 = Yes, and this severely impacts my quality of life.

5. Do you have seasonal or environmental allergies, asthma, eczema or other atopic conditions? (**Note**: we will focus on this in Chapter 13.)

   - O 0 = Not at all.
   - O 1 = I suffer mildly.
   - O 2 = I suffer a lot.
   - O 3 = Yes, and they severely impact my quality of life.

6. Have you been diagnosed with an autoimmune or auto-inflammatory disease? (**Note**: we will cover this in much more detail in Chapter 14.)

- O 0 = Not at all.
- O 1 = Yes, and I suffer mildly.
- O 2 = I suffer a lot.
- O 3 = Yes, and it severely impacts my quality of life.

Results for immunity and inflammation

- Under 1 = Great news! You seem to be doing really well. To continue in this vein, now is the time to implement preventative approaches.
- 1–3 = Some room for improvement. Throughout this book I'll highlight simple changes to target unwanted inflammation.
- 4–7 = Definitely areas to work on. Reflect on which ones might be contributing to inflammation so that you can move towards improvements.
- 8+ = Time to take action. Using the practical strategies in this book, we will get your immune system in tip-top condition and minimise that unwanted inflammation.

Nutrition, diet and gut-health assessment

You might think you have a great diet or this might be where you struggle the most. Either way, there is a lot that can be gained by taking an objective look:

Mark answers from 0 to 3, or as indicated.

1. Over the course of a week, what proportion of your meals is prepared from scratch using whole foods?

- O 0 = Almost all.
- O 1 = Most.
- O 2 = Less than half.
- O 3 = Barely any.

2. Do you think you are an emotional eater? (Do you tend to eat more when you feel stressed, angry or bored?) Do you eat until uncomfortably full? Do you feel that food controls you or do you often feel guilty after eating?

- O 0 = Barely at all.
- O 1 = Less than half the time.
- O 2 = Mostly.
- O 3 = Always.

3. Do you exclude any foods or food groups due to a perceived or suspected intolerance?

- O 0 = None.
- O 3 = Yes, I exclude foods or food groups.

4. How is your blood sugar? Do you feel tired, shaky or dizzy if you don't eat frequently? Do you crave sugar or experience an afternoon slump?

- O 0 = Barely at all.
- O 1 = Less than half the time.
- O 2 = Mostly.
- O 3 = Always.

5. How is your gut health – do you experience gut symptoms, such as bloating, reflux or constipation?

- O 0 = Barely at all.
- O 1 = Less than half the time.
- O 2 = Mostly.
- O 3 = Always.

6. How many different plant-based foods do you eat each week across the following groups: fruits, vegetables, legumes, nuts and seeds, herbs and spices?

- O 0 = Lots; more than 30.
- O 1 = 20–29 varieties per week.
- O 2 = 10–19 varieties.
- O 3 = Fewer than 10.

Results for nutrition, diet and gut health

- Under 2 = Great news! You seem to have your diet dialled in. Now you need to continue to be proactive.
- 2–7 = Some room for improvement. Using the practical strategies in Chapter 7, you can decide which small steps and minor tweaks to work on.

- 8–13 = Definitely areas to work on, but don't worry – Chapter 7 has you covered. Reflect on which areas of your diet and gut health are most problematic and put a plan in place to move towards better health.
- 14+ = Time to take action. Don't worry, though – we will get your nutrition and digestion back on track through small, consistent steps based on the knowledge and strategies in Chapter 7.

Mental wellbeing assessment

(Adapted from the Oxford Happiness questionnaire, which can be found at www.happiness-survey.com. In this instance the questionnaire was used as inspiration and is in Jenna's own words.)

Mark answers from 0 to 3.

1. How are your stress levels?

    - O 0 = I am not often stressed (in a negative sense).
    - O 1 = I am occasionally stressed.
    - O 2 = I am quite stressed.
    - O 3 = I am completely overwhelmed.

2. How often do you feel emotionally down? It can be hard to recognise or admit that you are not feeling 100 per cent, but try to look across an average week.

    - O 0 = I am rarely bothered by this.
    - O 1 = I am occasionally bothered by this.
    - O 2 = I am quite bothered by this.
    - O 3 = I am feeling this nearly all the time.

3. Do you have space in your week for activities that you enjoy?

- O 0 = I have plenty of time in my week for activities I enjoy.
- O 1 = I mostly have time in my week for activities I enjoy.
- O 2 = I sometimes have time in my week for activities I enjoy.
- O 3 = I rarely have time in my week for activities I enjoy.

4. Do you feel that you have people around you whom you have warm feelings towards – for example, a strong social or support network?

- O 0 = I definitely have people in my life who make me feel strongly supported.
- O 1 = I have some people in my life who make me feel strongly supported.
- O 2 = I have few people in my life who make me feel strongly supported.
- O 3 = I rarely feel supported by the people in my life.

5. I've been feeling optimistic about the future:

- O 0 = All the time.
- O 1 = Most of the time.
- O 2 = Sometimes
- O 3 = Almost never.

6. How satisfied do you feel with your life?

- O 0 = I am highly satisfied.
- O 1 = I am mostly satisfied.
- O 2 = I am not very satisfied.
- O 3 = I am very unsatisfied.

Results for mental wellbeing

- Under 1 = Great news! You seem to be doing really well. Now is the time to consider implementing preventative approaches.
- 1–3 = Some room for improvement. Using the practical strategies in Chapter 8 will help you work on your social wellbeing.
- 4–7 = Definitely some areas to work on. But don't worry – Chapter 8 has you covered with some helpful strategies to help you put a plan in place to move towards better social wellbeing.
- 8+ = Time to take action. It's not easy but your social wellbeing is worth investing in. We will get you back on track through small, consistent steps based on the information and strategies in Chapter 8.

Movement assessment

Mark answers from 0 to 3.

1. Do you frequently sit for long periods of time at home?

   - O 0 = Almost never.
   - O 1 = Occasionally.
   - O 2 = Most days.
   - O 3 = Daily.

2. Do you tire easily from exercise?

   - O 0 = Almost never.
   - O 1 = Occasionally.
   - O 2 = Most days.
   - O 3 = Daily.

3. Do you experience chronic musculoskeletal pain, or have swelling or stiffness in your body?

   - O 0 = Almost never.
   - O 1 = Occasionally.
   - O 2 = Most days.
   - O 3 = Daily.

4. Do you exercise regularly, yet have trouble recovering before your next exercise session?

   - O 0 = Almost never.
   - O 1 = Occasionally.
   - O 2 = Most days.
   - O 3 = Daily.

Results for movement

- Under 1 = Great news! You seem to be a regular mover and have your recovery dialled in. Now continue and use the strategies in this book to up the intensity if you want.
- 1–3 = Some room for improvement. Read Chapter 9 and plan some simple changes to increase the diversity and volume of your daily movement.
- 4–7 = Definitely areas to work on when it comes to moving your body. Read Chapter 9 and reflect on your barriers to daily movement, formulating strategies to overcome them.
- 8+ = Time to take action! The good news is that people who are moving the least have the most to gain by starting to increase their daily activity. Use the strategies in Chapter 9 to help you move towards your health goals.

Sleep and rest assessment

Mark answers from 0 to 3.

1. Do you go to bed and get up each day at the same times, including days not at work?

   - ○ 0 = Daily.
   - ○ 1 = Most days.
   - ○ 2 = Less than half the week.
   - ○ 3 = Barely at all.

2. How many hours of sleep do you get a night on average?

   - ○ 0 = 8–9 hours+.
   - ○ 1 = Roughly 6–7 hours.

- O 2 = Around 5 hours.
- O 3 = Consistently fewer than 5.

3. How often have you been bothered by trouble falling asleep, staying asleep or waking in the night?

- O 0 = Almost never.
- O 1 = Occasionally.
- O 2 = Frequently.
- O 3 = Every night.

4. Do you have trouble sleeping because you cannot breathe comfortably?

- O 0 = Almost never.
- O 1 = Occasionally.
- O 2 = Frequently.
- O 3 = Every night.

Results for sleep and rest

- Under 1 = Great news! You seem to be doing really well. Now you need to continue to support good-quality sleep.
- 1–3 = Some room for improvement. Read Chapter 10 to help you put in place some simple changes to improve the quality of your sleep.
- 4–7 = Definitely areas to work on when it comes to sleep. Read Chapter 10, reflect on what's stopping you getting better sleep and learn how to formulate strategies to overcome it.
- 8+ = Time to take action. The good news is that it can only get better. Use the strategies in Chapter 10 to take action and improve your sleep today.

Environment assessment

Mark answers from 0 to 3.

5. How often do you get out into green space?

 - ○ 0 = Daily.
 - ○ 1 = Most days.
 - ○ 2 = Less than half the week.
 - ○ 3 = Barely at all.

6. How often do you spend time in environments that feel pleasant?

 - ○ 0 = Daily.
 - ○ 1 = Most days.
 - ○ 2 = Less than half the week.
 - ○ 3 = Barely at all.

7. Is your home filled with more clutter or chaos than you would like?

 - ○ 0 = No, it's pretty organised.
 - ○ 1 = There is definitely some room for improvement.
 - ○ 2 = It's getting overwhelming.
 - ○ 3 = It is too much.

Results for environment

- Under 1 = Great news! You seem to be doing really well. Now you need to continue, ensuring that you spend lots of time in health-supporting environments.

- 1–3 = Some room for improvement. Follow the tips in Chapter 11 to ensure you keep on top of your clutter, curate a healthy home and get outside into healthy spaces.
- 4–7 = Definitely areas to work on. Read Chapter 11 to learn how your environment could be compromising your health and formulate your own strategies to improve it.
- 8+ = Time to take action. The good news is that it can only get better. Use the strategies in Chapter 11 to take action and improve your environment today.

Look at your total scores for each section to help identify the main areas of concern for you. There might be a lot you want to change, but this can be overwhelming, so set yourself up for success by prioritising where you would benefit from making changes first.

CHAPTER 4:

How Long Does it Take to Build Strong Immunity?

One thing I'm often asked is: how quickly do changes in your diet, lifestyle and environment improve your immune system? This is a very difficult question because each person reading this will have a different starting point based on their unique genetics and immunobiography, and there is no hard-and-fast answer that is applicable to all.

You make a million new immune cells every ten seconds, which means you have the possibility to rejuvenate some functions of your immune system quite quickly. Other cells of your immune system are very long lived, providing a library of memories around germs you were previously exposed to. There are several size and space checks in the immune system that maintain the number of immune cells permitted in your body at any given time. New cells are only let in if old ones are removed. Improving the quality of your diet and lifestyle will support this process. But how quickly that happens depends on where you are at baseline and the types of changes and interventions you are trying.

For some things, such as lowering baseline inflammation, you can often see some quite quick responses. A few weeks of lifestyle changes can dramatically change your unwanted inflammation levels. For example, three weeks of consuming excess sugar through beverages can raise inflammation,[1] and in healthy people, one week of a Western- style diet caused dramatic rises in inflammatory markers.[2] The good news is that negative changes are, by and large, reversible. However, old habits die hard and this can be the biggest hurdle to health. Positive changes may depend on how long you have been in a pattern of poor diet, lifestyle and environment.

Sure, supplements and diet might help you to begin feeling noticeably different, but the real changes come with time, dedication and consistency. The best thing you can do is to just start. Or restart. And be consistent.

SELF-EFFICACY: GET OUT OF YOUR OWN WAY

Making health-related changes is difficult. So the first thing I want you to do is to question any assumptions that you might find hard to let go of: think about your attitude to change and trying new things – are you wedded to particular ideas or beliefs about your health or your immune system? What if some of these are just not true? Or, worse still, even harmful? Our brains are biased towards the things we want to align with. This can be a huge hurdle, preventing us from making the changes needed to transform our immune systems. For example: hands up if you are a perfectionist and battle with an all-or-nothing mentality which prevents you from taking action or means you 'fail' at the first hurdle? Or maybe you believe that your illness is your identity? You have done a ton of research on Dr Google and decided nothing works. These are among the major reasons why people don't follow through with change. Start uncovering the beliefs that could be affecting your health by making brief notes on how you feel as you learn in each chapter.

Self-efficacy is your belief in your ability to succeed and is one of the most important factors in health psychology, determining how effectively you make changes to manage your health.[3] Thinking that you will fail will almost certainly mean that you do. Fortunately, self-efficacy is a psychological skill that you can foster and strengthen. Here are some key points that will help you to get out of your own way.

- **Focus on the why.** You won't feel driven every day, but you can always count on your personal 'why'. The thing that has led you to pick up this book and start taking significant and meaningful steps towards your long-term health.
- **It's not failure, it's life.** Life is tough. And it's not easy to have a healthy lifestyle, mostly because of your environment. So don't be hard on yourself.
- **Celebrate the small wins.** Honouring each small success – for example, getting to the end of a busy week and acknowledging that you have been consistent in implementing one small, positive change to your diet – is key to lasting change. It helps your brain associate the change with positive feelings that, in turn, nourish your health.
- **Fail to prepare, prepare to fail.** Preparation is the anchor against uncertainty, and routine provides structure to prepare. Of course, there are many things we cannot prepare for, and our brains (and bodies) hate not knowing. But in an atmosphere of anxiety and uncertainty, we can rely on established routines to cope.
- **Be accountable to others and surround yourself with those who are on a similar journey.** Knowing what to do is not an issue; it's *committing* to it that's the problem. Many of us lack the proper structures to support the behavioural changes our life goals require. Goals take time, hard work, perseverance and commitment. And results often do not

come as quickly as you would hope. Find someone you can trust to check in with, or explore virtual communities and be open to letting others help you.

- **Consistency is key.** When you consistently make choices that serve your health well, you are more able to buffer those days when you just can't, or don't want to. Consistent means regular, long-term, quality actions. Relying on willpower doesn't cut it in the long term. We have the best chance of success by increasing slowly and small enough for it to be unfailingly consistent from the very beginning.

ONE SMALL STEP!

Perhaps the COVID-19 pandemic has provided motivation to build strong immunity. Forced you to really consider just how critical immune health is to every aspect of your wellbeing and empowered you to start making positive changes in your diet, lifestyle and environment. If so, then you need to aim for sustainable changes using the tools and knowledge in this book. Try viewing each small step as a long-term investment, not a quick fix or an insurance policy against an immediate threat. Imagine you are building for the next pandemic, not just this one.

The results from the questionnaire you have just completed will guide you in choosing how to prioritise where you need to make each small change in the areas of concern for you. In Part 2, you will gain the knowledge and tools across each of the key pillars to improve your health. This might mean adding something new to your normal routine, removing something that no longer serves you, or changing something so that it better aligns with your needs.

IMPROVE YOUR CONSISTENCY TO CONSISTENTLY IMPROVE

Consider the key areas that shape your immune system like dials. How can you bump them up just a notch or two?

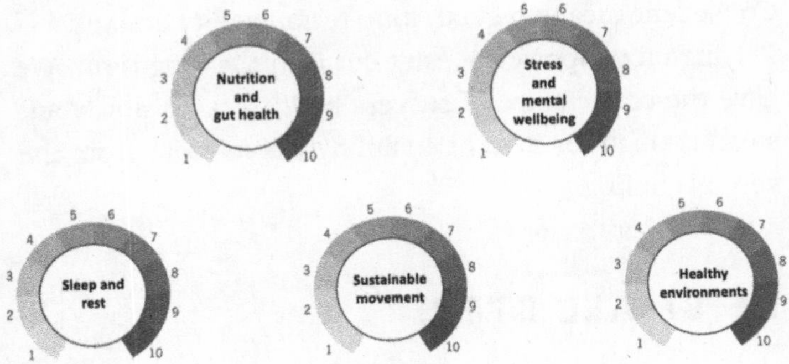

Figure 6 Most health practices are like dials; what does it feel like when you bump them up by just a notch or two?

It often feels like it's *never* the right time to make changes, least of all big ones. But to paraphrase Aristotle: wellbeing is not an act but a habit.

Think back to the last time you (or someone you know) made a New Year's resolution. You make a list of 'rules' that you aim to follow each day to meet your slightly unattainable goals. Either you manage to ace all that stuff . . . or you don't. Which means you either feel good about yourself and are therefore motivated to keep going, or you feel downright demotivated and ready to give up. We have all been there, right? But what if it doesn't have to be that way? What if you only have to get it half right or a little bit right?

Small steps can be empowering and easy to implement in a

sustainable way on a regular basis, leaving you more likely to feel accomplished without feeling overwhelmed or disappointed. Small changes can drive big results over the long term. By supporting your self-efficacy and self-esteem, they create an appetite for more positive changes, keeping you on your personal health journey and helping you to decide when to morph them into bigger and better endeavours. It's consistency that matters, not being 'on track' and getting everything right all the time.

Take the world-class powerhouse of talent that was the British cycling team at the Olympic Games in 2012, but was not always that way. Performance director Dave Brailsford shook things up when he was appointed in 2003. Aiming for gold was too daunting, so instead, he focused on the 'aggregation of marginal gains', whereby you make incremental improvements in everything you do.

We can all learn from this. Think small, not big, and adopt a philosophy of continuous improvement through the aggregation of marginal gains. Forget about perfection; focus on progression and compounding the improvements.

GOALS, HABITS AND RITUALS

You might have arrived at this book because you are highly motivated to educate yourself and discover the tools to build a strong immune system. It can be exhilarating to learn more about these things, but what is going to keep you going a month, a year or even ten years down the line? Motivation is a powerful, yet tricky beast. It may be really easy to get motivated, but it's a finite resource.

We've established that consistency is key to achieving long-term greatness in almost any category: your health, business, even relationships. The problem? It's the one thing we mortals can struggle with the most — especially when we're trying to improve, well, anything. It's hard to be consistent without a strong idea of where you are at and where you want to be. Completing the self-assessment questionnaire on pp. 41–53 will have given you a better idea of your starting point. Next, I'll let you into a secret: the special sauce to *achieving* consistency going forwards is not just learning what to do but turning that into habits and rituals guided by setting achievable incremental goals.

In the words of American Olympic athlete Jim Ryun: 'Motivation is what gets you started. Habit is what keeps you going.'

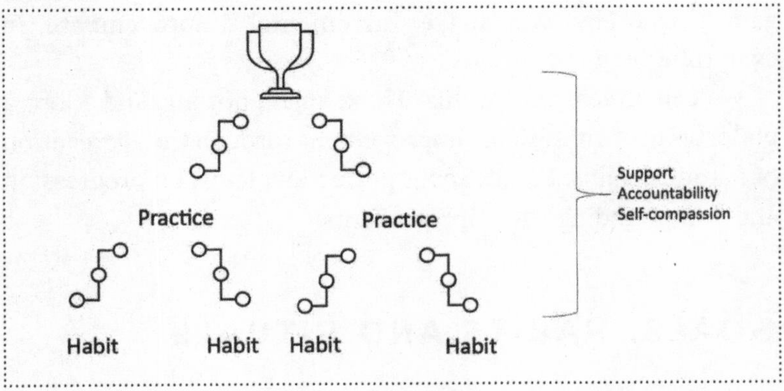

Figure 7 Building habits and practice help us to achieve our goals

Identify your goals – what you want to move towards. Break those goals down into the small, specific practices that are needed to move you in the desired direction. These eventually become habits – automatic behaviours that are seamlessly ingrained into everyday life. Goals are important, but nothing will change your future trajectory like your habits. Habits form when you repeatedly carry out a certain action or behaviour in response to a given situation.

An anchor habit is something you do every day without thinking about it. For example, brushing your teeth. Often, it's the first step in a bedtime routine. If you don't brush your teeth, it doesn't feel quite right (plus they won't turn out very well). To create that consistency in other areas of your life, you must change, start and evolve small daily practices and routines until habits become rituals – habits with soul.

This way, we begin to learn and form an association between anchor habits and new habits, so the behaviour in question (our response) becomes our default when faced with this situational context and its related cues (the stimulus). Every person and each habit, routine and ritual will be unique and contextual to their life, so there's no way to determine exactly how long and how many repetitions it will take for a particular behaviour to become a habit – it can take anywhere from 18 to 254 days, according to scientific research.[4] If the habit is strong enough, it can override the need for conscious motivation, reducing the burden on your brain's prefrontal cortex – your decision-making command centre. This means it requires less mental energy (i.e. motivation), which is a massive bonus when reclaiming your health amid the demands of life. If your prefrontal cortex was a muscle, it would probably be the weakest one in the body. The more decisions you make, the more fatigued this part of the brain becomes, making each successive decision a little bit harder. To make caring for your health more automatic, consider your day from top to bottom, including your daily schedule (if you have one) and your surroundings. What kind of support, planning and nudges might you be able to consider to make changes easier and more automatic? How might you stack healthy habits on top of something you already do? Build a system around your new habit: routines, tasks, people, rewards, consequences, events, tools.

Why not try using a habit tracker to provide tangible evidence of your progress? It will serve as a visual cue to remind you to act, give you motivation as you see the improvements you are making, and it will feel satisfying to record your success in the moment. Visit www.drjennamacciochi.com for inspiration.

Breaking habitual behaviours

Habits can be beneficial because of their automatic nature, but this can also be problematic when trying to change or break one that isn't serving us so well. There are three approaches to 'breaking' a habit, but only the third will be really effective in the long term:

- **Remove or reduce exposure to the cue.** This does not mean the habit will be gone when you are re-exposed and it won't, ultimately, change your behaviour.
- **Stop the response.** This means you choose not to act on the cue. This requires willpower, which is a finite resource. Plus, targeting the habitual behaviour may be challenging if the habit is strong enough for the behaviour to become automatic.
- **Substitute the association.** Your brain starts to make associations over time. Quite often, these are contextual; a good example is getting up from the computer to make a cup of tea. The tea is refreshing and creates a small break from computer work. But each time you boil the kettle you might open the fridge and eat something unhealthy while you wait,

even though you are not hungry. Then, at dinner time, you realise you are not hungry. The more you do this, the stronger the habit becomes, as summarised by the phrase 'neurons that fire together, wire together'. Understanding the trigger or stimulus (making a cup of tea) can help to change the behaviour that follows, preferably to something that also provides pleasure or benefit (pausing to look out the window or taking a moment to breathe or stretch instead of going to the fridge). The first few times feel hard, but then it becomes more automatic. This way, you are maintaining the habit, but swapping out the behaviour for a new (hopefully) more desirable one.

Throughout Part 2 of the book, I will guide you on how to identify habits you want to create or break before they break you!

Goal setting

A goal is the end result, whereas a habit can help us to get there. Goals are different from habits because they rely more on our finite supply of extrinsic motivation. Setting goals can have a number of benefits, including:

- helping us to focus on what's important
- providing motivation and increasing productivity
- giving us purpose
- helping us to develop resilience
- encouraging us to engage in beneficial practices that lead to achieving said goals.

Setting goals is a very effective technique for any health behavioural change if we design them correctly. There are two types of goal, depending on whether you focus on the process or the outcome:

- **Process goals (also known as behaviour goals):** a necessary step in achieving a desired outcome (i.e. the outcome goal).
- **Outcome goals:** this is the final target but doesn't address how you will reach it (that's what process goals are for).

When it comes to investing in our long-term health and caring for our immunity, long-term process goals are where we mostly want to focus. These can evolve as you get better. Use little steps to climb the ladder for more chance of success, building competency and self-efficacy, both of which are known to be important in building the power that is internal motivation.

SMART goals

To avoid failing at the first hurdle, adopt the traditional SMART goals [5] as follows:

- **S**pecific (**s**imple, **s**ustainable, **s**ensible, **s**ignificant)
- **M**easurable (**m**eaningful, **m**otivating)
- **A**chievable (**a**greed, **a**ttainable, **a**ccountable)
- **R**elevant (**r**easonable, **r**ealistic and **r**esourced, **r**esults-based)
- **T**ime-bound (**t**ime/cost limited, **t**ime-sensitive)

Your goals should also bring some challenge, but not too much. When implementing them, keep the following in mind:

Step 1: Choose your goal. Break down larger goals into smaller specific ones.
Step 2: Turn it into a SMART goal using the S-M-A-R-T bullet points on p. 64.
Step 3: Write it down and tell someone about it. Maybe they can join you.
Step 4: Keep track and record.
Step 5: Give yourself a break. Some days will be harder than others, some weeks busier than others. This is normal and part of the process. Be patient and compassionate with yourself. Take a deep breath and then start over the next day.

BE KIND TO YOURSELF

Habits can be difficult to change and goals challenging to achieve; both require a certain amount of mental energy that might be in low supply, depending on where you are with your health. How we deal with setbacks can condition us for how we approach change in the future. It's a feedback cycle that can sometimes go awry, causing the psychological response called learned helplessness – a mental belief that you are unable to change. If you believe you *can't*, then the science shows that this increases the likelihood that you *won't*. Self-doubt is the ultimate consistency destroyer.

Change also requires an open mind; a letting go of self-limiting beliefs. For example, have you labelled yourself with a particular identity? Or do you define yourself through the lens of your illness? The more you believe in this identity, the harder it becomes to be open to positive change. Your identity can become a barrier to self-improvement, resulting in a cycle of learned helplessness or feeling bound by a rigid regimen, identity or feelings of being deprived. It's like a psychological tug of war at every setback – a mental battle between what you want to do (for example, be more physically active, eat better) and your current habits (for example, eating too much unhealthy food).

Here are my tips for starting over:

- **Keep your eye on the why.** As before, making sure your goals come from the heart will get you halfway there.
- **Get educated.** Which is exactly why you are reading this book.
- **Identify the smallest possible goal to start.** It may be so small that it hardly seems 'worth doing' – but that's exactly where your starting point should be.
- **Schedule your priorities, rather than prioritising your schedule.** We all have our to-do lists and work concerns, but can you include time in your schedule to prioritise your health?
- **Learn from lapses.** Rather than seeing mistakes as a failure, use strategies to self-monitor. Take a moment to describe your 'lapse' and reflect on it as both a failure and success. This will help you to learn and grow from the experience.
- **Make it automatic.** Piggybacking new, healthy behaviours onto anchor habits (see p. 61) minimises the need for motivation and mental energy in the beginning. As your behaviours become habitual, new practices become second nature.
- **Hold steady.** Take it low and slow for best results.

- **Make it achievable on your worst days as well as your best.** This is something many of us struggle with, but consistency is so important. That means sometimes you just need to do it, even if you don't feel like it.

Reclaiming your health in today's world is not easy. Self-criticism is linked to procrastination, stress and rumination – none of which motivates people to continue pursuing a goal. Perhaps the most important thing we can do during the process is to practise self-compassion. We're far more likely to bounce back if we're kind to rather than critical of ourselves. This is not only good for the immune system (more on this in Chapter 8), but is key to your health transformation.

FUTURE-PROOF YOUR HEALTH: LESSONS FROM A POST-COVID WORLD

COVID-19 meant that we all had to adapt, stay home, work differently and juggle more, so some of our old behaviours and routines might have been forgotten. The gym, yoga and all the activities we loved became harder to do or stopped altogether. It's no wonder that so many people felt sluggish and tired, wondering just where and how to start improving their health.

In our post-COVID world, our health needs and expectations are changing. We have to help ourselves to stay healthy, happy and independent for as long as possible – because we never know when a pandemic might come along. We need to future-proof our wellbeing so that the next curveball doesn't throw it off:

1. **Wellness can no longer be location-dependent.** Fancy gym membership and expensive avo-on-toast healthy brunch hangouts? Wellbeing activities need to be designed so that they can be done in any location, at any time – even during a lockdown.
2. **A shift from treatment to prevention.** While no diet or wellbeing intervention could stop or cure COVID-19, a healthy lifestyle is an additional preventative measure. There never has been a more important time to focus on our immune systems.
3. **Health is societal.** Significant health inequalities exist (further exposed by COVID-19), and we can all do our bit to prevent them. The more we can do to help ourselves and each other, the healthier our societies will be, saving our previous healthcare resources for those most in need.
4. **Craving for interaction.** With so many workplaces switching to virtual, opting for an extended work-from-home policy, the real-life interaction that we all so badly need is set to disappear. We have to work hard to ensure that we feel sufficiently connected.
5. **Relationship with technology.** While it may at first have seemed like the ideal route to a flexible work–life balance – no commute, fewer office distractions and more time with family – with so many of us being forced to work from home in 2020/21, our reliance on technology soared as never before. In many cases, this has led to a loss of clear demarcation lines between work and home life, and increased pressure to always be online. This is a breeding ground for poor tech habits, bad posture and long sedentary periods. We need to be proactive in managing tech use so that the cons don't outweigh the pros.

6. **Taking illness seriously.** Sick days are no longer skivers' territory. We need to be alert to the signs that we need to rest, not suffer through our sniffles while simultaneously infecting all our colleagues or other commuters. Presenteeism – the problem of people showing up to work but, due to illness, not fully functioning – can cut individual productivity by a third or more. Allowing ourselves time to rest and recover and creating a culture in which it's ok to do so is imperative.

COVID-19, a collective trauma on an unprecedented scale, far worse than anyone could ever have imagined, has taught us that even in the best of health, we don't know what is around the corner. Life is messy and rarely goes to plan. But in any circumstances where health and wellbeing are challenged, we can be made hyper-aware of our strengths, as well as the aspects of our lifestyle that are not serving us well. We can grieve, reflect and cultivate positive change, increasing our capacity to thrive. We can adapt and create – because that is what our biology is designed to do.

Change can be difficult and uncomfortable. And it is definitely not linear. But it can also be necessary and energising. The route to successful achievement of goals lies in the habits we create and the consistent, small changes that add up to desired results. Read on to find out exactly how to go about this.

PART 2

Building Your Foundations

Your health is complex, and therefore solving the puzzle of better health and a stronger immune system calls for a broad and holistic approach. It requires addressing all aspects of your physical and mental health, as well as the environments you frequent. That is why here, in Part 2, we will be building sturdy foundations by exploring the five big lifestyle levers that are so strongly connected to your immune system and your relationship to them.

CHAPTER 5:

You and Food

Since COVID-19, more people than ever before are learning about the various ways food can support immune function. It's often viewed as an easy win – an accessible way to gain agency over our health, particularly when life feels chaotic. There are millions of scientific studies showing that what (and how) we eat matters for proper immune function, infection protection and reducing unwanted inflammation and chronic-disease risk. This makes diet a good starting point. But while food has a measurable impact on immune function, it is far from a quick fix. And it's not as simple as just taking more vitamin C or eating from a list of so-called immune-'boosting' foods. In fact, in today's modern world, eating – a biological necessity entangled with our social and emotional health, shaped by culture, memories and rituals – is anything but straightforward.

I am often asked how to 'boost' immunity with food, and people usually expect me to start with recommendations for what they should and shouldn't eat, and how to supplement. But when we drill down, this is not where help is needed. Most of us *kinda* know what we *should* be eating and are aware of resources, such as the Eatwell plate in the UK, which provides basic nutritional information.[1] In fact, 'I don't know *what* I should eat' doesn't even make it into the top ten biggest struggles reported by people who are trying to improve their diets.[2] Yet that is the thing we focus on the most. My point? Knowing what you should be eating probably isn't what's holding you back. Rather, it's things like emotional eating, cravings and social pressure to eat (or not eat) certain things.

YOUR RELATIONSHIP WITH FOOD

Food has always been its own language. And it turns out that it can be a translator, too – helping us to understand ourselves when nothing else can. Have you ever eaten because of how you were feeling, rather than because of hunger? Or maybe you have felt 'hangry', with hunger impacting how you feel? This is all normal, but what it means is that it's important to work on your relationship with food, building a deeper understanding of how you interact with it before getting down to the nutritional specifics around nourishing your immune system.

So many things drive us to eat – we're too polite, we're happy, we're busy, we're bored . . . No one hunger generator can be isolated from this complex experience. But, importantly, intensity of appetite is not directly and singularly correlated with the number of calories a person needs. Yes, it can be influenced by biological factors (i.e. the number of calories/satiety from food eaten), but hormones, circadian rhythms, stress, anxiety, expectations, preferences and social factors all play a part, too. So what are the factors besides hunger that compel us to eat?

Everyone overeats sometimes or turns to food to cope with life events on occasion. But when this is your only mechanism to cope, it can erode your relationship with food and put you in a vicious cycle. Emotional eating is different from the response to physical hunger and is characterised by a drive to eat as a reaction to an emotional trigger, such as boredom, anxiety, sadness or excitement, in an attempt to alleviate, reward or cope with a feeling. It is important to remember that emotional eating is not due to a lack of willpower or weakness. You have not failed. Emotional eating is an adaptive response and, with the right knowledge and support, you can learn new ways of coping.

Real-time tips for nurturing a good relationship with food

Do you think you are an emotional eater? Do you tend to eat more when you feel stressed, angry or bored? Do you eat until you're uncomfortably full? Do you feel that food controls you? Do you crave specific foods? Do you often feel guilty after eating? If any of these resonate with you, don't worry, we can break the cycle. To repair your relationship with food, you must be kind and curious, removing guilt and judgement from eating. Here are some strategies to put you back in touch with the internal cues that tell you when to eat and when to stop:

- **Know your triggers.** Be aware of external cues making you hungry. Ask yourself: 'Am I in full control of this eating decision, or am I being negatively influenced by an external cue outside my control?'
- **Know your hunger.** Check in with yourself before you eat and ask: 'How am I feeling? Am I actually hungry or am I eating to fill a deeper psychological need?'
- **Eat balanced meals.** Eat meals that will leave you feeling satisfied with less need for unhealthy snacks (see pp. 145–7 for how to build your plate).
- **Be self-compassionate.** Stop punishing yourself for what you ate yesterday. Dwelling on the past does not serve you or your body. All it does is cause stress and anxiety, which are not good for your immune system.

- **Practise mindful eating.** Put down your phone and engage with your senses at every meal. Eat more slowly to help digestion and regulate your feelings of fullness.
- **Be grateful.** This is about where your food has come from and how it got to your plate.
- **Stop black-and-white thinking.** If you just had one 'bad' meal, avoid stepping into a vicious all-or-nothing cycle, as this can lead to bingeing, guilt and shame.

Remember, good nutrition isn't about what you eat on your best days, but about making it sustainable for you on your worst days. Trust in the process and the results will follow.

Reconnect with hunger and fullness

To say eat when you are hungry and stop when you're full may seem obvious, but think over the past week: how many times did you eat when you weren't hungry?

Consider hunger and fullness on a 0–10 scale, where 0–1 is absolutely starving and 9–10 is painfully stuffed. You want to begin eating when you first get hungry (say, 3–4 on the scale) and stop when you first feel comfortably full (around 6–7). It's also wise to eat when you first get feelings of hunger because you're more likely to enjoy your food and to eat mindfully; when you let yourself get too hungry, chances are you'll eat really fast and not really pay attention to your food. In fact, one of the biggest predictors of overeating is letting yourself get too hungry in the first place. Of course, there will be times when you overindulge or get over-hungry because of the situation you are in (work, celebrations, disruption to routines), but these small deviations are pretty minimal compared to the overall pattern.

Nutritional agnosticism

Before we move on, there is another aspect of our relationship to food that we should address – our beliefs. Ask yourself if you have a belief system about a certain way of eating. For some it might be low-carb for the win, while others argue for low-fat or vegan. You might believe you need to eat little and often, while intermittent fasting might be the only way for others.

We all hold beliefs that complicate our diet choices, muddied further by the latest trends and the fact that we all eat but don't all have degrees in nutrition. This means it's easy to base our food choices on said beliefs, emotions and personal anecdotes, rather than on real evidence. The concept of 'healthy' foods can be particularly confusing due to frequent application of our belief systems. This stems, in part from the monetisation and marketing of food, but also from years of conflicting information from health information sources. But beliefs don't necessarily have anything to do with fact. When we believe something, we choose to accept that it's true, which may or may not have anything to do with factual certainty.

- **Accept there is no 'best' diet.** It's normal to have biases and it's natural to seek information that aligns with what we believe and ignores what doesn't. The question isn't whether we have set beliefs or biases, but that we pro-actively try to counter them and remain open to new and often-changing information.
- **Cast a critical eye.** You don't have to look very far online to find a sales pitch of someone's beliefs around a certain set of foods or supplements. 'Because it worked for me' isn't enough to mean it works for everyone. Explore the evidence and do your own experiments, documenting the effects.

- **Know about nuance.** Nutrition has become so complicated that many people are confused about how they should eat. 'Is alcohol bad for my immunity?' 'What about if I eat this piece of cake?' 'Tell me your top five immune-boosting foods.' I'm asked questions like these a lot. And the answer is always . . . it depends. I know you don't want to hear that, but no single finding applies to all people in all situations all the time. We know this from science. Younger people have different protein needs from older people. Ultra-processed foods (UPFs) pose different health risks depending on your socioeconomic and psychosocial status. Vegan might be a great choice for you to thrive, but others will struggle. We are all unique, and context matters.
- **Focus on the bigger picture.** A lot of these nutrition conversations focus on the disagreements and details that don't really make a whole lot of difference when you look at the bigger picture – that being the overall diet pattern (see p. 83).

TOXIC FOOD ENVIRONMENT

Our food choices are subtly shaped by the complex world in which we live, the so-called food environment, which takes in everything from the kinds of foods available to us in our homes, how far we live from the nearest supermarket or fast-food restaurant, social pressures to eat, aggressive food marketing and even the ways that governments support farmers.[3] Our current food environment has been called 'toxic' because of the way it corrodes healthy diets and promotes lifestyle-related disease. Key aspects currently under intense scientific scrutiny include the explosion of fast-food restaurants, the enormous increase in portion sizes, the power of food advertising and marketing and the ubiquity of unhealthy UPFs.

The problem with UPFs

A wealth of research consistently points to one resounding conclusion: humans are healthier when they consume minimally processed foods. But what do we mean by processing and how can this knowledge help us to nourish our bodies going forward?

The NOVA food classification devised in 2009 divides foods into categories from unprocessed to ultra-processed.[4] As food processing increases, nutrient density generally decreases, while additives, preservatives, fillers, sugar, sodium, unhealthy fats and/or refined starch tend to increase.[5]

More than half the calories the average person in the UK eats come from UPFs, the most processed category of foods,[6] and new research has linked them to early death and poor health.[7] UPFs are defined as 'industrial formulations . . . containing five or more ingredients and artificial additives, with no wholefood components'. Put simply, they are highly refined with large amounts of nutrients such as sugar, fat and salt in just the right combinations to make them irresistible.

So it's no surprise that we tend to overeat UPFs – their composition makes them easier to consume and simultaneously less able to trigger our normal satiety hormonal signals. One randomised controlled trial even found that people ate a stunning 500 more calories per day when they consumed a diet rich in UPFs compared to one rich in minimally processed whole foods. That's essentially the equivalent of consuming an extra meal a day.[8]

But it's not just our potential to overeat them that makes UPFs problematic. Even when we are not consuming a surplus of calories, which can lead to obesity and its associated health issues, UPFs seem to be problematic for our health. Usually low in all the immune-nourishing goodness discussed in this chapter, they contain little, if any, intact food and provide 'empty calories' that take up space from more healthful foods. They contribute to reduced microbiome diversity, which coincides with a bloom of digestive issues, such as irritable bowel and small intestinal bacterial overgrowth (SIBO), a serious condition affecting the small intestine.[9]

How processed is your food?

UPFs tend to be cheap and convenient, hence their ubiquity and popularity. But the degree of processing is not always clear when you're in the shops. It's also confusing because some processing of foods is beneficial – for example, tinned tomatoes or culinary ingredients, such as olive oil. Use this guide to help you recognise UPFs:

- Products containing a long list of ingredients (usually more than five), as well as ingredients you don't recognise or wouldn't add when cooking at home
- Mass-produced breads or fresh foods with an incredibly long shelf life
- Frozen and shelf-stable, ready-to-heat or ready-to-eat meals, including frozen pasta, pies and nuggets
- Fast-food dishes, including hamburgers, pizza and French fries from fast-food outlets
- Pastries, buns and cakes, breakfast cereals, crisps, biscuits, fruit drinks and confectionery

The moral of the story? Shop and eat smart. Remember, food companies are *not* public-health agencies. They are out to make a profit, and they spend an enormous sum of money on ensuring we can't stop buying UPFs. This is not about willpower but acknowledging the problematic food environment in which we live and acting on it. UPF manufacturers are currently still allowed to present their products as fun, as treats and even as 'healthy'. We need not only to become label detectives, but also to understand how we are being manipulated before we can see past the propaganda. Then we can make healthier choices, irrespective of our food environment and the advertising we are fed.

The food environment as a determinant of our health

We are all trying to figure out how to navigate the current food environment and even the science hasn't fully caught up yet on determining the extent to which it is impacting our health. We don't want to ban all UPFs, but rather find the right amount of them, so that life still has some pleasure (because food is more than nutrients, after all). Biological responses to 'junk food' depend on your total exposome (see p. 35), with each meal being part of that. This means, the percentage of UPFs in your diet is pushing or pulling your biology towards or away from poorer health, depending on the other areas of your diet and lifestyle. So those with a larger life load might be more easily pushed down a negative health trajectory by a lower dose of UPFs.[10]

There's a great word that describes what happens when we overdose on using our phones, whether it's Twitter doomscrolling or going down a YouTube rabbit hole: when you spend too much time staring at a device, you get screensick. You're grumpy and distracted by exposure to the underbelly of humanity on social media. You can't pay attention to anything else, yet feel guilty for not stopping. The notifications on the phone in your pocket steal your focus like an itch you just cannot scratch.

The social media algorithms that keep us hooked, like the people who make UPFs, don't care about our health, which is why they've spent so much time, energy and money engineering ways to keep us wanting more. We are living in less than healthy environments where less healthy food options are the default, leaving us the food equivalent of 'screensick'.

So if you are finding it challenging to eat healthily, that's because it is.

DIET PATTERNS – WHAT'S THE DEAL?

Did you know that there is a universal core to the optimal immune-nourishing diet? One that supports our ability to ward off infections effectively and protect against immunological ageing and chronic inflammatory disease? And, unsurprisingly, this goes way beyond just avoiding key deficiencies in micronutrients.

Michael Pollan, American author, journalist and Professor of Science and Environmental Journalism at The University of California, Berkeley, says everything he has learned about food and health can be summed up in seven words – 'Eat food, not too much, mostly plants'. I love the simplicity of this oft-quoted statement. But one detail that is often overlooked is that when Pollan states 'Eat food', he means 'real' food – i.e. unprocessed – because a plant-rich diet can also be a highly processed one. As can vegan, high-carb or low-carb diets, or pretty much any diet that purports to be the healthiest du jour.

It's easy to become trapped by thinking that individual foods and nutrients can make or break our health. But in reality, a diet can't be described by one food or meal in isolation. Rather, it's the overall quality of your diet and the pattern of foods you habitually eat over time that are a better indicator of the general healthfulness of your diet. Looking at your *diet pattern* allows you to take a step back and look at diet as the sum of all the foods you enjoy eating over many weeks and months. This has been shown scientifically to be a much more reliable indicator of health.[11]

It's all about obtaining the majority of macronutrients (proteins, carbs and fats) and micronutrients (vitamins and minerals) by consistently combining a diversity of whole foods into an overall healthful pattern. Taking the focus off specific foods allows room for flexibility in your diet. It allows food to be put in the context of culture, age, season, location and accessibility. It also enhances your relationship with food, enabling you to enjoy times of celebration and relaxation – when meals may be less nutrient-dense or more frequent than normal – without feeling guilty.

Health-promoting diet patterns all tend to have commonalities, including being anti-inflammatory in nature and promoting higher amounts of fresh produce, dietary fibre, adequate protein and healthy fats. They can be cultural (the Mediterranean diet) or devised using specific health outcomes (the DASH diet,[12] developed by the National Heart, Blood and Lung Institute to reduce the risk of heart disease). Among the anti-inflammatory diet patterns, the Mediterranean diet (MD) claims the lion's share of scientific research. Encompassing a variety of the traditional diets places that border the Mediterranean Sea, it is rich in fish, fruits, vegetables, whole grains, fibre-rich beans and pulses and healthy fats, and is known for its health benefits, including anti-inflammatory properties and healthy ageing, and associated health-promoting behaviours, such as being physically active.[13]

There isn't necessarily a single diet pattern that is superior (so I hope everyone can quit arguing about this on social media). This means that a healthy eating pattern can be adapted to meet your individual food preferences, environmental concerns, food-preparation capabilities and culture and traditions.

Despite this, many people still believe that particular nutrients should be the focus when it comes to diet. In this chapter, you will notice that I do mention specific nutrients with regard to their roles in supporting immunity, but there is no list of foods or one best diet for your immune system, and there is no one-size-fits all. I prefer to practise nutritional agnosticism – the philosophy that different people have different nutritional needs, and that these needs will change.

Moving your overall diet pattern towards an anti-inflammatory one should be your focus, and is now recommended by most professional bodies for optimal health, providing all our day-to-day nutrition and preventing chronic inflammatory disease. Adhering to a healthy overall diet pattern has been shown to reduce the risk of infection, inflammation and associated chronic disease risk, even after adjusting for age, BMI, smoking and ethnicity.[14] Diet patterns are a potent indicator of our health-related quality of life score (HRQOL) – a metric of happiness and life satisfaction.[15]

CHAPTER 6:

Metabolic Health – and Why it Matters

Metabolism refers to the set of chemical processes that collectively convert food into energy and then use that energy. Metabolism is occurring continuously inside your body – breathing, repairing cells, digesting food and, of course, sustaining the energy needs of your immune system.

The mitochondria are at the core of all metabolic processes. They are small organelles found in all our cells, helping us to turn our food into energy by generating something called ATP – the energy currency of our body.

THE NEW SCIENCE OF IMMUNOMETABOLISM

Metabolism and the immune system are deeply interconnected with the mitochondria as a central hub in the balance and regulation of immunity. Immune responses are demanding processes, requiring large amounts of energy and metabolic building blocks to fuel them. When our immune cells are not engaged in a particular activity, they are relatively 'quiet' metabolically. Under these circumstances, the mitochondria inside our immune cells are busy fulfilling the energy needs to maintain this quiet state. Mitochondria are also the metabolic switches needed to transform immune cells quickly into a metabolically active state to carry out specific functions, such as inflammation and fighting infection when needed. For example, fever in humans and other mammals is associated with increased metabolic demand. A rise of 1 degree celsius in body temperature corresponds to a 10–15 per cent increase in metabolic rate.[1] This association between metabolism and immune responses is called immunometabolism.[2]

Damaged mitochondria can trigger an inflammatory response. This has evolved as a protective mechanism but if we don't take care of our mitochondria it can also cause unwanted inflammation. They release various immune-cell-signalling molecules known as damage-associated molecular patterns (DAMPs), which activate inflammation via a system called the inflammasome within our innate immune cells. This is a danger signal that happens when we injure ourselves – for example, a sprained ankle with tissue damage releasing DAMPs, but no infection.

Whenever mitochondria produce energy, they also produce some oxidative stress. This is normal and is not a problem when we have sufficient antioxidant status. But certain lifestyle factors – such as smoking, stress, lack of sleep, environmental pollution and a nutritionally poor diet pattern – as well as the ageing process can drive a decline in mitochondrial quality and quantity. Damaged mitochondria release DAMPs that activate inflammation when it's not actually needed. They also end up producing less ATP and more oxidative stress, further perpetuating inflammation and damage that can snowball throughout the body. This means mitochondrial dysfunction plays a role in chronic inflammation, immune-mediated diseases and even many vague unexplained symptoms, such as fatigue, sluggishness, digestive disorders, brain fog, blood-sugar irregularities and pain. Sadly, it can become a self-fulfilling prophecy: when mitochondria are not functioning properly, this can lead to a build-up of cellular waste and further oxidative stress, accelerating biological ageing.

METABOLIC HEALTH AND IMMUNITY

Metabolic health exists on a spectrum. Recent estimates suggest that less than 20 per cent of adults in Western countries have optimal metabolic health.[3]

Metabolic syndrome is the collective term for a cluster of metabolic dysregulations including increased blood pressure, poor blood sugar control and excess body fat around the waist, increasing your risk of heart disease, stroke and type-2 diabetes. Metabolic syndrome impacts the immune system in a significant way,[4] including:

- disrupting the function of immune tissues and organs
- contributing to immunological ageing
- preventing production of fresh new immune cells and immune rejuvenation
- reducing infection protection and vaccine responses
- contributing to chronic inflammation and accelerating inflammatory disease.

Metabolic syndrome is also a risk factor for certain cancers, cognitive decline, allergies and autoimmune disease.

The importance of metabolic health to immunity has been acutely highlighted during the COVID-19 pandemic. Suboptimal metabolic health is associated with poor COVID-19 outcomes rooted in the immune dysregulation that occurs as a result of poor metabolic health. There are even calls for public-health interventions to include metabolic health as a cornerstone of future pandemic preparedness.[5]

We're discovering more and more ways to support our metabolic health, which has important knock-on effects in optimising immune function.[6] The ray of hope is that poor metabolic health is largely driven by diet and lifestyle factors, which means these are also tools we can use to treat, prevent and reverse it.

In this chapter, we are going to examine two of the parameters of our metabolic health over which we can have some leverage and which have significant implications for immune health: blood-sugar control and body composition. Your doctor can also test for things such as blood pressure, cholesterol and triglyceride levels for a more comprehensive assessment of your metabolic health.

IS YOUR BLOOD SUGAR BALANCED?

Sugar might be the nutritional demon du jour but there is a lot more to the story than meets the eye. A study in 2021 found that elevated blood sugar is the most likely single risk factor to explain why otherwise healthy patients with no other apparent risk factors get severe COVID-19.[7] Elevated blood glucose weakens antiviral defences and promotes viral replication. This causes dysregulations in the immune response, promoting a storm of inflammatory factors to be released, escalating disease severity towards multi-organ damage and failure. This finding gives us all the more reason to do as much as we can to reduce and stabilise blood-sugar levels. But let's first understand how these change.

Blood-sugar levels rise and fall after every meal or snack. This is normal and primarily down to the carbohydrate content of the food we eat. A healthy blood-sugar response is one where our bodies break down carbohydrates into simple sugar molecules, such as glucose, that are absorbed by the gut into the bloodstream, resulting in an increased blood-sugar level one to two hours after eating, which then normalises within three to four hours (see fig. 8). This is down to the actions of the hormone insulin, which rises after eating to help shunt sugar out of the blood and into the liver and muscle tissue, where it is stored for use when we need it. Our muscles are one of the biggest sinks for glucose, which is a primary reason to maintain a decent amount of muscle mass (see p. 101).

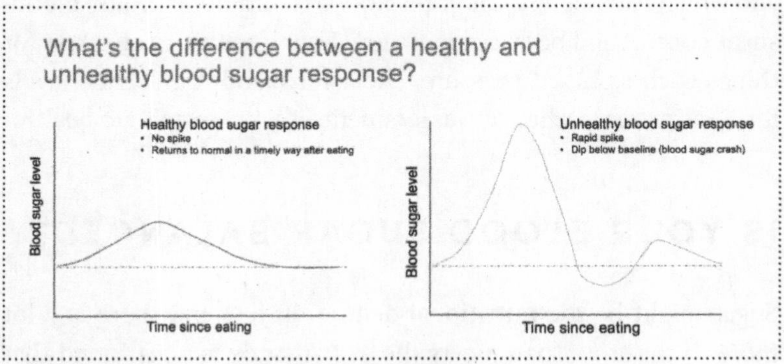

Figure 8 Healthy vs unhealthy blood sugar response

The key differences between a healthy post-eating blood-sugar response and the unhealthy 'roller coaster' are the size of the spike after eating, how long sugar is allowed to hang around in the bloodstream and whether it dips below baseline three to four hours after eating before stabilising again (known as a blood-sugar crash). This can affect not only energy levels, appetite and fat storage, but it's also a major problem for the immune system and levels of inflammation.

Let's learn more about how this blood-sugar roller coaster negatively affects the immune system:

- **Dietary inflammation** An exaggerated inflammatory response can occur after eating. This adds extra allostatic load to the immune system, so it is less able to deal with other threats, as all resources are triaged into putting up a sustained battle against the dietary inflammation.
- **Advanced glycaemic end products (AGEs)** Glycans are sugar molecules that surround and modify our immune cells, disrupting their function, triggering unruly inflammation and exacerbating inflamm-ageing.
- **Dicarbonyls** These breakdown products of blood sugar interfere with infection-controlling antimicrobial immune molecules called β-defensins.
- **Insulin dysregulation** Insulin is the hormone that removes sugar from the blood and helps it to enter our cells. When we are on the sugar roller coaster, insulin can become dysregulated and our cells desensitised to it. This can mess with the availability of energy to immune cells when they need it and can also increase oxidative stress in the body.
- **Methylation** Blood-sugar issues can affect how well our epigenetic methylation processes occur, accelerating ageing.

How to balance your blood sugar

Without using a blood-sugar monitor, how can you tell if your blood sugar is out of whack? I'm sure we have all been there: the post-lunch slump? Feeling tired, irritable and often still hungry an hour or two after eating? Craving carbohydrates? If any of these sounds like you, it's possible that your blood sugar rises too high too fast, then your insulin overcompensates, causing your blood sugar to drop rapidly. You might also feel shaky, sweaty, lightheaded or even experience 'brain fog'. Constantly riding the blood-sugar roller coaster can push up insulin levels, which can drive the sex hormones oestrogen, progesterone and testosterone wild. This, in turn, can further disrupt our blood-sugar response and cause a suite of issues relating to hormone imbalance.

First, know that everybody is different in their blood-sugar response to food. There are some key things that are known to affect blood sugar, as I'll describe, but findings from the PREDICT studies show that normal, healthy people eating identical foods can show up to an eight-fold difference in blood-sugar response, as well as the accompanying unhealthy effects of a post-eating rise in inflammation called dietary-inflammation.[8] Even identical twins – who share all their genes and much of their environment – can experience vastly different responses when they eat the same meal.

What's causing these huge variations? Blood-sugar control is impacted by things such as exercise and stress because they signal to the body to liberate sugar into the blood from the tissues to prepare us for movement or fight or flight (the physiological reaction that happens in response to a threat). As we age, we become more susceptible to poor blood-sugar control after meals, in part because we tend to be less active, but also because the output of insulin from the pancreas tends to become slower and lower. Ageing and hormones combined have a serious impact, but by far the biggest factor is down to the unique collection of bugs in our gut, known as the gut microbiota. So when you see someone online telling you what to eat to 'fix' your blood sugar, remember that just because it works for someone else, doesn't mean it's going to work for you.

But if there is no one-size-fits all, is there anything we can do? The good news is yes, but it requires a short-term investment in time as you play around and experiment with different foods to find what works best for you, gives you the most stable energy and keeps you satisfied for longer.

Practical tips for good blood-sugar control

Finding a blood-sugar balance might feel like an impossible task. Carbohydrates have the biggest impact on blood sugar, but it would be impossible (and unhealthy) to cut ties with carbs entirely. What you can do, though, is to be sugar aware and aim to stick within the recommended dietary guidelines which advocate limiting *added* sugars to 10 per cent of daily calories (this may differ for children of different ages). Sugar is more ubiquitous than ever, and with over 200 names (including barley malt, cane juice, glucose, sucrose, maltose, dextrin and fructose), it is hard to spot. Become a sugar detective so you can dodge the refined grains, added sugars and sugar-sweetened beverages.

Consider the quality of carbs over quantity. The total amount of carbohydrate is less important than its quality. This means there is no need to cut them out or go low carb, unless you have been advised to do so by a nutrition professional for a specific condition, such as diabetes. Instead, replace the highly processed carbs with minimally processed whole grains, legumes and whole fruits and veg. Remember, carbs contain fibre, the unsung blood-sugar-balancing diet hero we are not eating enough. Fibre fertilises our gut microbiota, which also help to regulate those blood-sugar roller coasters. Use the carb:fibre ratio – at least 1g fibre to every 10g carbs on the food label (divide total carbs in grams by fibre in grams).

Aside from carbs, proteins and fats can also play a role in how sugar is absorbed in the body. Adding protein to each meal is one of the simplest dietary changes to improve blood sugar. It helps stabilise blood sugar in healthy people and those with type-2 diabetes, even in the absence of weight loss – especially if you eat the protein in your meal first.

And here are some other small tweaks:

- **Add cinnamon and ginger to your meals.** These flavours might not work for all dishes, but have a plethora of scientific data to support their blood-sugar balancing effects.
- **Keep a food diary (see p. 142).** This will help you to notice how you feel in those hours after a meal. Look for patterns when you tend to hit the post-eating slump and nail down foods that send your blood sugar wild.
- **Move your body.** Short walks of only fifteen minutes after each meal are as effective at reducing blood sugar over twenty-four hours as a single forty-five-minute walk at the same moderate pace.[9] If you can't walk, try standing or doing some things around the house. Just remember that irrespective of any other blood-sugar stabilising tips you try, too much sedentary behaviour can blunt your efforts.[10] Keeping a healthy muscle mass through regular resistance exercise also works to lower blood sugar after eating.
- **Play around with meal timings.** Eating on a pretty consistent meal schedule helps to keep your blood sugar stable and you feeling energised throughout the day. It can help prevent you from becoming over-hungry and eating more than you need, which can result in a significant blood-sugar spike.[11]
- **Add vinegar to your meals.** Some studies have shown that acetic acid, the main acid in kitchen vinegar, has beneficial effects on blood sugar.[12] Dietary acetic acid is well tolerated with no adverse side effects; it can be found in many forms, including apple cider, rice, balsamic and white wine vinegars. Many pickled foods, including kimchi, pickled cucumbers and kombucha, are also good dietary sources.

'Natural' sugars and sugar substitutes

Sugar is still sugar, whether it's the white stuff or something with an organic and healthy-sounding name, such as brown rice syrup, honey, agave nectar and maple syrup (although some of these do offer marginally more nutrition). Should you replace added sugar with these? Perhaps, if you like the taste – but you should still consider them added sugars and include them in your daily calorie allowance.

Non-nutritive sweeteners (NNS) are low-calorie or calorie-free natural or chemical substances used to substitute sugar. They are pretty controversial in the nutrition world.[13] Although they may be deemed safe by the European Food Safety Authority, they are not necessarily healthy. Many of us might be swapping sugar for NNS because they don't have the calories, but they might still have negative effects on the body. Evidence suggests they can impact our ability to handle sugar normally, causing blood-sugar spikes and lowering blood-sugar tolerance (a precursor to type-2 diabetes). They are linked to increased appetite and cravings for sweet foods, as they don't satisfy biological sugar cravings, and may play a role in weight gain and obesity.[14, 15] So although they might not be overtly harmful, they interfere with metabolism and increase the risk of unhealthy responses to foods. And almost all of them have an undefined impact on the gut microbiome.

BODY COMPOSITION

I touched on obesity as having a significant impact on metabolic health and immune function. But it's important to be a little more specific here: our body composition matters more. Because of societal ideals around body shape and the influence of diet culture, exercise and gyms have evolved around weight loss, leaving a lot of confusion as to what a healthy body composition actually is. Just because your body weight isn't changing doesn't mean that your hard work isn't paying off. Your body composition may even be improving, especially if you are exercising.

Unlike body weight, which is your total body mass and the number when you step on the scale, body composition is what that mass is made up of: fat, bones, muscle, water, organs, etc. Put simply, there are two main areas of focus: sufficiently developed muscle mass (around 40 per cent of your body mass, depending on age and gender) and a body-fat percentage in a healthy range (10–20 per cent for men; 18–28 per cent for women). Why are these two parameters so important? Because each plays a different role in your inflammatory balance and their relative proportions can even impact immune rejuvenation. Muscle and fat really are the yin and yang of immune balance (see also p. 101). The relative amounts of each in your body composition give a clear picture of your health and can be an indicator of your risk of an infection or for developing a chronic inflammatory disease.

The wonderful organ called fat

Fat! It can seem like a dirty word, but it is, in fact, hugely misunderstood. Fat is not just a convenient place to store energy – it is now considered an organ in its own right (yes, it is an organ system within our bodies) because of all the jobs it carries out. Over half of the human brain is made of fat, and fatty acids contribute to nerve development and function. We also need fat to develop hormones, which serve as the body's chemical signals between different types of tissues. It behaves like a shock absorber, while we do things like run or jump, and some kinds of fat can act as insulation from the cold. It's also a depot for immune cells and a key player in inflammation/immune-regulation balance.[16]

Whether fat is used for energy or stored in the body depends primarily on our energy balance. When we are consistently in a calorie excess (either through overconsuming calories or a movement deficit), this energy will be stored in fat (adipose) cells, rather than used. To a certain extent, our body fat is related to both the number and the size of our fat cells. It's now thought that each person has a unique and individual, genetically determined number of fat cells and therefore capacity to store body fat. This number doesn't waver much throughout our lives.

When we gain weight, we store the excess energy we don't use in our fat cells. Once we surpass our personal fat-storage capacity, this excess impacts the ability of fat to function properly as the important immune-balancing organ it is. Fat cells become metabolically unbalanced as they struggle to store the excess energy and primarily grow in size rather than number. The body then has no choice but to accumulate fat around the muscles and vital organs. This type of fat becomes immunologically imbalanced, which can lead to (or perpetuate) inflammation and metabolic dysregulation.

Obesity is a stark demonstration of the immune-imbalancing effects of a poor body composition. Global obesity rates have increased nearly threefold over the past four decades.[17] Obesity can also be called a gateway disease to other conditions because it's linked to hundreds of complications, but it also changes the communication between the immune system and fat cells, disrupting the balance and increasing the likelihood of:

- poor metabolic health
- developing a vast array of inflammatory conditions
- susceptibility to infection and reduced response to vaccines
- poor health-related quality of life[18]
- susceptibility to thirteen different cancers.[19]

Obesity can also impair quality of life in a number of other ways: isolation, weight stigmatism and social exclusion, feelings of shame and vulnerability, plus an increased risk of developing anxiety and depression.[20] A calorie imbalance and lack of physical activity may be mechanisms that lead to obesity, but they're not the 'cause'. The reason behind the calorie imbalance is much more complicated. Nutritional habits, stress, sleep and a host of complex socioeconomics play into this. We live in a world where we are surrounded by a constant supply of tasty, high-calorie UPFs that are very easy to overconsume. These foods are also incredibly cheap, convenient and widely available, meaning that those with lower incomes rely on them more. That countries with the highest income disparity also have the highest rates of obesity really speaks to the complex socioeconomic issue that this is. Understanding these forces can help us to confront them and cultivate confidence in challenging food environments.

It's important to note that even in the absence of obesity, people can end up metabolically unhealthy. Subcutaneous fat is considered the more metabolically healthy type which occurs under the skin. Visceral fat is that around the internal organs and often seen as abdominal fat. It can be hazardous to your health and is associated with poor metabolic health, even in the absence of obesity.

Assess your body composition

Body mass index (BMI) is a person's weight in kilograms divided by the square of their height in metres. It is an inexpensive and easy screening method for large population-based studies, but it's flawed in that it doesn't take into account distribution of fat or overall body composition.

One way to determine if your body composition might be putting you at risk of unwanted inflammation or compromising your immune system is to have your body composition analysed. The most accurate methods are usually expensive and only available in special clinics. But at home you can track the circumference of body parts, such as waist, hips, arms, legs or chest. A decrease in waist circumference is typically a sign that you are losing belly fat. The waist-to-hip ratio (WHR) is a quick measure of fat distribution that may help indicate a person's overall health. People who carry more weight around their middle than their hips may be at higher risk of developing certain inflammatory conditions. To calculate the WHR, divide waist circumference by hip circumference; 0.85 or 0.9 or less for women and men respectively is considered healthy. A person's waist-to-height ratio (WHtR), also called waist-to-stature ratio (WSR), is a measure of distribution of body fat and is calculated as waist circumference divided by height, both measured in the same units. Higher values of WHtR indicate higher risk of obesity-related cardiovascular diseases; it is correlated with abdominal visceral obesity. For people under forty, the WHtR should be under 0.5; for people aged forty to fifty, it should be between 0.5 and 0.6; and for people over fifty it should be around 0.6.

A DEXA (dual-energy X-ray absorptiometry) scan is a piece of equipment found in some gyms and healthcare settings that can be used to determine the percentage of lean muscle and fat. Although not 100 per cent accurate, it can give an indication. For men, you'll want to be no higher than about 20 per cent body fat; for women, try to stay under about 28 per cent. This assessment will reveal your body-fat percentage, a number that you can use to understand if the amount of fat you have is healthy or excessive for someone of your size. A more accurate way would be a skin-fold assessment, which needs to be done by a trained practitioner.

Improve your body composition

A lot of people wrongly assume that they are not in control of their body composition. Certainly, genetics play a part, but your body composition is very heavily impacted by what you eat and how you exercise. This means that you can be in control of these two primary levers. Of course, it is a lot more nuanced than this, but these should be your starting points. Read on to find out more.

Hunger and satiety hormones

We make over 200 food choices per day and many of these can become automatic.[21] Our fat produces hundreds of hormones, many of which influence satiety and hunger and play a significant role in how much we eat and overall body energy balance regulation. Leptin and ghrelin are two key players in this. These opposing hormones are released rhythmically based on habitual food intake. Leptin signals to the brain to lower appetite after we have eaten (although we can, of course, eat through it, and our food environment plays a huge part in this). Leptin is dramatically altered by changes in our body fat, with high body fat leading to more of it. Ghrelin is a peptide that plays an important role in short-term appetite regulation. It is released when our stomachs are empty and we start to grow hungry, but it can also be influenced by food marketing and our mental wellbeing.[22]

When blood sugar, body composition and eating schedules go awry, leptin and ghrelin follow suit. For some of us, this can result in an inability to distinguish between real and perceived hunger. But it can also have knock-on effects to the immune system. Leptin can have pro-inflammatory effects, while ghrelin is anti-inflammatory.

Muscle: the yang to fat's yin

Unless you are a body builder, you may not have given your muscle mass or muscle strength much thought. But here is why you should: muscle cells require more energy to maintain than fat cells, so they contribute to a healthy metabolism and blood-sugar control.[23] Strong muscles improve balance and decrease the risk of falls. You don't need to be a competitive weight lifter, but the stronger your muscles become, the better your health will be. When it comes to your immune system, muscle is non-negotiable. I'd go as far as to say that this is perhaps one of the least recognised ways in which we can care for our immune system. Muscle tissue is preventative against some of the most common and increasingly rampant inflammatory health conditions.[24] In fact, muscle correlates with reduced metabolic disease, better outcomes from cancer therapy, better infection protection and a decrease in all-cause mortality. Simply put, more muscle mass and muscle strength = less risk of dying.

Muscle mass and strength are in a constant state of flux. Our bodies are continually breaking down muscle protein (muscle protein breakdown – MPB) and rebuilding or synthesising it (muscle protein synthesis – MPS), depending on what we are doing. When MPB exceeds MPS, we start to lose muscle mass. This occurs on a micro level (daily shifts) and a macro level (long-term shifts). These macro losses as we age are the biggest challenge to our health. Sarcopenia (the science-y term given to this age-related decline) begins as early as our forties, ramping up dramatically as we enter our sixties, with up to 50 per cent of mass being lost by our eighties.[25]

The causes and consequences of sarcopenia are many and complex, including neurological decline, hormonal changes, chronic inflammation and long-term illness, mitochondria dysfunction, sedentary behaviour and poor nutrition with a lack of protein – all related and contributing to the decline. Your muscles also stop using protein as efficiently with ageing and are less able to repair themselves. Sarcopenia might seem far into your future and not something you need to worry about just yet, but you need to be building that muscle bank account now, through exercise – because if you don't use it, you lose it. That said, however, because you lose it, doesn't mean it is gone for ever.

But before you get too hung up on how much muscle and fat you have, remember they are only one part of the picture. Just make sure you are dedicating some time to them; I'll detail the ways in which you can work on body composition to protect your muscle a bit later on (see pp. 117–121).

CHAPTER 7:

Immune-Nourishing Nutrition

We have looked at *how* you eat, and now it's time to consider *what* you eat. I will guide you on how to make small dietary tweaks, ensuring that your diet supports all your immunity needs, is nutritious, fits your lifestyle *and* is enjoyable. (**Note**: this might mean forgoing the latest craze!) This will be not a restrictive dietary protocol but, rather, the knowledge and tools to curate a sustainable diet pattern around diversity, abundance and variety, all supported by clinical scientific evidence. Consider food to be a tool – physically, socially and emotionally nourishing – to build up your immune resilience, raise immune rejuvenation and lower unnecessary inflammation. The best diet for you depends on your physiology, food preferences, age, health, budget, cooking skills and personal beliefs. Simply, it's any healthy diet pattern you can sustain in the long term.

THE BASICS

Food does several important things to support proper immune function, protect your body from infection and maintain balance and resilience to chronic disease:

- It provides the raw materials to make new antibodies, cells and molecules.

- It provides energy to fuel an immune response, which is energetically very costly.
- It provides key nutrients that are co-factors in hundreds of key reactions in the body.
- It has its own antioxidant, anti-inflammatory and anti-microbial superpowers to reduce your risk of illness.
- It prevents malnutrition and overnutrition.

Your immune system depends on energy in the form of calories to fuel its function. Before we get into the specifics of what foods and nutrients make up your diet, it is important to note that the simple fact of consistently eating either too many calories (over-nutrition) or too few (malnutrition) will impair your immune system: too many are inflammatory and can compromise important antioxidant mechanisms, as well as potentially altering muscle–fat balance and, consequently, baseline inflammation; too few and it won't have all the necessary materials to make antibodies and cells.

The principles of nutritional immunology (that things we eat can influence the immune response) arose many decades ago from treating diseases of deficiency and malnutrition by 'supplementing' with micronutrients (vitamins and minerals) which would 'cure' disease and restore infection protection. This means we know the importance of specific micronutrients (including vitamins A, B, C, D, E and K, and certain minerals, including copper, iron, selenium, and zinc) in supporting the body's immune defences.[1]

The immune system is complex, with its needs dictated by age, sex and life stage. Generally speaking, RDAs (recommended dietary allowances) are designed to avoid deficiency in the general population aged between nineteen and sixty-five. Individual RDA will vary depending on age, lifestyle, underlying conditions and dietary choices. Of course, avoiding deficiencies in any of the essential micronutrients is key to supporting proper immune function and reducing risk of infection. Deficiencies, even mild, 'sub-clinical' ones, can happen unintentionally as certain dietary choices leave one or another nutrient in short supply. But today's health challenges in the UK are less about malnutrition and micronutrient deficiencies, and more about our complicated relationship with food and our food environment.

Food first . . . but sometimes supplement

Who doesn't like a quick fix? Imagine taking a few supplements and never having to worry about your immune system again. I'll be the first to say that a 'quick' immunity fix *might* be achieved through time, consistency and a 360-degree lifestyle approach. (Well, not exactly quick, but not out of reach either.) Pre- COVID-19, 59 per cent of UK adults reported taking a vitamin or mineral supplement. Since the start of the pandemic, interest in supplements supporting immunity has skyrocketed, but recent data actually shows only modest effects of supplementing against COVID-19 symptoms.[2]

So the supplement aisle doesn't necessarily offer a quick panacea (although I don't doubt that it provides a sense of agency over health, and there is something to be said for the placebo effect). And results from large, randomised, controlled trials on micronutrient supplements on everything from infection to inflammation and all-cause mortality (a measure of anything that causes death) generally show no beneficial effects unless you have a deficiency. Also, studies showing the 'advantage' of vitamins and minerals for our health come mainly from studies of food, not supplements.

Aim to strengthen your immunity nutritionally with the food you eat. If you are thinking about a supplement, consider these key principles:

- **Supplements should be there to, well, 'supplement'.** They do have a place – for example, to replace something missing in a diet, such as vitamin B12 for those following a vegan lifestyle, or as part of a treatment for a particular condition. But it's highly personal and you need to be well informed before you spend your money.
- **Can you get it from your diet?** I am often asked what vitamins I take, and people are surprised by my answer: vitamin D and not a lot else. Sure, vitamins are 'good' when it's been shown that you need them (i.e. you don't have enough), but they are generally best found in food (with the exception of vitamin D) and taking more won't necessarily make your immune system work better than baseline.
- **What additional ingredients are lurking in your supplements?** Read the labels and consider the inactive ingredients, such as sugar, fillers, binders, bulking agents, coatings, colourings, carriers and other harmful, unnecessary and sometimes, quite frankly, terrifying ingredients. Look for full transparency on any brand's product.
- **Do your homework.** Weigh up the evidence supporting health claims of a supplement you are considering. Do you have any circumstances that may affect your micronutrient requirements – for example, following a specific diet, going through a period of stress, an underlying condition, chronic alcohol consumption or pregnancy? Talk to a healthcare professional if you are confused, or seek advice from a credible online resource, such as the National Health Service in the UK or National Institutes for Health Office of Dietary Supplements.
- **It takes a 360-degree approach.** No single supplement (or food) will support every aspect of your health if you

haven't sorted out the reasons why overall diet and lifestyle might not be supporting you as needed.

- **Check the formulation.** Sometimes it's not as simple as taking a multivitamin, because your body prefers – in some cases, requires – the active forms of vitamins, which are rare in most supplements. Examples include folate in the form of 5-methyltetrahydrofolate (called MTHF) and B12 as methylcobalamin to aid healthy methylation.
- **More is not always better.** Vitamin and mineral supplements tend to cause little or no harm in the short term. Negative consequences can come from long-term consumption of micronutrients that we don't need (although there are always exceptions).[3] In some cases, this can even slightly increase adverse effects on health due to high doses. One example is reports of health hazards from taking beta-carotene (pro-vitmain A).[4] Another key example is toxic effects from excessive intake of antioxidant supplements, showing they promote rather than prevent oxidative damage – a phenomenon termed the 'antioxidant paradox'.[5] Eating plenty of antioxidant-rich whole food is a much better idea than supplements and is proven more effective in reducing oxidative damage.[6]

Vitamin D

Vitamin D is fat-soluble and regulates calcium and phosphate balance for healthy bones. But it's also a hormone and immune modulator, acting directly on our immune cells to shape their function. Vitamin D is produced when the skin is exposed to UVB radiation from sunlight. Getting out in the sun has a stack of benefits for our wellbeing, but there are many reasons why we might not get enough to maintain good levels. Food sources include oily fish, eggs, butter and fortified foods. Vegan dietary sources of vitamin D, such as mushrooms, provide the D2 form of the vitamin which needs further conversion to D3 by the body, so is less bioavailable. It can be hard to obtain enough from diet alone. Public Health England now recommends that everyone should supplement with 10mg per day of vitamin D during the winter months (October–March), but those with darker skin, the elderly and those who spend a lot of time inside and are at greater risk of deficiency are advised to supplement all year round. Opt for a regular intake daily and use the D3 form rather than D2.[7]

HIGH-VALUE EATING: AN IMMUNE-FOCUSED ~~DIET~~ WAY OF EATING

A healthy diet pattern is one that encompasses 'high-value eating'. This is not only about having a good relationship with food but choosing foods that are nourishing and satisfying. It's about eating in a way that's doable, sustainable, customisable and doesn't come with strict rules. It adds to your life, instead of taking away (which also means that one bad meal does not poor health make). It is centred on whole, unprocessed or minimally processed foods – such as vegetables, fruits, whole grains, nuts and legumes – retaining the fibre, as well as the whole portfolio of beneficial phytochemicals and nutrients.

Cumulatively, a high-value eating pattern will pay into your **protective** immune health bank account, **strengthen** your body's defences and **fuel** your body to meet all the demands that life places on it.

Protective nutrition

All fruits and vegetables are important, and studies show that increased consumption improves inflammation and immune-cell profile.[8] But some have more powerful immune-protective properties than others. Protective nutrition is about including a variety of produce with your meals, while ensuring you include specific groups on the regular because of their special compounds that have particular benefits. These include direct effects on the immune system like supporting antioxidants, epigenetically activating beneficial genes and silencing less favourable ones to dampen unwanted inflammation.

****IMMUNITY TIP**** Before we dive into the details, remember: higher fruit and veg consumption is scientifically shown to give us better protection against infections. The minimum daily requirement in the UK is at least five portions a day to support general health. To prevent chronic disease, we should consume at least eight portions a day. And there may be benefits to eating more if you have an underlying condition. We don't know the optimal intake for your immune system because those studies haven't been done, but it makes sense that more is likely better. However, the most important thing is to start where you are and slowly and incrementally increase, trying not to limit variety.

Phytonutrients

Phyto is the Greek word for 'plant'. Phytonutrients are the chemicals produced by the immune systems of plants (as mentioned previously, everything on this planet has an immune system). They serve to protect plants from environmental challenges, including the damaging rays of the sun, insects, disease and other possible threats to their survival. Phytonutrients, unlike the vitamins and minerals we are familiar with, do not meet the classic definition of 'essential' nutrients. Amazingly, however, these compounds have profound effects on our bodies, from upregulating our internal immune defences, to helping us fight infections and tame inflammation, and even supporting healthy immune rejuvenation of our immune cells from the bone marrow. These 'longevity compounds' even help to neutralise the oxidative stress associated with the daily wear and tear on our bodies. There may not be a recommended daily amount, but not getting enough of these is known as 'long-latency deficiency'. In order to understand what this means, we need to talk about the opposite: 'short-latency deficiency'. Examples of short-latency-deficiency diseases are pellagra, beri-beri, scurvy and rickets. These are conditions that arise quickly after a person becomes overtly deficient in a single essential nutrient. Vitamin C deficiency leads to scurvy, vitamin B3 deficiency leads to pellagra and vitamin B1 deficiency leads to beri beri. In the UK, these short-latency-deficiency diseases are thankfully rare, in the most part eliminated through nutritional policies, guidelines and fortification of foods. The timeframe to developing them is short enough to make the benefits of correcting the deficiency perceptible. But this has also led to the presumption that if the intake of a nutrient is sufficient to prevent the expression of a short-latency-deficiency disease (i.e. vitamin C and scurvy), then it is adequate for our optimal long-term health. By contrast, long-latency deficiency diseases are, in part, the result of subtle nutritional shortfalls over long periods of time, leading to things such as heart disease, inflammatory conditions, certain cancers and poorer overall health as we age. They don't have one single indicator, and it may take twenty years or more to suffer the ill-effects.

The power of vitamin P

Vitamin P is a term that was once used to refer to flavanoids, a specific group of phytonutrients that belong to the polyphenol family, because they were originally thought to be another type of vitamin. These nutrients not only quench free radicals, but also induce our own protection mechanism against oxidative stress and inflammation, enhancing immune resilience. Large studies have even found that flavonoids and other phytonutrients can significantly reduce the risk of getting infections, such as the common cold, and stave off chronic disease. Even more exciting is their emerging role in epigenetics – modifying our genes to significantly benefit our health.[9] Although a lot of the exciting scientific research on vitamin P typically uses high doses of phytonutrients, you don't necessarily need to take supplements, as your intake can be substantial in a diet rich in plant diversity. Plants often provide the most bioavailable way to consume these amazing phytonutrients – another great reason to aim for a food-first approach.[10]

Thousands of different types of phytonutrients exist and are responsible for the flavours, colours and smells of fresh produce. They are divided into six main subclasses:

- **Flavonols,** including kaempferol, quercetin, myricetin and fisetin. These compounds are found in olive oil, berries, onions, kale, grapes, tomatoes, red wine and teas.

- **Flavones**, found in parsley, thyme, mint, celery and chamomile.
- **Flavanols and flavan-3-ols**, including catechins, such as epicatechin and epigallocatechin, which are found in high concentrations in black, green and oolong tea, as well as cocoa, apples, grapes and red wine.
- **Flavanones**, such as hesperitin, naringenin and eriodictyol; found in citrus fruits, flavanones are responsible for the bitter taste of orange, lemon and other citrus peels.
- **Isoflavones**, such as genistin and daidzin, which are found in soybeans and soy products.
- **Anthocyanidins** are the phytonutrients responsible for the red, blue and purple colour of plants; they are present in blueberries, blackcurrants, strawberries, pomegranates and plums.

The simplest way to add vitamin P to your plate is to add plants to each meal, think about colour and aim to eat a rainbow of diversity where possible.

IMMUNITY TIP Scientific studies have shown that cacao is packed with flavonoids. Opt for dark chocolate to enjoy this vitamin- P-rich food.

Antioxidant tips

Free radicals cause oxidative stress, which hurts the immune system. They form during the digestion of food and general day-to-day running of our bodies, as well as from exposure to things in our environment, such as pollution. Our ability to fight oxidative stress depends on our overall diet and lifestyle, and it decreases as we age, so it's important to balance out free radicals with sufficient numbers of antioxidants. But where can we find them? In all the colourful, phytonutrient-loaded fruits and veggies. My easy tip to up the antioxidants in your diet is to add herbs and spices, as they pack the biggest antioxidant punch per unit of weight. That means you don't have to add a lot to benefit from them. Herbs that are easy to grow on a windowsill include sage, parsley, basil, oregano, thyme, mint and dill. But since not all of us will have a herb garden, keeping dried herbs in your cupboard is a convenient and quick way to enhance the antioxidant content (not to mention flavour) of dishes.

Load up on leafy greens

Dark green vegetables – such as kale, chard, spinach, rocket, Brussels sprouts and sprouting broccoli – all provide a variety of beneficial micronutrients, such as vitamin A and magnesium, but also folate, an important nutrient in supporting methylation. They also carry many phytonutrients and chlorophyll, shown to reduce oxidative stress and stimulate production of new immune cells from the bone marrow.

Another thing that makes these so special is that they are packed with nitrates, which are converted to nitric oxide (NO) in the body. NO is antimicrobial, it inactivates viruses and is being explored as a treatment in COVID-19.[11] It's also crucial in relaxing blood vessels, improving blood flow and maintaining healthy blood pressure, and supporting physical activity and brain function.[12] If there is one thing to add to our diets, it is this group of vegetables. Aim for at least one portion per day (remembering that some of them shrink considerably in terms of volume when cooked, making it easier to achieve this target).

Stock up on sulphur-rich crucifers and alliums

Sulphur is an essential mineral that the body cannot make on its own. By weight, it is one of the most abundant minerals in the human body, coming in at around 140g for the average person, and this is no accident. It assists in numerous processes involved in protecting your body.

While there is no RDA for sulphur, the health benefits are clear, and eating sulphur-rich foods is the best way to ensure you're consuming adequate amounts through your diet. Sulphur is found in a range of animal and plant foods, including:

- allium vegetables such as garlic, leeks and onions
- cruciferous vegetables such as rocket, broccoli, cabbage, cauliflower and kale
- eggs, dairy, meat and seafood
- legumes such as chickpeas, lentils and beans
- nuts and seeds.

Although sulphur is found in animal foods, research has identified that several of its key health benefits come specifically from sulphur-rich plants. This is because they are abundant sources of sulphur-containing compounds known as glucosinolates, which are hydrolysed to isothiocyanates.[13] Many isothiocyanates, particularly sulphoraphane, are instrumental in optimising immune function. They induce the expression of antioxidant enzymes,[14] as well as reducing inflammation and the risk of developing chronic health conditions, such as heart disease and certain cancers.[15, 16]

Cruciferous and allium vegetables are unique in that they are particularly rich sources of isothiocyanates. To maximise the benefits of these compounds when consuming allium and cruciferous veggies, slice them, then leave to sit for a few minutes before steaming to liberate and activate the compounds prior to consuming. These compounds are also particularly enriched in the sprout during the germination process, making sprouted seeds a great way to enjoy the benefits.

Another good reason to eat these sulphur-rich vegetables is that they are a source of a chemical signal called indole-3-carbinol (I3C) that is important for a fully functioning immune system. IC3 triggers the Aryl hydrocarbon Receptor (AhR) on specialist immune cells known as intra-epithelial lymphocytes (IELs). IELs patrol our body barriers like the gut and the skin, IC3 helps IELs do their job effectively, regulating our body barriers and preventing unfavourable germs and toxins getting into our bodies.

IMMUNITY TIP Aim to include at least one portion of cooked crucifers and/or alliums per day.

Myconutrients

A myconutrient is the fungi and yeast version of a plant phytonutrient. Myconutrients have an array of bioactive properties, including antiviral effects, plus antioxidant and anti-inflammatory power to nourish and support many functions of your immune system.[17,18] β-glucans are particularly well-studied myconutrients, with many established immune-enhancing effects. Several immune cells have receptors that specifically recognise β-glucans, leading to enhanced resistance to infection and possibly cancer too.[19]

Mushrooms have a cherished place in culinary traditions all over the world. There's hardly a human culture on this planet that does not eat mushrooms of one sort or another, and now we have the science to support why. Mushroom-based wellness products are everywhere these days, from tinctures and pills to coffee and moisturisers. Their unique myconutrients also contribute to their savoury umami flavour profile, making them a very desirable culinary ingredient that can be readily added to soups, stews, sauces and more. Their fibres produce a dense, meaty texture that provides a great alternative to meat, especially when grilled. They couldn't be easier to incorporate into your diet.

IMMUNITY TIP Mushrooms can be an acquired taste and some people dislike the texture. Try adding them into meals you already enjoy two or three times per week. Chop them small or experiment with some of the functional mushroom powders now available. Keep mushrooms upside down on your windowsill to boost their vitamin D content.

For a myconutrient-rich alternative to cheese, sprinkle nutritional yeast onto foods or add to dishes for a nutty and unique savoury flavour.

Zoonutrients

Zoonutrients are found in animal sources and help to support your immune system. Astaxanthin – the reddish pigment that gives the pink colour to salmon, trout and seafood – is a great example. It has potent antioxidative and anti-inflammatory effects, and through these and other mechanisms, astaxanthin can enhance and improve how your immune system functions.[20] Don't overlook tinned fish, which tend to be smaller, mercury-free varieties loaded with essential omega-3 fats.

Strengthening nutrition

Strengthening nutrition is all about giving the immune system the building blocks to keep our bodies strong – from building new immune cells and antibodies and enhancing our barriers (such as the skin, lungs and gut) to protecting our muscle mass and supporting a healthy body composition.

Protein and pulses

One of the biggest myths about protein is that you only need to worry about it if you work out and have specific physical goals with regard to muscles. Protein is a critical cornerstone of a strong immune system, and protein energy malnutrition is one of the leading causes of immune deficiency worldwide.[21]

Protein provides the building blocks that enable the immune system to mount an appropriate immune response and produce new immune cells and antibodies, as well as being essential for the repair and growth of our bodies' tissues. Research also consistently shows it helps with satiety, appetite regulation and, importantly, blood-sugar control, which means it can play an important role in your relationship with food. If your body is the house, protein is the bricks. And the more active, stressed and older you are, the more bricks your body needs.

You can get protein from many food sources, including both animal foods and plants. Irrespective of where you get it from, protein is broken down into its constituent amino acids. When choosing between plant and animal sources, it is important to factor in the other nutrients that the foods provide. Animal sources also contain important micronutrients, such as vitamin B12, and zoonutrients, such as astaxanthin in fish and seafood. Animal protein in its untouched form is also a NOVA Group 1 classified unprocessed or minimally processed food. Animal sources tend to contain all the essential amino acids needed to support the body.

Plant sources of protein, such as beans and pulses, are conveniently packed with lots of gut-loving fibre. Aim to have roughly a palm-sized portion of protein at each meal of the day. I buy pulses in bulk in jars and add them to soups, make them into hummus and other dips, throw them into curries and stews, or eat them cold with some olive oil, lemon and a few chopped herbs.

Not all protein sources are created equal in terms of their amino-acid composition. Historically, animal proteins were considered superior, but a closer look tells us that this is due to animal sources generally being higher in the amino acid leucine, which is the most important for muscle protein synthesis.[22] (See p. 101 for more on the importance of muscle for immunity.) Leucine is also found in plant-based sources, just in more variable amounts. Be judicious with plant-based protein, diversifying your sources to ensure you meet your leucine needs. Animal-based foods that are high in leucine include chicken, beef, pork, fish, cheese, milk and eggs. Plant-based examples include soy-based foods (for example, tofu, tempeh and edamame), legume-based (lentils, beans, rice, chickpeas) and whole- grain-based (seitan), as well as nuts, seeds, mushrooms or vegan protein powders, such as a pea/hemp-blend.

How much protein do you need per day?

As with most things in nutrition, there is no simple answer. The right amount of protein for each person depends on a number of factors, such as age, gender and fitness goals, as well as the protein source. For adults in the UK, its estimated that we need around 75g of protein per kilogram of body weight per day. For simplicity's sake, this equates to approximately 56g and 45g per day for men and women aged nineteen to fifty respectively. Sixty grams of protein per kilogram of body weight per day is the minimum to prevent protein energy malnutrition, but my suggestion is to aim for more, mixing up your sources to ensure you meet the threshold for each essential amino acid and spreading it across each of your meals in the day. Not only does this become particularly important as you get older for mitigating sarcopenia (see p. 102), but it also helps with satiety and blood-sugar balance. There is an extra requirement for growth in infants and children, and for pregnant and breastfeeding women.

Test the power of protein: one day increase the amount at each meal. Note down your hunger and satiety. Then compare to a day when you eat protein-poor meals.

Fuelling nutrition

Fuelling nutrition is all about providing the fuel for the work your immune system has to carry out – and remember, even when you are not aware of it, your immune system is always working hard in the background. Fats and carbs are the two key macronutrients that our bodies use for fuel. But these labels actually cover a huge diversity of foods, many of which have been vilified at one time or another, making it a little sticky and confusing. Read on to find out my simple take on fuelling your immunity.

Fuelling fats

Once vilified, are dietary fats healthy when it comes to your immune system? And, if so, which ones and how much?

First, fats play lots of important roles not only in our immunity, but also more broadly in our general health. They:

- are needed for absorption of vitamins A, D, E and K
- can help with blood-sugar regulation (see p. 93)
- are part of our cells' structure
- are needed for the production of some hormones that play a key role in the immune system
- are involved in the resolution of inflammation
- make food taste good.

Fat is not one thing. There are many different types, some more healthy than others. Some fats are essential, and others are non-essential. Foods will generally contain a mixture of the different types of fats, so look for ones lower in trans/saturated fats and higher in poly- and monounsaturated fats.

Here is my quick guide:

- **Essential** Both omega-3 and omega-6 polyunsaturated fats are considered essential because you can't live without them and your body doesn't have the ability to make them naturally. Omega-3s have a known protective function and are key to resolving inflammation, preventing unnecessary collateral damage to our delicate tissues.[23] Look for a combination of eicosapentaenoic acid (EPA) and docosahexaenoic acid (DHA), which are found in oily fish or supplements, rather than alpha-linolenic acid (ALA) from vegan sources, which gets poorly converted to the active EPA and DHA. If you are not regularly eating oily fish, you should supplement with omega-3s.

- **Include regularly** Monounsaturated fats found in oily fish, nuts and seeds, olive oil and avocados.[24]
- **Reduce** Saturated fats, which tend to be found in fatty or processed meats, as well sources such as butter, lard, ghee, palm oil and coconut oil. They have direct pro-inflammatory properties, and are also absorbed directly into the lymphatic system, which can increase the volume of lymph fluid, impairing immune-system function and the removal of toxins from the body.[25]
- **Avoid** Trans fats arise from processing oils at high temperatures (called hydrogenation). Luckily, in the UK, trans fats have been largely removed from the food chain but can still be found in small amounts in pastries and other baked goods.[26]

****IMMUNITY TIP**** Some ingredients stand the test of time, and olive oil is definitely one of them. Olive oil is not only a great source of healthy monounsaturated fats, but it's packed with polyphenols such as oleic acid, oleuropein, hydroxytyrosol, tyrosol and olecanthal and – unlike some other vegetable oils – it has been shown to have particular benefits on the immune system. Extra virgin olive oil (EVOO) has the highest levels of these amazing phytonutrients, as well as the best taste and a pretty good shelf life, too, making it one to always have in your cupboard (although it never lasts long in our house). Look for mono-varieties (Arbequina, Hojiblanca, Manzanilla or Picual), if possible. Despite the myth that we shouldn't cook with EVOO, there is no real evidence for this and it is perfectly fine to use for most types of home cooking (although it shouldn't be re-used).

Considered carbs

Just like the other macronutrients (protein and fat), not all carbs are created equal. Low-quality carbs from processed foods high in added sugars represent more than 40 per cent of our daily calories.[27] When we instead choose high-quality carbs from whole grains, nuts, fruits, and vegetables, we not only enjoy a greater variety of foods, but also many health benefits (such as increased fibre) that help support a happy and healthy microbiome. Carbohydrates are found in all plant-based foods. The best way to consider them is through eating lots of delicious plant-based foods, which provide a source of fibre to keep our gut bugs happy. I've got a lot to say on the topic of fibre-rich carbs, gut bugs and our immune system, but for now, it's about quality (unrefined, minimally processed plants) and quantity (approximately a fistful on your plate).

The bitter taste of infection

When it comes to our diet pattern, we must consider taste as part of the equation. We have five basic types of tastes: salty, sweet, bitter, sour and umami. And we have around twenty-five different kinds of taste receptors for bitter –

way more than for the other tastes. But bitter flavours often get neglected. Examples of bitter plants include radicchio, endive, dark leafy greens such as kale and collards, ginger, aniseed, fennel, citrus peel and dandelion greens. Perhaps you remember the first time you tasted the bitterness of leafy greens as a child? Vowing never to eat the stuff again because it was just too bitter?

The bitterness comes from the phytonutrients as part of their own immune defence – to discourage insects from eating them, for example. When we consume them, they make important contributions to our health through their digestion-enhancing properties, helping to control appetite and blood sugar.[28] They also have an especially profound influence on the immune system, providing antioxidants, anti-inflammatory effects and even prebiotic properties.

Bitter taste receptors aren't just on our tongues. They are more or less all over the body, even in our immune cells, where they play an essential role in our immune defence by responding to bitter molecules released by germs.[29] People who are genetically more sensitive to bitter tastes have been shown to be more likely to attain longevity[30] and are better able to mount a strong immune response to oral and upper-respiratory infections.[31]

The food industry puts a lot of work into removing bitterness from plants by selective breeding and debittering processes in response to consumer demand. The less we eat bitter foods, the less we want to. Perhaps it's one reason why the advice to eat more veggies often goes unheeded when there are more palatable UPFs on offer.

We each have varying sensitivity to bitter flavours and this plays a central role in influencing which foods we consume.

Even if you are not a genetic bitter supertaster, it turns out taste buds are reprogrammable. This means, if you really want to, you can slowly work towards enjoying those initially less palatable bitter veggies and one day actually enjoy them.

HYDRATION

It would be remiss not to mention hydration and the immune system. Hydration keeps our lymphatic fluid flowing, helping immune cells to move around the body and perform their functions. When we are hydrated, we produce adequate mucus of the right consistency which helps protect the delicate barriers of our airways and gut.

It's impossible to give a precise guideline, but aim for a minimum of 1.5–2 litres per day – maybe more if you're drinking coffee and/or alcohol, or sweating more due to heat or exercise. And don't forget, herbal teas are rich sources of phytonutrients and can contribute to overall intake of antioxidants and management of unwanted inflammation. When it comes to alcohol, many of us are familiar with the phrase 'drinking in moderation'; you may even have heard this can bring health benefits and that abstaining from alcohol is less beneficial than drinking a little (this flawed conclusion is thought to be due to abstinence by people with chronic diseases).[32] But sadly, alcohol, even in moderation, can interfere with the immune system. Alcohol disrupts our body barriers, including the airways and the gut barrier, as well as the beneficial microbes that live there. It can have negative effects on sleep, stress, eating habits and the absorption of nutrients; it also requires micronutrients for its removal, leaving fewer available for other body systems.

GUT HEALTH IS IMMUNE HEALTH

Microbes inhabit all surfaces of the body (that's any surface that interfaces with the environment – most obviously our skin, but also our lungs, digestive, reproductive and urinary tracts). The greatest density and diversity of microbes is within the gut. This means your gut it not only a digestive tube, but an ecosystem of trillions of microbes known collectively as your gut microbiota (GM). As our knowledge of the GM grows, so do the health claims associated with it. This ecosystem is now considered to influence the development and function of all systems of our bodies.[33]

Although deep inside us, the gut is outward-facing – in direct contact with our environment, via all the things we put into our mouths and swallow. And it is where we are most vulnerable and need the most protection. This is why an impressive 70 per cent of the body's immune system is housed in the gut. This means it's right up close alongside your GM. In fact, these bugs outnumber your immune cells by 200,000:1, which makes your gut and all its microbes and marvellous digestive processes a massive part of your immune-health journey. One reason so much of the immune system is located in the gut is to defend this long and delicate barrier, the largest surface in the body exposed to the outside world. This close proximity is no accident. The immune cells are lone security guards of the entire digestive tract, while our good gut bugs are a helpful neighbourhood watch, surveilling this barrier, helping crowd out the bad guys and raising signals for the immune system to respond. These microbes are so important to our health that we immunologists very much consider them a part of our immune defences – a supportive organ inseparable from overall physical and mental health.

THE GUT-IMMUNE AXIS

The inner gut ecosystem functions as the immune system's control tower in a two-way relationship known as the gut-immune axis. Bacteria seem to get the most attention as they are by far the best understood microbes, though fungi, viruses and other microorganisms claim a place in this complex ecosystem, too. Their collective genetic material is estimated to contain 100 times more genes than our own human genome. Although sometimes used interchangeably, the term microbiota refers to the collection of microbes, whereas the term microbiome refers to these microbes and all the potential functions that their genes provide.

There are multiple lines of communication through which the GM influences our immune cells, supporting the health of body and mind:

- **Indirectly, by eating your food for you** We humans have very few fibre-digesting gut capabilities, unlike our gut microbes, which have an estimated 60,000 digestive enzymes.[34] This means we have largely outsourced digestion of carbs to our gut bugs. Why? Because it allows us to be extremely adaptable and resilient to our changing environment. In this way, our GM indirectly supports the immune system through ensuring effective digestion and absorption of nutrients. It also supports production of hormones that influence feelings of satiety, regulating gut motility and a healthy metabolism. It even contributes to the production of some key micronutrients, such as biotin, folate and vitamin B12, and how many calories we absorb from our food.
- **Educating and training immune cells** Much of our immune development occurs after we are born, and continues to a

certain extent for the rest of our lives. The GM is a key trainer and educator of immune cells. In fact, without a GM, you wouldn't even have a functioning immune system.[35]

- **Producing powerful postbiotics** 'Postbiotics' are the metabolic by-products released when our GMs help us to digest plant fibres in our food. They may be underrated GM metabolic 'waste' products, but they play a huge role in both gut and overall immune health.[36] Short-chain fatty acids (SCFAs) acetate, butyrate and propionate are among the best-studied postbiotics (see box overleaf).[37]
- **Maintaining gut barrier health and integrity** Signals between the microbes and their postbiotics support gut barrier cells and help to maintain layers of mucus and antibodies called secretory IgA to prevent unwanted gut contents from entering the bloodstream.[38]
- **Colonisation resistance** It outcompetes infectious germs and uses antimicrobial postbiotics to prevent any one niche group of microbes from overpowering the rest of the population.[39]
- **Toxin biotransformation** Biotransformation is a process by which toxic chemicals that we inadvertently consume are transformed into a less toxic form to help us remove them or reduce their persistence and toxicity. This process is aided by the microbes in the gut.[40]

A good relationship with your GM is a ticket to a fit, strong and resilient immune system. This puts a new slant on the words 'You are what you eat'; or, more accurately, you are what your microbes digest *and* how well they support your gut. Even if you have the 'healthiest' diet, you can only really get the full nutritional benefits if you care for your microbes. In fact, *the* single most effective dietary strategy that you can adopt to build strong immunity is to take care of your gut microbes. If they're happy, you'll probably be happy, too. Happy, because they can also *literally* make you happier via the 'gut-brain axis' that you will meet in the next chapter.

Short-chain fatty acids in a nutshell

SCFAs are like the magic currency of both gut health and whole-body health. Not only do they nourish your gut, protecting and healing its barrier and managing gut inflammation and immune defences, but they are absorbed into the blood and travel around the body dispensing their powerful benefits everywhere from the brain to your airways and beyond. Collectively, SCFAs do many beneficial things, including inhibiting the most powerful pro-inflammatory signals in the body. They also play a role in generating regulatory T-cell production and function for the entire body, which is kind of a big deal in terms of maintaining that immunological balance I mentioned earlier.[41]

- Acetate helps regulate your gut's pH, deterring opportunistic infectious germs, and stopping them from invading the delicate gut barrier. Acetate also helps control appetite and nourishes beneficial bacteria that produce butyrate.
- Butyrate is the main fuel for the cells of the gut, providing up to 70 per cent of their energy needs and supporting the integrity of this essential barrier.[42] Butyrate also has epigenetic effects, supporting anti-

inflammatory gene expression, combating inflammation and turning off cancer genes.

- Propionate helps regulate appetite, but also combats inflammation and protects against cancer.
- Lactate is a less appreciated SCFA that helps maintain immune health, combats opportunistic bacteria and is food for other beneficial bacteria that produce butyrate.

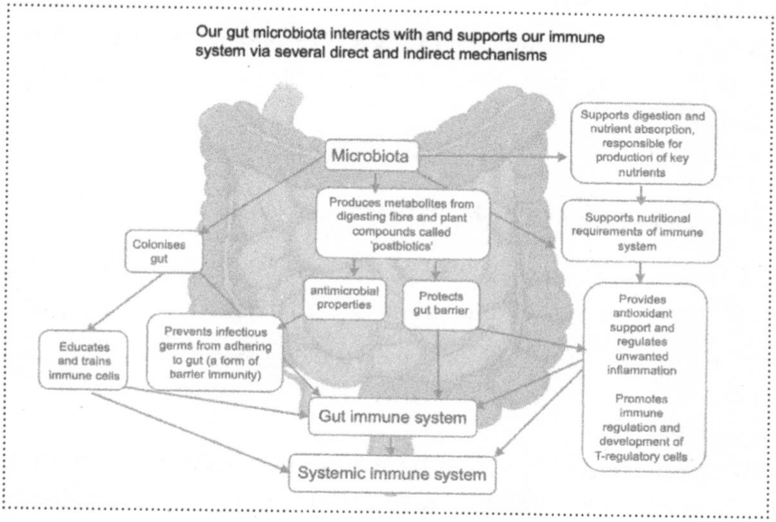
Our gut microbiota interacts with and supports our immune system via several direct and indirect mechanisms
Microbiota
Supports digestion and nutrient absorption, responsible for production of key nutrients
Produces metabolites from digesting fibre and plant compounds called 'postbiotics'
Supports nutritional requirements of immune system
Colonises gut
antimicrobial properties
Protects gut barrier
Provides antioxidant support and regulates unwanted inflammation
Promotes immune regulation and development of T-regulatory cells
Educates and trains immune cells
Prevents infectious germs from adhering to gut (a form of barrier immunity)
Gut immune system
Systemic immune system

Figure 9 How the gut microbiota supports the immune system

WHAT IS A HEALTHY GUT MICROBIOME?

The small but mighty microbes in our gut are both personal and unique to us. Their types and quantities can change over our lifespan, so how do we know if we have a healthy GM?

It's diverse!

Full disclosure: scientists don't exactly know which microbes do what within any given individual's microbiome, and there is, as yet, no such thing as a clear definition of a 'healthy GM'. So while the scientists are still unravelling all the details, the best way to conserve and nourish your inner ecosystem is to approach it from a large-scale gut-health viewpoint, the magic word here being 'biodiversity'. Whether you're talking about a large ecosystem like the Amazon rainforest or one on the microscopic level inside you right now, a more diverse microbiome is generally a healthier one.[43]

The gut and chronic inflammation

As I mentioned earlier (see p. 23), chronic inflammation is a real issue, playing a role in almost all health conditions and symptoms. Sadly, the gut can be a standout contributor.[44]

Dysbiosis

An imbalance in microbial communities that leads to a disruption in how our inner ecosystem functions is known as 'dysbiosis', from the ancient Greek, *dys-* (bad or ill) and *biosis* (way of living).[45] Your entire gut mucosal immune system is compromised when there is dysbiosis, which is often a reflection of a diet poor in plant diversity and fibre, medications such as antibiotics, anti-inflammatories and proton-pump inhibitors, and lifestyle factors – such as stress, smoking and being sedentary.[46] And alcohol makes this list, too.[47] People with a number of different diagnosed diseases, such as allergy and autoimmunity, have also been shown to suffer dysbiosis.

Dysbiosis may be associated with a depletion in the amount

of secretory IgA antibodies – our immunological gatekeeper that helps protect the gut barrier. This, in turn, can increase our risk of infection. Dysbiosis can lead to small intestinal bacterial overgrowth (SIBO), in which some of the bugs from the lower bowel find their way up into the small intestine where they can produce excess methane or hydrogen, causing issues like bloating and digestive upset.[48] Candida dysbiosis occurs when a harmless yeast that normally inhabits the gut grows out of control and takes over the local microbiome with uncomfortable consequences known as candidiasis.[49] And it doesn't just affect your gut. It can affect any body part that has its own special ecosystem of microbes. For example, oral dysbiosis, which presents as gum disease and poor oral health, is linked to gut dysbiosis.

Dysbiosis can affect seemingly well people, and we are often unaware that our GM is less than healthy. In other situations, a wide range of persistent digestive disturbance symptoms occurs, including diarrhoea, cramping, constipation, bloating and indigestion, telling you something is a little off with your GM. This means you won't get the full benefits of all the wonderful things the GM does for your health, such as training your immune cells, liberating vital nutrients from your food, lowering inflammation, programming your immune cells and providing beneficial SCFAs.

Leaky gut

The gut barrier is incredibly thin and held together by special junctions that play a crucial role in regulating what is allowed to cross the intestinal barrier.[50]

The gut barrier is naturally dynamic, and 'leakiness' is not always bad news. Think of it more as a sliding scale than a binary switch. It occurs to a certain degree each time you eat, and in some ways is useful. Phytic acid (a substance found in many plant-based foods that binds micronutrients), for example, has been shown to transiently increase intestinal permeability, allowing for greater absorption of beneficial phytonutrients.[51]

In a dysbiotic gut, certain unfavourable microbes releasing lots of harmful compounds can gain a foothold. An over-abundance of these harmful bacterial components like endotoxins are directly toxic to the gut barrier, causing it to become more permeable. Bacterial endotoxins can then leak into your bloodstream. These activate immune sensors called toll-like receptors around the body. Your immune system then recognises these foreign molecules and attacks them, resulting in inflammation rising up and immune regulation breaking down. This puts an increased burden on the liver, which has to detoxify these microbial endotoxins, thus depleting important micronutrients. This is why an imbalanced GM can have body-wide effects, including activation of immune cells in the brain, resulting in mental ill health or increased sensitisation to pain.

Remember, there is no 'perfect' microbiome, and we cannot undo things that may have harmed our gut microbes in the past. But feeding your GM with all the foods it needs to flourish can restore balance in your inner ecosystem. This is particularly important to be aware of if you suffer from an underlying inflammatory condition such as autoimmunity. Even a transient shift towards increased permeability in someone who, say, has an autoimmune condition, might exacerbate symptoms.

Improve your inner biodiversity

In today's environment, our gut is continually challenged by things that undermine its integrity. Below are just some of the culprits:

- Consistently snacking, grazing and overeating
- Lack of dietary fibre
- Eating very large meals, or meals heavy in excessive saturated fat or high in fructose (fruit sugar) in the absence of fibre
- Lack of rhythmicity and mindfulness (your circadian rhythm, when you eat and how you eat)
- Specific nutrient deficiencies, including zinc and vitamins A and D
- High doses of vitamin C (over 2g)
- Gut-meddling medications, including aspirin or NSAIDs, antibiotics and chemotherapy
- Pesticides and environmental toxins
- Alcohol overuse
- The menstrual cycle (in the weeks from ovulation to menstruation)
- Heavy exercise, particularly in hot climates
- Getting older
- Feeling chronically stressed
- Persistent acoustic stress from noise pollution
- Poor sleep

If you want to improve your GM, you have to be prepared to change both your diet and lifestyle. No matter where you are at right now, there are some basic general rules that you can follow to achieve a healthier gut.

Stop the destruction

The first step is to stop the destruction by reviewing the list on p. 133 and identifying GM-harming practices that you can control. Now you are aware of what might be damaging your GM and gut barrier, you can start to improve the diversity of your inner ecosystem. Just as we need to work together to conserve the habitats and biodiversity on our planet, the key aim of good gut health is to protect your delicate gut ecosystem and support the diversity of microbial communities living there.

Fibre fuel your SCFAs

The most practical way to nourish your gut microbiota is by fertilising and cultivating your inner ecosystem with the right foods. Two different groups of plant compounds are key for gut health, SCFA production and supporting a diverse microbiome: fibre and phytonutrients. Food can also nurture your GM in other ways: it can be a source of live, helpful bugs, which can support the gut environment, keeping it favourable for a healthy microbiome.

Fibre-famished gut microbes are linked to poorer immune systems. Fibre is fodder for your GM, providing the raw materials for production of beneficial SCFA and other helpful postbiotics. (see p. 128). It's the fraction of the edible part of plants that your digestive enzymes cannot break down in the first part of your intestine (called the small intestine). These fibres then arrive intact at the colon, ready to be digested by gut bugs, helping to stimulate their growth, diversity and immune-supporting activities.

To encourage lots of different types of microbes, we need to eat lots of different types of plant fibre. A diet rich in fibre is scientifically associated with improved health and wellbeing across a whole host of parameters, including supporting a strong immune system.[52]

However, chances are you are not getting enough. Fibre is the essential dietary nutrient that almost the entire UK population is not eating enough of. Did you know you should aim for more than 30g of fibre per day? Most of us are not even hitting half of that. Our diets have slowly become more and more fibre-poor over the past fifty years,[53]and not only are we eating less fibre, but also fewer varieties of it, favouring a limited diversity of gut bugs.

Fibre is not one molecule; it is many different types, all with different characteristics. So to achieve as much diversity as possible, you need to focus on eating a plant-rich, minimally processed diet. Some plant fibre confers a 'prebiotic effect', essentially fertilising the gut microbiome.[54] By increasing the number of prebiotics in your diet, you can nourish and optimise production of immune-nourishing SCFAs. Aromatic vegetables, such as onions, leeks, celery, asparagus, garlic, chicory, dandelion greens and Jerusalem artichokes, are all rich in prebiotics such as fructans and inulin. Legumes such as kidney beans and chickpeas, as well as nuts and soy, contain the prebiotic galactooligosaccharides (GOS). And buckwheat, unpeeled apples and figs are good sources of rutin, a prebiotic bioflavanoid.

Mind the mucus

The gut lining has mucus layers that separate microbes from gut-barrier cells. If the integrity of these layers is compromised – for example, by a poor diet or dysbiosis of the GM – it can lead to inflammatory changes in the gut, followed by widespread immune activation throughout the body, affecting all the organs. Some microbes live within this specific mucus niche, where they act as guardians of the gut barrier.

Akkermansia muciniphila is one very important gut microbe that thrives on the mucus lining.[55] This means that, unlike other gut bugs, *Akkermansia* doesn't rely on you to feed it via your diet because it feeds on the mucus. This is an example of a symbiotic relationship: by eating the mucus in your gut barrier, it encourages your gut-barrier cells to make more, which, reciprocally, strengthens the barrier. *Akkermansia* turns mucus into specific SCFAs, including acetate (see pp. 128-9). Collectively, this helps to cultivate a rich and healthy ecosystem supporting overall microbiome health and gut-barrier integrity. This, in turn, supports the immune system and reduces unwanted inflammation.[56]

Akkermansia should account for up to 4 per cent of intestinal bacteria in healthy individuals. But it has been seen to be less abundant in certain disease states, including metabolic dysfunction and type-2 diabetes, as well as irritable bowel syndrome.[57] You won't find it in any probiotic supplements (yet!), but this beneficial bug is a good gut guardian that you definitely want to cultivate. Certain foods can support the mucosal lining and help these gut guardians thrive. *Akkermansia* has a special relationship with polyphenols, the colourful compounds found in fruits and veggies. In particular, there is evidence for the proanthocyanidins found in cranberries, rhubarb, red grapes, pomegranate and green tea.[58, 59, 60]

SO YOU HAVE A SENSITIVE GUT?

I'm sure there are a few of you shouting, 'I can't do this. I feel horrible when I eat legumes or other fibre-rich foods!' Up to 80 per cent of UK adults say that fibre-rich foods bring out the worst in their gut symptoms – such as gas bloating, poor digestion or an irritated bowel.

You may well have taken foods out of your diet over the years, including foods you used to enjoy, or excluded foods that you know are nourishing because of a fear that your sensitive tummy symptoms are a sign that they are harming you. Many naturally occurring prebiotics in foods can aggravate gut symptoms in the short term, but please don't restrict plant diversity in the long term without seeking support from a gut-specialist nutrition professional. Because the great irony is that excluding these foods might be worse for you in the long run as you risk starving off more of your good bugs, depriving yourself of their health benefits and entering a vicious cycle. But with some active recovery, you have a good chance of improving your tolerance. Perhaps you can think of some root causes that may have damaged the diversity of your gut in the first place. It might take some trial and error to discover your ideal diet. Work up slowly to the sweet spot, where you are getting in maximum plants with minimum gut distress. And remember, you can give your gut a helping hand by starting that digestive process in the mouth, by chewing your food thoroughly.

We all suffer with gut issues from time to time, but this isn't about perfection; the goal is to keep them to a level where they are not impacting your quality of life.

CAN PROBIOTICS DRIVE RE-*FLORA*-STATION OF A DAMAGED GUT?

Probiotics, by definition, are live microorganisms that are beneficial to gut health. They occur naturally in some fermented foods and can also be taken as supplements.

So if you suspect your gut health is less than great, can't you simply repopulate with 'live and active' bugs from probiotic sources? Sounds simple, right? Sadly, there isn't enough evidence to say that a healthy person should be taking a probiotic to stay healthy. The whole point of taking a probiotic is to benefit from the many ways these microbes support you – for example, SCFA production. But your GM is unique, so at present it's virtually impossible to prescribe probiotics to a healthy individual and guarantee a positive effect. (However, certain probiotics have been shown to be beneficial for a handful of specific health concerns, some of which are covered in Part 3.)

Many probiotics sold have more than twenty strains, which can lead us to think that more is better. But probiotics are both strain- and population-specific – an extremely important point that is so often overlooked, meaning that probiotic bacteria of the same genus and species can have different unique functions, depending on their strain. Let's take the example of *Lactobacillus reuteri* DSM17938:

- The first word, *Lactobacillus*, is the genus.
- The second word, *reuteri*, is the species.
- The additional numbers or letters on the end refer to the strain.

You have to be taking the right strain for the job, and there has to be some evidence that the strain can actually do that job.

Even then, there's no guarantee a probiotic will help you as an individual. My best advice would be to go upstream of the bugs themselves and just work on cultivating the microbes you have through feeding them the right diet.

If you do wish to try a probiotic, use my quick guide below to help you decide.

A quick guide to probiotics

- **Is it safe?** Has it passed tests from the European Food Safety Authority to show the microbes are fit to consume?
- **Which one?** Most probiotics will contain species in the *Lactobacillus* and *Bifidobacterium* categories or a mix of both. Controlled, randomised studies suggest that specific strains of *Lactobacilli* and *Bifidobacteria* supplements may be effective in supporting proper immune function.[61] Healthy levels of *Bifidobacteria* and *Lactobacillus* tend to drop, so may be useful as we get older. *Saccharomyces boulardii* is another well-researched probiotic. A type of yeast, its benefits apply mainly to direct support of the gut-immune environment. One of the best things about it is that it cares for the good bacteria in your gut, which support your digestive and overall health, and positive effects have been reported.[62] It stops germs and their toxins from infecting the gut, and increases important immune defences, such as the antibody Immunoglobulin A, as well as decreasing inflammation in a wide range of disorders. Just remember that within each species there are different strains, which may have strain-specific effects. Talk to a

gut-health specialist to help you find out which might be right for you.

- **How are they taken?** In order to withstand the harsh conditions of processing and acid in the human gut, bacteria can be freeze-dried (lyophilised) or they may be wrapped in a resistant coating (encapsulated). They don't generally need to be refrigerated, as they return to their active state in the gut. Capsules need to be kept away from moisture to maintain viability, and food products usually need refrigeration to keep them safe. If a probiotic food product has been pasteurised, it will no longer contain any of the live bacteria.
- **How long for?** If you feel you have an irritable or sensitive tummy, NICE (the National Institute for Health and Care Excellence) and The British Dietetic Association recommend trying probiotics for a minimum of four weeks, which is a useful rule of thumb, unless you have been advised otherwise by your healthcare professional.
- **How do I know it is working?** First, be really clear on what you hope to achieve by taking probiotics. Then set up a little experiment to monitor and evaluate whether they are helping. Start by asking: what would 'improvement' look like? Don't make any other drastic changes at the same time, and track what you notice over a few weeks.

FERMENTED FOODS

Naturally fermented foods are amazing for your gut microbial diversity. These live-culture foods and drinks – such as kefir, yoghurt, kombucha, kimchi, sauerkraut and natto – naturally contain probiotic bacteria such as *Lactobacillus*, which break down and transform the foods, giving a distinctive texture and flavour, as well as delivering lots of live beneficial microbes to the gut when eaten.

While they might have a long-standing history of being healthy, the scientific research is only just catching up. The largest body of evidence is in support of fermented dairy products, in particular kefir, which has many more 'live and active' bugs than its dairy cousin yoghurt. Microbes found in kimchi have been shown to be protective against influenza[63] and kill cancer cells in test tubes,[64] while a study has demonstrated that a ten-week diet high in fermented foods, both dairy and vegetable, enhanced the diversity of gut microbes, reducing unwanted inflammation.[65] In the same study, people who started out with higher levels of microbial diversity had reductions in inflammation when given a high-fibre diet, while those with the least microbial diversity had slight increases in inflammation when they ate more fibre. This suggests that people with low microbiome diversity may lack the right microbes to digest all that fibre and need more time for their microbes to adapt. So fermented foods could be a good option while you slowly increase fibre.

Fermented foods also have an abundance of additional benefits, including improving the taste, texture and digestibility of our food. Many contain fibre, have an enhanced nutritional profile and can be easier to digest. Aim for those that are not pasteurised to get the most benefit from those live bugs, and always read the label to check for unnecessary ingredients, such as sugar and sweeteners.

YOUR IMMUNONUTRITION BLUEPRINT

Now that you have a bellyful of knowledge and self-awareness around food and immunity, you'll start to notice your relationship with food and apply the key principles when it comes to planning your meals and improving your diet pattern. Eating well can set off a virtuous cycle of other health-promoting behaviours

Short-term change; long-term gains

Simple tweaks can make a big difference you may start to see beneficial alterations in your GM just twenty-four hours after switching to a more plant-rich diet,[66] but cultivating a sustainable, immune-nourishing diet pattern matters most. I like to think of it as an insurance policy – paying into your immunity pension plan for the long game, crowding out the foods that may not be supporting your health. To explore and benefit from these marginal gains with an open mind, you need to know your starting point. Self-monitoring with a food diary is a great first step on the path. Remember, we all can and should be doing things better, but it all begins from a place of self-compassion.

Keep a food diary

Write everything down, but don't overcomplicate it. When you pay attention to something and measure it, you're more likely to find ways to personalise and improve it, and to know whether any changes you then implement really work for you. You don't need to do it indefinitely – seven to ten days should provide useful insights to help you explore your relationship with food, understand your eating habits and support you through any changes you want to implement. The secret is accuracy and consistency. Follow these principles for a basic food diary:

- Write down everything you eat and drink (be specific), while keeping your diet and lifestyle as normal as possible. Don't wait until the end of the day, as you are likely to forget.

- Note down roughly how much you are eating.
- Note down when you are eating. This can be very helpful in understanding behaviour patterns linked to eating, such as late-night snacking.
- Note down where you are eating. Is it in front of your computer or while scrolling on your phone?
- Note down who you are eating with – family or household members, alone, with colleagues?
- Note down how you feel – both physically and emotionally (see p. 38) – each time you eat to help you to identify 'triggers' that shape your food choices.
- Note down any symptoms experienced following eating. It can also be useful to track bowel habits, since it can take three to four days for foods to move through your digestive tract.
- Record other events and activities, including exercise, stressors, sleep, life events and so on.

Food-diary reflections

By recording your behaviour around food, you can establish whether you are on track to reach your goals. After completing it, search for any trends, patterns, or habits. You might want to consider the number of servings of fruits and vegetables, whether you are including enough diversity, or if your mood is affecting your eating behaviours. Once you've identified areas for improvement, set one or two healthy-eating goals for yourself – small, realistic and personal ones you can implement for positive diet changes that stick. Remember self-compassion and keep in mind that the overarching goal should be to find a diet pattern that is sustainable in the long term for you.

Here are some points to reflect on:

- How many different plant-based foods do you eat each week?
- Are you having regular meals?
- Are you having two portions of oily fish per week (or supplementing with omega-3s if not)?
- Are 'treat' foods taking up too much space in your diet?
- Is most of what you are eating following the principles learned in this chapter?
- What common obstacles keep cropping up (lack of time, workload, family duties, feeling tired).

An awareness of what you are eating and what's shaping your eating behaviour in relation to your goals will prompt you either to continue if you are already on the right track (positive reinforcement) or to adjust your behaviours if your progress has been hindered. For example, if you plan to increase daily vegetable intake, but get to the end of the week and haven't achieved this, your food diary can illuminate why: poor meal planning, lack of time, snacking, stress, work environment, etc. You can also spot patterns of behaviour. For example, you might eat poorer-quality meals at certain times of the day or in particular settings. You can't always control when life gets in the way, but you can think a few steps ahead and plan for it, which means less reliance on willpower and motivation (which can be lowest at the times you need them most).

****TOP TIP!**** Remember, eating healthily is important, but not at the cost of your mental health.

Build a sustainable, immunity-focused plate

If your head is swimming with all this new information, or you are struggling for inspiration for how to put your new knowledge into action, don't worry – I've created the simple steps below to give you a helpful nudge onto the right track. But the specifics – foods, frequency and how much, and which nutrients you might be lacking in – will differ from person to person.

A balanced plate

- **A palmful of protein (roughly 20g):** aim for protein at each meal (or more, if you exercise hard or are aged forty or over). Include plant-based protein sources for that important gut-loving fibre.
- **Add a finger of healthy fats:** focus on poly- and monounsaturated fats (avocado, nuts, seeds, olive oil, oily fish) and keep saturated fats to a minimum.
- **A fistful of considered carbs:** consider the quality and quantity of carbs, aiming for minimally processed and full of fibre (such as whole grains and legumes).
- **Plant up your plate with colourful vitamin P:** fill the rest of your plate with fruits and veggies (roughly two palms' worth).
- **Include leafy and sulphur-rich greens:** try to add these on a regular basis, even if just a small amount. It all adds up to a big difference.
- **Lean on ferments:** if you don't have time to cook or prepare veggies, keep some fermented ones in your fridge so you can easily add some tasty diversity to each meal.
- **Don't forget the flavour:** herbs and spices bring flavour to liven up your meals, while also packing a phytonutrient punch.
- **Don't overthink it:** gauge portions based on foods that are cooked, and guesstimate mixed dishes, such as chilli.

- **Cook from scratch where possible:** aim for whole foods and plant up your favourite dishes to reduce the volume of UPFs you consume.
- **Reduce or swap meat for plants:** serve smaller portions of meat and add lentils to things such as bolognese sauce.
- **Eat fruits and veggies with the skins on where possible:** if you like fruit smoothies, try to add some vegetables or different greens, too.

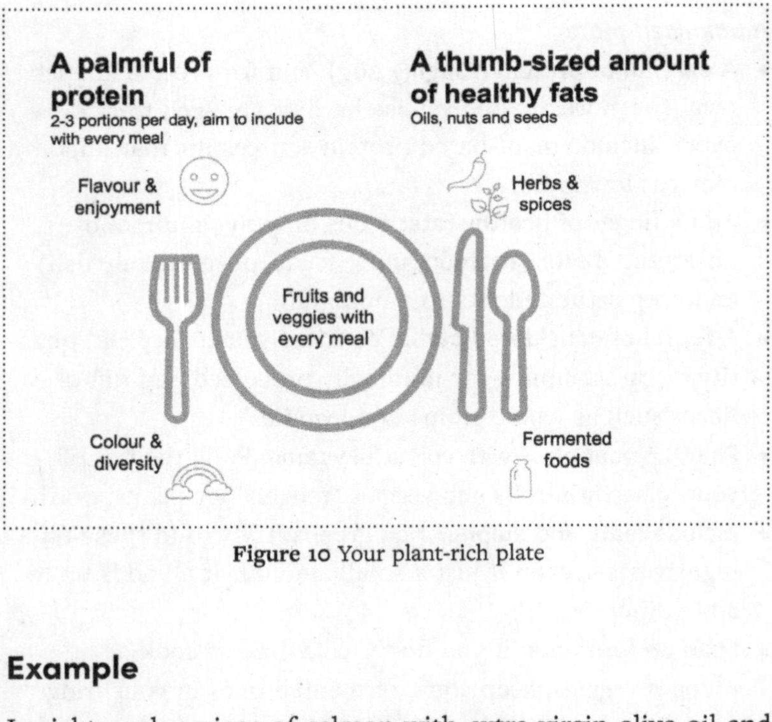

Figure 10 Your plant-rich plate

Example

I might cook a piece of salmon with extra virgin olive oil and lemon for dinner (protein and healthy fats). I could add lemon zest for citrus bioflavonols, steam some greens, adding as many different types of veggies as I can, and roast a few roots or sometimes tinned butter beans or chickpeas in the oven, seasoned with lots of herbs or spices. Then I'd think of how to enhance the fibre (a sprinkling of seeds or nuts), or add some diversity (chopped herbs or microgreens, such as sprouts).

If your current diet is a long way from what I've just described, you might want to introduce a protein-rich snack mid-morning or midway between lunch and your evening meal to help regulate your blood sugar while your body adjusts. Focus on getting the good stuff in, rather than worrying about excluding the bad stuff. If you feel deprived of specific foods, that's guaranteed to bring on cycles of a poor relationship with food.

Top tips across the week

Remember, it's overall patterns that matter the most. One bad meal does not a bad diet make.

- **It's about more than five-a-day:** familiar with the current UK recommendations to eat at least five a day of fruit and vegetables? Well, think of this as a baseline. In reality, the more, the better. Currently ten x 80g portions of fruit and veg each day give the best gains against inflammation and poor health.[67] Just start by eating more and don't worry about diversity *yet*. Aim to build up to two fruits, five portions of vegetables, three portions of whole grains, and one to two portions of nuts, seeds and legumes per day.
- **Fibre up!** Aim to eat thirty different plants per week (that's thirty different plant foods across seven days) to help you to meet the recommended minimum fibre intake of 30g per day. The higher the number of plant-based foods you eat each week, the more diverse your gut bugs will typically be, each with different skills to train and maintain your immune system.

Eat the rainbow!

Colour is the trademark sign of phytonutrients. Once you have got into the swing of using more fresh produce on your plate, start to bump up the nutrient quality by adding as many varieties, textures and tastes as possible at each meal. Each colour will have additive and synergistic effects.

Reds	apples, tomatoes, strawberries, chillies
Yellows	bananas, lemons, sweetcorn
Oranges	peaches, carrots, oranges
Leafy greens	kale, cucumber, broccoli, avocado
Blacks/deep purples	aubergines, grapes, plums
Whites/browns	coconut, tea, onions, mushrooms, wheat

Goal setting

Time to set some goals. Refer back to p. 64 to recap on how to set SMART goals, remembering to focus on *your* why, no one else's. This will help you to kickstart and maintain positive changes. Remember also, making changes isn't easy, especially against the tide of easily accessible UPFs in our current food environment.

Reflect on your food diary and use what you have learned in this chapter. Focus on the process, not the outcome, and prioritise sustaining new behaviour changes to get you there. Anchor your goals to automatic behaviours you have in your life and keep it positive. Choose a convenient period to start, avoiding stressful times at work or busy social weeks. Share your goals with those close to you, or find like-minded individuals who share similar ones. Social support creates accountability, making you more likely to stick to your goals.

Be honest with yourself. Is your diet where you want it to be? Not yet? Then make a change, starting today. Grab a pen and use the template below to dive into setting some goals.

Short-term goals What would you like to achieve over the next 2–4 weeks?	**Medium-term goals** What would you like to achieve over the next 2–4 months?	**Long-term goals** What would you like to achieve over the next 6–12 months?
1. 2. 3.	1. 2. 3.	1. 2. 3.
Start date:	Start date:	Start date:

What will you need to do to accomplish your goals?		
In the short term...	In the medium term...	In the long term...

- Consider what has gone well: notice your wins, no matter how small. Pick out the positives and note down what you enjoyed.
- What has not gone so well? Take stock, note what you

disliked most. Identify barriers to help you work towards overcoming them.

- Keep reflecting on your immunobiography: what do you want its next chapter to look like?

Turning obstacles into superpowers

Limiting factors are the things that stand in the way of you achieving your goals; common ones include not having enough time or a busy work schedule. Identify your limiting factors and use them to formulate possible next actions. This might mean adjusting a goal to make it more achievable, for example, or minimising any barriers highlighted. Then turn your biggest obstacles into superpowers with the IF → THEN approach:

- If I work late → then I'll use a meal prep or . . .
- If I don't have time to prepare food in advance → then I'll start prepping more food on my days off.

Finding ways to make your goals more achievable involves problem solving and experimenting. And if at any stage you are really struggling, refresh your knowledge by refamiliarising yourself with the details in this chapter.

Remember, the key is to work towards an eating pattern that you can consistently sustain for life without feelings of frustration and defeat. And think beyond the food. Food is important, but it's not the only thing that matters.

Recipes

The decline in home cooking in our hectic world closely tracks the rise in obesity and all the chronic diseases linked to inflammation and lifestyle. Cooking, in and of itself, promotes health. Meals prepared at home tend to be associated with lower consumption of UPFs and are less likely to lead to overeating.[68] It also makes you the producer as well as the consumer: you are controlling the food environment, rather than it controlling you.

As a young girl, I was taught the basics and inspired to get creative in the kitchen by my mother, who trained in cookery and worked in catering. She had the art of frugality, provenance and indulgence down to a fine art. For me, cooking brings joy. I savour the pleasure of the process and relish the sense of accomplishment. It's also a great way to relieve stress, a social and emotional activity and, of course, a wonderful tool for immune-nourishing health and wellbeing. I've fused my passion for immunology with my farm-to-table Scottish–Italian heritage, and through my recipes, inspired by traditional healthful eating patterns, my goal is to give you a helping hand and inspire you, too.

FLAVOUR AT ITS BEST

The natural cycle of produce is perfectly designed to support our health. Building a lifestyle around seasonal foods helps to facilitate the body's natural needs. But there are other benefits, too. Food grown outside its season or natural environment needs a lot more human input (in the form of pesticides, for example), to grow and look appealing. So by choosing local and seasonal food, you are more likely to get produce grown with minimal artificial support. And although there might not be much difference between the vitamin and mineral content, organic produce grown without pesticides can have up to 100 times more phytonutrients.

Research has also found that organic produce is home to a significantly more diverse bacteria population, which is good news for gut health. One study found that organic apples also contained the 'good' bacteria *Lactobacillus*, a common healthy probiotic, while conventional apples were more likely to have potentially pathogenic bacteria, such as *Escherichia* and *Shigella*, which are known to cause food-poisoning symptoms.[69]

Seasonal produce will differ depending on where you are. Here is my guide to what to look out for in the UK:

- **Spring:** artichokes, beetroot, cabbage, carrots, cucumber, leeks, parsnips, purple sprouting broccoli, radishes, rhubarb, spring greens, spring onions, watercress
- **Summer:** apricots, bell peppers, cherries, corn, cucumber, garlic, lemons, limes, melon, nectarines, peaches, plums, radishes, strawberries, tomatoes
- **Autumn:** apples, aubergines, blackberries, cabbage, celery, kale, onions, parsnips, pears, potatoes, pumpkins, runner beans, spinach, turnips
- **Winter:** Brussels sprouts, butternut squash, leeks, onions, potatoes, sweet potatoes, Swiss chard, wild mushrooms, winter squash

DO A PURGE . . .

Before you stock up, you need to clear out. Go through your pantry, fridge and freezer. The best way is to take everything out, then toss out anything that's expired or you just don't use. Now is also the time to clean out your cupboards by vacuuming and wiping down before everything goes back in. Be on the lookout for UPFs by checking ingredient labels. You don't need to completely purge your kitchen of these foods, but you do need to become label aware so that you can gauge the volume of these foods your household is eating.

. . . then stock your store cupboard

Keep the ingredients below to hand so that you always have the means to knock up something delish, even when life is busy:

- Oils, vinegars and condiments: extra virgin olive oil (EVOO) is a must, and choose good-quality vinegars (red wine, white wine and cider); beyond the basics, I'd go for Dijon mustard and maybe sriracha (chilli sauce)
- Tomato purée (adds a flavour punch to lots of different dishes)
- Nutritional yeast
- Capers and olives – an easy way to plant up a meal or a delicious savoury snack
- A selection of dried herbs and spices; honey
- Tinned fish, such as salmon, sardines and mackerel
- Tinned tomatoes
- Coconut milk
- Beans and pulses

- Unrefined oats
- Rice, pasta and grains
- Nuts and seeds

HOW (AND WHY) TO SPROUT

Sprouts are seeds that have germinated to become very young plants. This process begins with the seeds being soaked for several hours, followed by exposing them to the right combination of sunlight and moisture for several days. Many different types of seeds can be sprouted, including bean, lentil, pea, grain and vegetable, like my own personal favourite – broccoli seeds (see below).

Cruciferous vegetables like broccoli contain compounds called glucosinolates which are transformed into powerful phytonutrients, such as sulforaphane, from the isothiocyanate family.[70] Sulforaphane acts on our genes as a beneficial epigenetic regulator (see p. 34). The health benefits attributed to sulforaphane are many, and include reducing the risk of cancer, supporting our bodies' own internal detox and antioxidant mechanisms and reducing unwanted inflammation.[71]

Broccoli sprouts are a particularly rich source of sulforaphane, but the power of this phytonutrient is only released through the action of an enzyme known as myrosinase, also contained within the broccoli plant and activated when the plants are chopped, crushed or chewed (see tip opposite). As well as broccoli sprouts (and adult broccoli), other crucifers, such as kale and cauliflower, also contain these compounds, but at lower levels.

To sprout broccoli seeds, I use a glass sprouting jar that has a special lid, but you can use any jar and cover the top with gauze and leave at an angle so the seeds can drain after rinsing.

- Take 2 tablespoons broccoli seeds and soak for twenty-four hours.
- Rinse and drain the seeds daily (normally for four to five days), until you see them sprout.
- Keep them in the fridge, covered with an airtight lid.
- Add them to anything and everything!

> **TOP TIP** Steaming broccoli, kale and cauliflower for up to five minutes is scientifically the best way to retain myrosinase enzyme activity and optimise sulforaphane production.[72] Other cooking methods may deactivate myrosinase. But don't worry – if you are concerned about cooking for optimal sulforaphane, serve your crucifers with mustard seeds (which contain myrosinase) instead.

HOW (AND WHY) TO FERMENT

Fermenting veggies to make sauerkraut and kimchi involves brining (salting) the vegetables to draw out their water content. This helps to preserve them and allows the seasonings to penetrate the food over time; the final salt concentration ranges from 2–5 per cent. Probiotic strains (such as *Lactobacillus*) in fermented foods contribute to their health potential.

- Choose your veggies – Chinese leaves and mooli for a classic kimchi, or red cabbage, carrots, cauli, etc for pickling – and add extra herbs, spices and botanicals (e.g. dill, garlic, coriander, juniper berries and turmeric).

- Finely slice and place in a mixing bowl and measure the weight of the veggies. Calculate 2 per cent of that weight by multiplying by 0.02 and measure it out in salt.
- Sprinkle the salt on the veggies and get to work, massaging it in.
- Leave to sit at room temperature for 30 minutes.
- Pack into sterilised glass jars, ensuring that the brine covers the veggies.
- Cover and leave at room temperature for 1–2 days, checking that the contents remain submerged. Add a little brine if needed to keep them immersed.
- Start tasting after 7 days; once you have the perfect tangy flavour, store in the fridge for 2–3 weeks.

COOK'S NOTES

Unless stated otherwise in the recipes:

- All spoon measures are level.
- All eggs are medium, preferably free-range and organic.
- All vegetables (including garlic and ginger) are medium-sized and should be peeled or trimmed.
- All herbs and leaves should be washed and trimmed, as necessary.
- Bunches of herbs are 30g if small, 60g if large.
- All canned beans should be drained and rinsed before use.

Soups and Sides

***Note:** all recipes serve 4*

Feel-better brodo

For me, slow-simmered brodo di pollo (Italian for chicken broth) is the richness that underpins sauces, stews, curries and soups. It also makes a great standalone consommé. Probably the ultimate old-fashioned feel-better elixir, this is a hybrid reflecting my family's Scottish–Italian heritage. We don't eat very much meat at all, but I do still make big batches of chicken broth, so I always have portions in the freezer. There are many traditional ways to prepare it, but this is my quick and effective method. Non-meat eaters can create a boneless version using wild seaweeds (such as dulse and wakame), functional mushrooms (such as shiitake) and season with a mineral-rich sea salt and generous amounts of black pepper.

INGREDIENTS

- 1 whole chicken carcass, including meaty and collagenous parts
- 2 large sprigs of rosemary
- 1 tbsp cider vinegar
- Handful of bay leaves
- Generous seasoning of salt and pepper
- Optional: grate in some fresh turmeric or any other combination of your favourite herbs and spices

METHOD

1. Place the chicken carcass in your slow cooker or a large saucepan. Add enough water to three-quarters cover (or an equal weight to the chicken).
2. Add the remaining ingredients, bring to the boil, then simmer slowly for 8–24 hours to extract the most nutrients and flavour from each ingredient.
3. Once cooled, drain the liquid through a sieve and set aside, discarding all the solids.
4. The liquid will naturally gel, forming a layer of fat and impurities that float to the surface. These can be easily skimmed off and the remaining brodo used or stored in the fridge or freezer.

Nonna's roasted tomato soup

This is a deep, rich, velvety soup made with roasted vegetables. I always start with a base of tomatoes and chicken stock, but then add whatever other Mediterranean-style veg I have in. I find adding a few chickpeas helps to thicken the soup and adds some more fibre.

Although many diets have been noted for their anti-inflammatory and longevity properties, the Mediterranean diet is probably the most studied eating pattern. With my hybrid Italian family, extra virgin olive oil is the lifeblood of my home cooking, while tomatoes are a Mediterranean staple – rich in vitamin C and releasing an anti-cancer compound called lycopene when cooked.

INGREDIENTS

- ½ butternut squash, roughly chopped
- 4 garlic cloves, roughly chopped
- 1 red onion, roughly chopped
- 2 tbsp good-quality olive oil
- 2 litres chicken stock
- 1 x 400g tin chopped tomatoes
- 2 tbsp tomato purée
- Dried Italian herb mix
- Sprig of fresh oregano
- Handful of chickpeas
- A swirl of cream (I sometimes use coconut cream, but dairy or vegan cream work quite well)
- Sea salt and black pepper

METHOD

1. Preheat the oven to 200°C.
2. Place the butternut squash, garlic and onion in a baking tray.
3. Coat with olive oil and roast until softened (approximately 15–20 minutes).
4. Simmer the chicken stock gently, adding the tinned tomatoes, tomato purée, herbs, chickpeas and roasted squash, garlic and onion.
5. Season with salt and pepper, then cook over a medium-low heat for 30 minutes, stirring occasionally.
6. Blend together, adjusting the liquid to suit your preference, adding more chicken stock or water as needed.
7. Swirl in the cream and serve.

Watercress, pea and artichoke soup

I love watercress and welcome its seasonal return in the UK each spring, making the most of it with fresh and fast recipe ideas. Watercress packs a super-nutritional punch, being rich in beta-carotene (the plant form of vitamin A), vitamins C, E, K and B, as well as calcium, iron, potassium and iodine. It's also high in dietary nitrate, which is heart healthy, and reduces blood pressure and inflammation by supporting nitric-oxide production. Peas are a household classic, with most of us having a bag in the freezer. They are a fantastic source of plant-based protein, a key macro-nutrient to support immunity. I've added prebiotic-rich artichokes to give the soup more body and texture, as well as to fertilise our gut bugs. For anyone suffering with hay fever or histamine issues, watercress is a low-histamine green full of flavonols that have been shown to be helpful with symptoms.

INGREDIENTS

- ½ onion, chopped
- 2 garlic cloves, roughly chopped
- Sprig of thyme
- 1 tbsp extra virgin olive oil
- 800ml chicken stock (I use my own chicken stock – see my website – but you can use any)
- 300g frozen peas
- 1 × 80g bag watercress (keep some aside to garnish)
- Handful of artichoke hearts (ideally cooked from fresh, but a jar is fine – just be sure to drain off any excess oil)
- Sea salt and black pepper
- Crème fraîche to serve
- Parsley and home-grown broccoli sprouts (see p. 154), to garnish

METHOD

1. In a wide pan, fry off the onion, garlic and thyme in the olive oil, seasoned with salt and pepper, until soft.
2. Add the chicken stock, peas and watercress.
3. Simmer for 10 minutes, then leave to cool before adding the artichoke hearts. Transfer to a blender and whizz until smooth.
4. Return the soup to the pan and warm through until piping hot.
5. Serve the soup with a little crème fraîche, garnished with more watercress, parsley and home-grown broccoli sprouts.

Broccoli, garlic, almonds and preserved lemons

Ever since I was a kid, broccoli has been one of my favourite veggies. I never get bored with it and mix it up between regular and sprouting varieties, even using the stalks in some recipes. I sprout my own broccoli seeds (see p. 154), which are known to contain higher levels of the phytonutrient sulforaphane.

I regularly prepare this as a side dish, but you could add some good protein sources, such as fish, boiled eggs or tofu, and make it into a salad.

INGREDIENTS

- 1 large head of broccoli, chopped into florets, or 200g Tenderstem broccoli
- 2 garlic cloves, sliced
- Extra virgin olive oil, for frying
- Handful of almonds
- 2 preserved lemons
- Sea salt and black pepper

For the dressing:

- 1 tbsp Dijon mustard
- 1 tbsp extra virgin olive oil
- 2 tbsp lemon juice
- 2 heaped tbsp chopped parsley, to garnish

METHOD

1. Steam the broccoli for under 5 minutes until al dente.
2. Fry the garlic cloves with a little olive oil for a few minutes over a high heat. Set aside.
3. Toast the almonds in the same pan as the garlic.

4. Drain, dry and thinly slice the preserved lemons.
5. Combine the broccoli, garlic and preserved lemons and transfer to a serving dish. Top with the toasted almonds.
6. Prepare the dressing by combining the mustard with the olive oil and lemon juice. Season with salt and pepper.
7. Drizzle the dressing over the broccoli and garnish with chopped parsley.

Potato dischetti with anchovy capers

In Italy, antipasti is a critical part of a meal, being seen to prime the stomach and signifying the start of enjoying the full experience of a meal. Although growing up in Scotland was a far cry from the Mediterranean, I still find myself daydreaming of recipes that remind me of being there.

Potatoes are a staple in Scotland, so I am always looking for ways to include them in a meal and give them a Mediterranean twist. This simple antipasto recipe uses potato discs (dischetti), drizzled with a flavourful mixture of capers, anchovies, oregano and parsley. It's gluten-free, and cooking and cooling the potatoes increases their resistant starch, giving your gut microbes lots of important fibre to chow down and producing important postbiotics to nurture your gut and, therefore, your immunity.

Low on the food chain, anchovies are one of the most nutritious and sustainable fish. They're not only a complete protein source, but also notably rich in anti-inflammatory omega-3s. They are also fairly cheap to buy tinned. Tiny capers, used for centuries in Mediterranean cuisine, pack a big punch as they are an unexpectedly big source of natural antioxidants.

INGREDIENTS

- 4 potatoes
- ½ tbsp salted capers
- 30g black olives
- 80ml olive oil
- Juice of ½ lemon
- 1 tbsp chopped parsley
- 1 tbsp chopped oregano
- 20 anchovy fillets in oil (roughly one for each slice of potato)
- Sea salt and black pepper

METHOD

1. Boil the potatoes until cooked, but not overly soft. When cooled, carefully peel and slice them into circles 5mm thick.
2. Rinse the capers and roughly chop them together with the olives. Set aside.
3. Make a dressing by blending the olive oil, lemon juice, parsley, oregano, salt and pepper.
4. Place the potato slices on a large platter and lay an anchovy on each slice. When the platter is covered, sprinkle the olive and caper mixture on top of the dischetti.
5. Drizzle over the herb dressing and serve slightly warm or at room temperature.

Root veggies four ways

On my family's tiny wee farm in rural Scotland we grew *a lot* of root veggies, especially turnips. In fact, at times I think we probably ate turnips with at least two meals each day!

Turnips are part of the brassica family, and both the root and leaves can be eaten, which means they're really versatile. Not only are they cheap, but they are also an undervalued source of fibre, phytochemicals and essential micronutrients. Here are four ways to use turnips – or any root veggies – as accompaniments to a meal.

CHAMPIT

Neeps is the Scottish word for turnips, and champit means mashed. Mashed turnip has historically been the classic accompaniment to haggis, but any mashed root can make a tasty twist on the classic mashed potato. Steam your turnip or other root until soft, mash with a generous serving of butter and season with salt and pepper. Use as an accompaniment to a meal or to top a winter pie. A crowd-pleaser with my kids, for sure!

ROASTED AND SPICY

Roots are a great addition to any tray of roasted veg, but I like to make them spicy and combine with cavolo nero. Place diced turnip, chopped chilli and cavolo nero in a roasting tray. Rub with olive oil and season with salt and pepper before roasting in the oven at 180°C, until softened and crispy around the edges.

CURRIED

Slowly simmer turnip cubes with an Indian-inspired gravy made from onion, garlic, ground ginger, turmeric, coriander, cumin and chilli. Add some stock and tomato purée, until the consistency is just right. Top with freshly chopped coriander and serve.

BABY TURNIP SALAD

Baby turnips (or other baby roots) are sweeter and more delicate in flavour than the fully grown ones, which tend to be more pungent and peppery. Baby turnips can be eaten raw, and their mild flavour and crunchy texture are fantastic in winter salads. Just wash and slice off the roots, then shave them into a salad bowl, combining them with the chopped turnip tops and your favourite salad ingredients.

MAINS

Fresh anchovy fritto misto

Fresh anchovies have a deliciously mild, fresh flavour compared to the salted, tinned variety. They're amazing served like this, quick-fried and piping hot – a real taste of the Mediterranean. Traditionally, small, fresh anchovies can be eaten whole, but ask your fishmonger to gut and debone any larger ones.

INGREDIENTS

- 400g fresh anchovies
- 2 lemons
- Bunch of flat-leaf parsley, finely chopped
- 150g chickpea (gram) flour
- 50g polenta
- Pinch of cayenne pepper
- 1 tbsp olive oil
- Sea salt and black pepper

METHOD

1. Preheat the oven to 150°C and line a large baking tray with baking parchment.
2. Place the anchovies in a shallow dish, squeeze over the juice of one lemon and sprinkle over two-thirds of the parsley.

3. In another shallow dish, mix together the flour, polenta and cayenne pepper. Season well with salt and pepper.
4. In a large pan, heat the olive oil.
5. Coat the anchovies in the flour mixture, shake off any excess and add to the oil in batches, frying for 1 minute, until crisp.
6. Transfer the anchovies to the baking tray and place in the oven to keep warm while you cook the rest.
7. Serve scattered with the remaining parsley and the remaining lemon cut into wedges.

Artichoke tart

This prebiotic-packed pastry-less tart is both time-saving and tasty. The combination of flavours makes it an incredible dish for lunch or supper any time of the year.

INGREDIENTS

- 4 tbsp olive oil, plus extra for greasing
- 1 onion, finely chopped
- 2 tsp dried Mediterranean herbs
- 2 garlic cloves, grated
- 3 large eggs
- 1 x 400g tin artichoke hearts, drained and quartered
- 100g green olives
- 100g Parmesan cheese (vegans can use nutritional yeast or vegan Parmesan)
- 2 tbsp milk (or plant alternative)
- 30g breadcrumbs
- 2 tbsp chopped parsley
- Sea salt and black pepper

METHOD

1. Preheat the oven to 190°C.
2. In a large frying pan, heat the oil and add the onion. Season with salt and pepper and add the herbs. Fry over a medium heat for 10 minutes, until the onions are soft and translucent.
3. Add the garlic and continue cooking for 5 minutes.
4. Beat the eggs in a large bowl, add the cooked onion and garlic, along with the artichoke hearts, olives, three-quarters of the Parmesan and the milk.

5. Grease a 20cm tart tin and pour the mixture into it.
6. Sprinkle with the breadcrumbs, remaining Parmesan and the chopped parsley.
7. Bake for 35–40 minutes, until golden. Serve hot or cold with a simple green salad.

Pan-fried salmon or trout with lemon oatmeal

Buying frozen fish is a great way to save money. It's also handy for whipping up a great meal if you don't have much else around.

This recipe is based on a traditional Scottish one that I grew up with. Wild salmon can be expensive, but trout makes a cheaper, and no less tasty alternative. Also, nutritionally speaking, trout packs a real punch. It's a great way to get vitamin D, plus it's rich in good fats, such as omega-3s, which quench inflammation and keep our cells and tissues supple. Oats add crunch, and are a good source of beta glucan, beloved by our microbiomes; it also has great immune-nourishing effects for fending off those winter bugs.

Serve with a fresh salad in spring or summer, or with jewelled leeks in winter (see overleaf).

INGREDIENTS

For the fish:

- 2 salmon or trout fillets (about 150g each)
- 1 egg, beaten
- 70g oatmeal (I normally buy the big, chunky oats, as I use them for porridge, but for this recipe I give them a quick blitz in the blender so they cling to the fish better)
- Few sprigs of fresh thyme
- Zest of 1 lemon
- 1 tbsp olive oil
- Sea salt and black pepper

For the summer salad:

- 200g Jersey Royal potatoes
- 4 tbsp extra virgin olive oil
- 2 tbsp apple cider vinegar
- 1 tsp wholegrain mustard
- Juice and zest of 2 lemons
- Handful of radishes, sliced
- ¼ cucumber, deseeded and thickly sliced
- 1 × 80g bag watercress, roughly chopped

For the jewelled leeks:

- Extra virgin olive oil, for frying
- 2 leeks, trimmed and chopped
- Seeds from 1 pomegranate

METHOD

1. Preheat the oven to 180°C.
2. Pat the fish fillets dry with kitchen paper.
3. Blitz the oatmeal briefly with the thyme and lemon zest.
4. Dip the fish into the beaten egg and then into the oat mix, pressing to coat thoroughly. Place on a plate, cover with cling film and leave in the fridge for 20 minutes.
5. Heat the olive oil in a deep, non-stick frying pan.
6. Place the fish in the pan and cook for 3–5 minutes (or until golden brown), then flip and cook for a further 3–5 minutes.
7. Remove from the pan and rest in the warm oven.
8. Boil the potatoes in salted water until tender.
9. Whisk together the olive oil, apple cider vinegar, mustard, lemon zest and juice to make the dressing.
10. Combine the potatoes, radishes, cucumber and watercress in a salad bowl, then toss in the dressing.

11. Place the leeks in a frying pan with a little olive oil and fry off for a few minutes, until softened.
12. Transfer to a serving dish and sprinkle with the jewel-like pomegranate seeds. Serve with the fish and the salad.

Slow-cooker curry (vegan)

I don't think slow cookers will ever be sexy, but mine just might be one of my most used cooking appliances, particularly in winter. I can simply chop, set and forget!

Butternut squash with its sweet-flavoured, brightly coloured flesh is a great source of immune-nourishing vitamins and minerals, but, more importantly, includes a host of phytonutrients and fibre, providing fodder for our good bacteria to ferment and creating 'postbiotics' – our own personalised pharmacy of bioactive compounds.

The science on the health benefits of turmeric is growing, and we now know that there is an exponential improvement in digestive uptake when it is eaten with a source of fat (for example, coconut milk) and a pinch of black pepper (due to the function of piperine). This recipe meets both these requirements.

INGREDIENTS

- 190g red lentils
- Dash of apple cider vinegar
- 700ml chicken stock or vegan stock
- 1 x 400ml tin coconut milk
- 1 x 400g tin cannellini beans (or beans of your choice)
- 1 tbsp freshly grated root turmeric
- 1 tsp ground turmeric
- 1 tsp ground cumin
- 3 garlic cloves, grated
- 2 red onions, chopped
- 200g baby corn, chopped
- 1 butternut squash, seeds reserved, flesh chopped (pumpkin and sweet potato also work well)
- High-mineral sea salt and freshly ground black pepper

- 2 tbsp extra virgin olive oil, to serve
- Fresh coriander, to garnish

METHOD

1. Soak the lentils in the apple cider vinegar with a pinch of salt; rinse well before using.
2. Chuck everything into the slow cooker (except the squash seeds, olive oil and coriander). Mix well and cook for 8 hours on the lowest setting. If you don't have a slow cooker, use a large casserole and cook in the oven at 180°C for about 1 hour.
3. About 15 minutes before serving, preheat the oven to 180°C (if it's not already on).
4. Rinse the squash seeds, then roast for 15 minutes.
5. Serve the curry, topped with the roasted squash seeds, a drizzle of extra virgin olive oil and a generous sprinkling of coriander.

Cottage pie with a twist

Cottage pie is a classic mince and potato combo that was my favourite as a child. I've given it a healthy spin by adding antioxidant-packed spices and replacing some of the meat with prebiotic fibre-packed beans.

INGREDIENTS

For the filling:

- Olive oil, for frying
- 400g organic minced beef
- 2 red onions, chopped
- 2 garlic cloves, chopped
- 2 tsp ground cumin
- 2 tsp ground coriander
- 2 tsp ground turmeric
- 2cm piece of fresh root turmeric, grated
- 200ml chicken bone broth
- 1 x 400g tin kidney beans, rinsed
- 1 x 400g tin chopped tomatoes
- Sea salt and black pepper

For the root veg mash:

- 150g sweet potatoes, roughly chopped
- 150g white potatoes, roughly chopped
- 5 large carrots, sliced
- 5 large parsnips, chopped
- 50g butter, chopped

METHOD

1. Throw all the ingredients for the filling into a slow cooker. Cook on low for 6–8 hours.
2. This can also be cooked in a heavy saucepan. Heat 1 tablespoon of olive oil in the pan over a medium–high heat and cook the beef for 5 minutes or until browned. Transfer to a bowl. Heat another tablespoon of oil in the pan. Add the onions, garlic, cumin, coriander and turmeric. Cook, stirring, for 1 minute or until fragrant. Return the beef to the pan. Add the broth, kidney beans and tomatoes. Season and cover, then bring to the boil. Reduce the heat to low and simmer for 1 hour.
3. To make the topping, put the sweet potatoes, white potatoes, carrots and parsnips in a large saucepan. Cover with water and bring to the boil, then reduce the heat slightly and simmer until soft. Drain and return to the pan before adding the butter and mashing. Season with salt and pepper.
4. Preheat the oven to 200°C. Place the beef mixture in an ovenproof dish, top with the mash and bake for 20 minutes.

Kitchari (vegan)

Kitchari means mixture, usually of two grains, and is one of the staple healing foods in Ayurveda medicine. This one is particularly nourishing and easy to digest, combining basmati rice and split yellow mung beans (thought to be the only legume not to produce intestinal gas). They are also soaked well in advance here, which further adds to their digestibility. Lentils in general are a fabulous source of dietary fibre. Combined with white rice, split yellow mung beans make a complete protein.

INGREDIENTS

- 100g basmati rice (I prefer to use white basmati, but brown also works; just remember that it has a higher nutritional value but is not as easy to digest – if using, be sure to soak overnight, rinse well and overcook)
- 200g split yellow mung beans (mung dal), soaked overnight
- 2 tsp olive oil
- 1 tsp whole cumin seeds
- 1 tsp mustard seeds
- 1 tsp ground coriander
- 1 tsp ground cumin
- 1–2cm fresh ginger, chopped or grated
- 1 tsp ground turmeric
- 1 litre vegetable stock (I use my vegan seaweed version of my brodo recipe – see p. 157)
- Pinch of salt

To serve:

- Handful of fresh coriander leaves, chopped
- Juice of 1 lime
- Coconut yoghurt

METHOD

1. Rinse the soaked rice and mung beans under running water for a few minutes.
2. In a large saucepan, heat the olive oil over a medium heat and add the cumin and mustard seeds, until they start to pop.
3. Add the ground coriander and cumin, fresh ginger and turmeric, stirring occasionally for about 30 seconds.
4. Add the drained rice and mung beans and stir until they are coated with the spice mixture.
5. Add the stock and bring to the boil. Lower the heat to a simmer and cover. Cook until the beans and rice are soft but not mushy.
6. Add the salt, then serve with a generous handful of chopped coriander, a squeeze of lime juice and a generous scoop of coconut yoghurt.

Savoury crepes

Upping the plant diversity and fibre in your diet shouldn't be time-consuming or expensive, nor should it mean compromising on taste.

This simple crepe batter is made using chickpea flour (also known as gram flour), which contains more fibre per gram than wheat flour, so it's a great swap. Switch up your fillings to add greater diversity. Try artichokes for prebiotic fibre (to feed your 'good' bacteria), as well as good plant chemicals (polyphenols); they also pair well with rainbow colours and Mediterranean tastes, such as tomato and avocado. Or for a probiotic hit, try adding a lemon kefir drizzle; kefir contains even more beneficial bugs than live yoghurt.

INGREDIENTS

- 3 eggs
- 50g chickpea (gram) flour
- 50ml water or kefir
- Small handful of spinach
- 2 tbsp olive oil
- Sea salt and black pepper

For the fillings:

- Pre-cooked artichoke hearts, plus chopped tomatoes and avocado, kefir and lemon juice
- Watercress and hummus
- Spicy kimchi and home-grown broccoli sprouts

METHOD

1. Crack the eggs into a blender. Add the flour, water and spinach and season with salt and pepper. Blitz until smooth.
2. Heat the olive oil in a frying pan over a high heat.
3. Add a quarter of the batter to the frying pan, ensuring it covers the entire bottom of the pan.
4. After a few minutes (you will see bubbles appearing), flip to the other side and cook for a further 3–4 minutes before setting aside and keeping warm. Make 3 more crepes in the same way.
5. Arrange the fillings on the table and let people fill their crepe as they wish.

Less-meat meatballs

There are many ways to make meatballs, but I like to use this quick and easy variation on the traditional panade method. I also use less meat and add extra fibre, and find the sauce is a great way to use up bits of veg to avoid #foodwaste.

INGREDIENTS

For the meatballs:

- 4 tbsp breadcrumbs (blitz up leftover bread)
- A little milk (plant-based, if you prefer)
- 200g minced beef
- 200g lentils
- 1 onion, finely chopped
- 1 tsp Italian herbs (fresh or dried)
- 3 garlic cloves, grated
- 85g Parmesan cheese, grated
- 1 egg, beaten
- Plain flour, for dusting
- 2 tbsp olive oil
- Sea salt and black pepper

For the sauce:

- See step 7 opposite

METHOD

1. Preheat the oven to 200°C.
2. Make a panade – this is a binder that helps keep the meatballs' shape and moisture. Soak the breadcrumbs in milk for 15 minutes, then squeeze out excess liquid.
3. Mix together the beef and lentils with the onion, herbs,

garlic, salt, pepper and a little Parmesan.

4. Stir in the egg and the panade mixture and gently combine.
5. Form into balls, approximately the size of a walnut and dust with flour.
6. Heat the olive oil in a pan and, when hot, fry off the meatballs for a few minutes to sear all over.
7. To make the sauce, I've got into the habit of using onion, garlic, tinned tomatoes and Italian herbs as a base, also adding veggies, such as roasted peppers or carrots, depending on what I have in.
8. Place your sauce in an ovenproof dish, add the meatballs, cover with the remaining Parmesan and place in the oven for 20 minutes. Serve with your favourite pasta, garlic bread or a green salad.

SNACKS

Roasted chickpeas

Most of the time I am known as the 'anti-snacker', but sometimes you just need or want a snack. And for me, it's almost always got to be savoury, quick and nutritious.

As much as I like to use chickpeas in recipes, sometimes I'll just open a tin, rinse, dry and roast them. Eat these within a couple of hours of making them. They may last a few days, but tend to lose their crunch over time.

INGREDIENTS

- 1 x 400g tin chickpeas
- Olive oil
- Sea salt and black pepper

Flavouring ideas:

- Ground dulse (dulse is a type of Scottish seaweed with a salty umami flavour, which reduces the need for added salt)
- Cinnamon and brown sugar
- Turmeric and black pepper
- Smoky paprika

METHOD

1. Preheat the oven to 200°C.
2. Rinse and dry the chickpeas thoroughly, then place in a baking tray. Coat with a little olive oil and seasoning of choice. Roast in the oven for around 20 minutes.
3. When they are nearly done, coat them in a light dusting of salt and pepper plus your chosen flavourings, then return to the oven for a few more minutes, ensuring that the seasonings don't burn.

Oatcakes

High in fibre with minimal ingredients, these are my go-to on-the-go snack. Growing up in Scotland, oatcakes were a staple (like pretty much everything else with oats).

INGREDIENTS

- 100g oatmeal
- 100g rolled porridge oats
- 2 tsp chia seeds
- 30g butter
- 1 tbsp water or a milk alternative
- Pinch of sea salt

Topping ideas:

- Hummus mixed with tinned wild salmon (this is a tasty source of protein, providing the amino acids needed to repair and build new muscles, plus other benefits for the immune system, including omega-3s, a host of vitamins and minerals and the antioxidant astaxanthin); top it off with cucumber and broccoli sprouts or any of your favourite veg
- As above, but add tomato or avocado instead of cucumber
- Smoked salmon, cream cheese, dill and a sprinkling of seeds
- Nut butter, banana and cinnamon

METHOD

1. Preheat the oven to 180°C.
2. Combine the ingredients to form a dough. Place between two sheets of baking paper and flatten with a rolling pin until 5mm thick.
3. Cut into shapes and bake for 10 minutes.

Granola florentines

Homemade treats like these give you more control over portion size and ingredients. Chocolate is full of beneficial cocoa flavonoids, so aim for dark and good-quality to maximise the benefits of these phytonutrients.

INGREDIENTS

- 200g chopped nuts and seeds (any combination you like)
- 300g jumbo oats
- 1 heaped tsp cinnamon
- 2 tbsp honey (or maple syrup)
- 2 tbsp olive oil
- 150g dark cooking chocolate

METHOD

1. Heat the oven to 170°C.
2. Mix the nuts and seeds, jumbo oats, cinnamon, honey and olive oil in a large bowl and mix well.
3. Tip onto a baking sheet, spread evenly and bake for about 10 minutes until golden brown.
4. Leave to cool completely before crumbling. (The granola can be stored in an airtight glass container for up to 1 month).
5. Place the dark chocolate in a small bowl and set over a pan of barely simmering water. When melted, pour a small amount into silicone muffin moulds or similar.
6. Sprinkle over the granola and place in the fridge to set.

Cranachan

Cranachan is a traditional oat-based Scottish dish made with whisky and usually served as a dessert at celebrations, such as Hogmanay, weddings or Burns suppers; but I think it's too tasty to save for special occasions, so here is my healthy version with thick and creamy yoghurt.

INGREDIENTS

- 40g whole, unrefined oats: either on their own or with nuts, seeds and other whole grains (quick tip: use muesli instead, aiming for those without added sugar; or, if you don't fancy toasting oats or muesli, use a homemade granola – see p. 189 – or a low-sugar shop-bought one)
- Fresh or frozen berries and seasonal fruits (I use frozen mixed berries as a cheaper and convenient alternative; adding seasonal fruits to a dish is a great way to eat fresh produce at its best and ensure you get important nutrients, such as fibre and vitamin C, for the immune system)
- 250g natural or vanilla yoghurt (or a plant-based yoghurt alternative); look for ones made with live cultures and without added sugar

To serve (optional):

- Honey
- Extra fresh seasonal fruits

METHOD

1. If using granola, there is no need to toast it, otherwise place oats (and any additional grains, seeds, nuts or muesli) in a dry frying pan and toast over a low heat,

stirring regularly for around 3 minutes, until golden. Set aside to cool.

2. Mash the berries and chopped seasonal fruits together with a fork.
3. Place a layer of oats in the bottom of your serving dish, followed by a layer of mashed fruit, then yoghurt. Repeat to use up all the ingredients, finishing with a layer of yoghurt.
4. Top with a drizzle of honey and sliced fresh fruit (if desired).

CHAPTER 8:

The Immune–Brain Romance

As I mentioned earlier, the biopsychosocial model of health suggests that our wellbeing is the product of a dynamic interaction between mind, body and environment. None of these factors in isolation leads definitively to health or illness – rather, it's the deep interconnection between them. If we are to build strong immune systems, then we cannot do so by diet alone; by focusing solely on food, we risk ignoring the other big levers of our physical and mental wellbeing. The tools and tips in this chapter may not give you immediate results, but they should help you to identify triggers of poor mental health and develop future-proofing skills to help you cope with and navigate life's challenges.

The brain and the immune system are exquisitely connected. Both are involved in how we interact with ourselves and the outside world, picking up signals and translating them into our bodies. Our thoughts, feelings, emotions and relationships all literally speak to the immune system in real time, regulating the function of immune cells, either for better or worse.

That bad memory you have, the post-traumatic stress, years of resentment or anger – they're all archived and locked into your immune system, deregulating its delicate balance, shifting you into an inflammatory state. This is why your mental wellbeing is associated with almost all health concerns known to medicine; everything from being more vulnerable to infections, impaired wound healing, poor metabolic health, elevated inflammation and even your risk of developing some cancers.

In this chapter, I'll help you get acquainted with your brain and its own unique communication with your immune system and provide the tools and knowledge to help you improve this relationship. Even if you don't feel you suffer from poor mental health, there is still a lot of utility in these practices. The COVID-19 pandemic has tightened the grip of the current poor mental-health crisis; none of us is immune to mental ill health, making this something really worth investing in. Good mental health is not an optional extra.

INFLAMMATION

Inflammation causes the junctions of the barrier between your brain and the rest of your body to become loose, allowing entry to inflammatory cytokines and other constituents of the blood and prompting inflammatory brain cells called microglia into action.[1] The resulting neuroinflammation has a negative effect on learning, memory and cognition (the scientific term for brain power needed for thinking, knowing, remembering and problem solving).

Inflammation can alter the activity or availability of serotonin, known as a 'feelgood' hormone, but also the molecule of willpower and calm.[2] This can lead to an inability to create and act on well-formed plans. That can mean difficulty with finishing things, feeling a little down, getting annoyed easily or being unable to control impulses. It can also affect sleep patterns, appetite, body temperature and hormonal activity, such as the menstrual cycle.

Inflammation can also upregulate dopamine. Dopamine activates brain areas involved in energy and motivation. It generally works with epinephrine to generate a sense of urgency or agitation, providing the fuel to get going. Together, these can make you feel excitement. But there can be too much of a good thing. Dopamine can modulate the function of microglial cells, which may result in neuroinflammation and, in turn, negatively impact the dopamine system, depleting your motivation.

Switching off inflammation

Acetylcholine (Ach) – a key component in learning and memory in the brain, as well as motor-neuron function – is the chief neurotransmitter involved in the regulation of the parasympathetic anti-inflammatory pathway, and its release in response to inflammation is known as the inflammatory reflex. Stimulating the vagus nerve elevates Ach, leading to this anti-inflammatory effect.[3] The pathway from the vagus nerve (the longest and perhaps most complex of cranial nerves – a key communication channel between the brain and all the other tissues and organs of the body) to its anti-inflammatory action is complex and incompletely understood, but Ach is the key communicating molecule relaying information between immune cells in the body and the central nervous system (CNS).

Knowledge of the inflammatory reflex provides us with possibilities to activate this powerful anti-inflammatory pathway. Hypnosis, acupuncture and meditation can significantly increase vagus-nerve output and reduce inflammation, as can behavioural conditioning using learned association and motor activity of the diaphragm, which is accessible through breathwork or singing.[4]

Track your immune health with HRV

Heart rate variability (HRV) is a function of the heart but originates in the autonomic nervous system (ANS). HRV is the variation in the time interval between one heartbeat and the next and is an excellent estimator of your overall immune health: decrease in variability means the heart is less responsive to signalling from the ANS, indicating elevated sympathetic nervous system (SNS) activity, i.e. stress; an increase in variability means the heart is responsive to cues from the parasympathetic nervous system (PNS) arm of the ANS. In a low-HRV state, your system is working overtime to maintain the processes required for physiological homeostasis. As a result, your body is less capable of adapting to acute stressors. Suppression of your HRV relative to your baseline is a sign of under-recovery and greater susceptibility to illness. It can even indicate the early stages of infection or inflammation before you have symptoms.[5] This is because HRV is very sensitive to inflammatory pathways – including changes driven by the innate immune system – as it ramps up to combat runaway viral replication. Often, your morning HRV will change abruptly and surprisingly, signalling the onset of illness. HRV is easily trackable using wearable devices and free smartphone apps. Read on for ways to nurture your emotional and social health, which enhance HRV via your ANS.

IS IT JUST YOUR PERSONALITY?

Personality can be defined as a collection of distinct psychological traits that remain fairly constant over time and therefore shape the way we react to the world around us. These traits include extroversion/introversion (how sociable we are), neuroticism (the tendency towards negativity) and conscientiousness (which includes how cautious we are and how carefully we plan). We know these can influence things such as job choices and friendships, but they can also impact the immune system, inflammation levels and ability to fight off disease.[6]

Extroverts tend to have increased expression of pro-inflammatory genes. While this could mean a greater ability to deal with infection, there are downsides, including a higher probability of developing autoimmune diseases. More conscientious personality types, on the other hand, have decreased pro-inflammatory gene expression. We are still making sense of this, but one of the most interesting questions is what is influencing what?

What happens in our heads and in our lives is connected to what happens in our health and sense of wellbeing. It is difficult to change our personalities, but an understanding of how they influence our susceptibility to disease might become a clinical tool in the future, guiding medications or teaching people to manage risky behaviours and adopt healthier ones. An extrovert might adopt a more altruistic outlook on life, for instance, since happiness that comes from having a deep sense of purpose has been shown to reduce inflammation.

Our nervous systems integrate and translate our emotions into a language the immune system can 'read' through their shared channels of communication. The ability to feel, express and perceive emotions is evolutionary. There is a varied menu of emotions designed to influence behaviour, linked to the immune system via the CNS. Emotions can be mapped onto neurochemicals and specific neurological patterns in the brain. More than fifty different neurochemicals and hormones work collectively to orchestrate our emotional brain chemistry.

Emotional wellbeing may serve as a safety signal, re-ordering the immune system's priorities, depending on how we are feeling, affecting the body's ability to remain or become healthy, or to resist or overcome disease.

HEALTHCARE STARTS WITH MENTAL SELF-CARE

The tight connections between the brain and immune system means that good mental health supports good immune health and vice versa. This means self-care of your own emotional and social wellbeing is part of your personal blueprint to strong immunity. Good mental health means being generally able to think, feel and react in the ways that you need and want to live your life. I think of it as the ability to surf well, making those constant tiny adjustments that bring you back to a good sense of your own wellbeing, no matter how the waves flow.

Did you know that your subjective view of your quality of life is one of the best predictors of future health – both mental and physical – even in those with long-term conditions?[7] Here are the most ground-breaking outcomes from studies:

- A good subjective sense of wellbeing leads to having a stronger immune system and being better protected against developing illnesses, improved recovery and healing.[8,9]

- A good subjective sense of wellbeing helps to build mental resilience to the effects of negative emotions on health.[10]

Subjective wellbeing refers in part to your emotions, moods and feelings and living in accordance with your 'true self'. Social relationships, self-care and finding meaning in life's experiences are all important ways to nurture your DOSE neurochemicals (dopamine, oxytocin, serotonin and endorphins), improving your own personal sense of wellbeing, which filters down to immunological wellness.

Let's define self-care

There is a strong positive correlation between self-care and subjective wellbeing,[11] indicating a strong need for self-care practices to support wellbeing. That said, if you are anything like me, holding down more responsibilities than you can manage, self-care advice can feel like an absurd and annoying paradox – both much needed and impossible.

Let's first give an alternative perspective to 'self-care'. It doesn't mean a spa day, exotic holiday or even a bubble bath. It can be as simple as showing up for yourself, being observant of how you are feeling as you move through different tasks in your day, or being mindful as you eat a meal or take a walk. At its most powerful, self-care is a continuous process, not a destination. And it looks different for everyone. The best bit? The by-product of an effective self-care routine is resilience – being able, both mentally and physically, to realise your abilities, strategically buffer and recover from the stresses of life, work productively and contribute to your community.

Life generally seems to make self-care incredibly hard and riddled with guilt. Just remember, this is not personal to you, it's systemic. However, you're feeling today, you don't have to wait for external factors to change in order to live better; your life doesn't have to resemble the craziness, chaos and confusion of the world around you. When you are facing challenges in life, it's about small steps, not an all-or-nothing mindset. And there are so many easy practices you can incorporate into your daily routine to nurture emotional and social wellbeing – from learning how to be an optimist, journalling and ecotherapy, to acquiring new skills, breathwork and practising gratitude.

I'd encourage you to explore a few emotional and social well-being tools that help you get to the next moment and be more effective in showing up for yourself and those around you. But above all, I recommend you try self-compassion.

Practise self-compassion

Self-compassion functions through both biological and behavioural pathways to promote health *and* improve the immune system, reducing the extent to which we suffer from challenging situations. There is a scientifically documented relationship between low self-compassion and stress-induced inflammatory cytokine production by immune cells. Practising self-compassion significantly reduced the cytokine IL-6, even when controlling for self-esteem, depressive symptoms, age, gender, ethnicity, BMI and post-traumatic stress syndrome, telling us that self-compassion holds huge immunological potential.[12] Self-compassionate people are also more motivated to take care of their health by engaging in healthy lifestyle behaviours and activities aligned with long-term goals.[13] By providing a consistent feeling of self-worth, self-compassion creates a foundation on which to see ourselves clearly, cope with negative emotions in healthy ways and reduce self-criticism. Importantly, it's separate from self-esteem, meaning we can still have compassion for ourselves, even if we aren't feeling good about ourselves. It's our modern-day superpower.

You can evaluate how self-compassionate you are via the following statements:

- I am judgmental of myself and fixate on flaws and inadequacies.
- I tend to feel more separate and cut off when I think about my inadequacies.
- I find it hard to be loving towards myself when I am feeling emotional pain.
- When I fail at something, I become consumed by feelings of inadequacy.
- When I see aspects of myself I don't like, I get down on myself.

There are many self-compassion interventions that are effective in reducing feelings of shame and self-criticism and can make you less emotionally reactive in stressful situations.[14, 15] There's no need to reinvent the wheel, but in addition to things you already do, you can raise self-compassion levels by cultivating each of the following daily:

- **Mindfulness** Practising mindfulness can naturally increase self-compassion. Mindfulness is an umbrella term that covers a huge number of practices, including meditation. Although there is no universally accepted definition, the consensus is that mindful moments should focus on being consciously aware or present in a given moment. For example, taking a self-compassion break in the middle of the day (stick it in your work calendar or set an alert on your phone, or while you boil the kettle to make a tea). Use the break to focus on taking a few deep breaths and non-judgementally try to sense your internal state of both body and mind.

- **Self-kindness** Remind yourself to act wisely in the face of negative behaviours but also forgive yourself.
- **Common humanity** Remind yourself that this is what it's like to struggle with challenges and that you are not the only one to feel this way.

STRESS

Most of us think we know what stress feels like: our hearts race, our palms get sweaty, we toss and turn in the small hours, with no end in sight, a temper bomb explodes when the smallest thing goes wrong . . . But some of the effects of stress can be more subtle, lurking beneath the surface, accumulating over time. Let's take a closer look at what happens.

A stress response – whether it's from a biological, psychological or environmental stressor – is orchestrated by the hypothalamic-pituitary-adrenal (HPA) axis:

- An area of the brain, called the hypothalamus, interprets stress, secreting corticotropin-secreting hormone (CRH).
- CRH tells the pituitary gland to release adrenocorticotropin hormone (ACTH).
- ACTH instructs the adrenal glands to make the stress hormones cortisol and adrenalin – the cornerstones of our stress response.

- Short-term stress can last from minutes to hours, causing: elevated heart rate and breathing increases, pumping oxygen to major muscles (supporting fight or flight)

- blood being drawn away from the digestive tract and other organs ('butterflies in tummy' or digestive upset)
- a rise in blood-sugar levels to provide fast energy
- short-term immune activation – when we are in fight-or-flight mode, we expose ourselves increasingly to injury; sustaining a wound could also risk infection, so the HPA axis induces a short-term immune activation to prevent this from happening.

The body's stress-response system should be self-limiting. Once the perceived threat has passed, and the adrenals have pumped out some cortisol, they tell the brain 'We did our job', and the brain flips off the stress response. Adrenalin and cortisol levels drop, heart rate and blood pressure return to baseline levels, and other systems resume their regular activities. At least, that's how it's supposed to work. But sometimes the adrenals don't give the brain the message or the brain doesn't hear it. The result? Cortisol production stays on when it should be off.

Chronic stress sends the HPA axis into overdrive, with effects felt throughout the body, sometimes even serving as further sources of stress. One of the most pronounced effects of long-term cortisol release is glucocorticoid resistance,[16] when cells in the immune system become less sensitive to the anti-inflammatory effects of cortisol. As a result, cortisol starts to increase inflammation throughout the body and brain, causing both physical and psychological symptoms, such as itchiness and rashes[17] or feelings of depression or loneliness.[18]

The following are some of the serious long-term effects of stress:

- Altered metabolism
- High blood pressure
- Blood-sugar spikes

- Suppression of immunity and uncontrolled inflammation
- Susceptibility to infection and chronic disease
- Fatigue, as energy and nutrients are 'triaged' to help with immediate stress response
- Sleep disturbances
- Changes in appetite
- Negative mood, poor concentration or irritability

Understanding why the body reacts in these ways can help us to develop strategies for preventing stress from getting under our skin. Without a system in place, we're nudged in a direction we don't want to go in.

Note: symptoms of chronic stress are diffuse and overlap with hundreds of other potentially serious conditions, so always talk to your doctor to rule out other causes.

Managing stress

The first step to managing stress is to redefine it. *Eu*stress is the term used for beneficial stress. For example, the coronavirus pandemic is a real concern, and an appropriate and realistic level of stress can help to prompt vigilance around helpful behaviours, such as handwashing and, where necessary, containment. A certain amount of stress has even been identified to influence optimal sports performance and, ultimately, we stress because we care. We want to be safe.

*Dis*tress is the opposite of eustress. It's the negative form of stress and, perhaps, the one we are more familiar with. Chronic or intermittent stress can evolve into distress, possibly the single biggest threat to immunity from our busy lives. Research shows we either have a stress-enhancing or stress-debilitating mindset, based on how we view our stress. Some factors that shape this are intrinsic, but most you have some control over.[19] This opens up possibilities for coping better with stress and reaping the unexpected benefits it can bring in the form of personal growth. But how?

1. **See your stress. Name it, label it. Don't deny it.** Recognise the power of your mindset in how you respond.
2. **Pause. Be mindful.** Proactively seek to view stressful situations not through your old pattern and defaulted negative ways, but from new, positive angles and possibilities.
3. **Own it.** Recognise that you tend to stress more (and more intensely) about things that matter to you. Stress shows you care – that the stakes matter.
4. **Use it as a good thing.** Contrary to what you might think, the body's stress response was not designed to kill you, but to help you grow and meet the demands you face.

STRESS-MANAGEMENT TOOLS

Helpful coping mechanisms act like a tap that lets stress flow out from your stress container, and a variety of strategies are needed for this. When you're in the middle of a stressful situation, you need easy, 'real-time' tools to pull out just when you need them most (because let's face it, you're unlikely to meditate when you have a moment of anxiety in the supermarket, remembering a work deadline you've missed). But even when you don't *feel* stressed, it's important to engage in regular stress management with what I call 'future-proofing tools' that can be practised when you're calm (like that meditation I just mentioned). These act to reduce the probability that a stressor will overwhelm you, by emptying your container or changing your relationship to stress. Finally, 'hormetic' tools are techniques that actually induce stress in a short-term, 'safe', regulated way, raising your threshold to get you comfortable with being uncomfortable.

Real-time stress tools

The following can be deployed to deal with stress any time, anywhere:

- **Use your eyes.** When you feel stressed, not only do your heart rate and breathing increase, but you also tend to narrow your field of vision. This further activates the fight-or-flight arm of the SNS and adds to the feeling of agitation. By widening your gaze and observing the periphery of your vision, you provide a signal to the brain to dampen the stress response. This is also important if you spend many hours gazing at a screen or smartphone. Try to get outside into green space and go for a walk, taking in the panoramic view, or just look out of the window if you can't get outside.

Top tip 1: Combine this with the rule of three: take in a broad vista, pause and name *three* things you see, then stop and name *three* sounds you hear, then, finally, take a moment to notice and wiggle *three* parts of your body.

Top tip 2: Experience 'optic flow' when going for a walk to further a sense of calm. Optic flow is the motion pattern created by your eyes as you move through any environment; it quiets some of the circuits responsible for stress and resets cortisol levels in a healthy way.

- **Use your breath.** Remember when I said that the breath is anchored to the diaphragm (see p. 194)? Well, consciously changing your breathing can immediately antagonise stress. When you exhale, your diaphragm rises, creating less space for the heart, which causes the blood to flow more quickly through it and, as a result, the brain sends a signal to slow down the heart rate. Start by extending your outbreath to slow down your heart rate and reduce your sympathetic-nervous arousal.

Top tip 3: reduce stress with a physiological sigh. A physiological sigh is a pattern of breathing you can deliberately employ to give you real-time control of your stress response. It consists of a double inhale followed by an exhale: take a long inhale through the nose, pause, then take a short inhale through the nose, followed by a long exhale through the mouth. In addition to balancing the ratio of carbon dioxide and oxygen in the bloodstream, this activates a neural circuit via the phrenic nerve that goes from the diaphragm back to the brainstem and informs the brain about the status of the body, helping you to get into a relaxed parasympathetic state.

Future-proofing stress tools

Future-proofing is all about practising techniques to incrementally manage stress over the long term by accessing the parasympathetic (rest-and-digest) arm of the nervous system as a counterweight to a stressed-out world.

Meditation and mindfulness are, of course, great tools to have in your mental-health toolkit. Meditation also has direct immunological benefits, raising your first line of defence: the IgA antibodies that protect mucosal barriers, such as the lungs and gut. But training the mind in mindfulness and meditation can be daunting, one of the biggest drawbacks being that they take time, training and skilled guidance.[20]

If meditation is just not your cup of tea or you find it tricky to master, don't despair. Here are a few simple, evidence-based alternatives for you to access your nervous system and calm your stress response:

- **Reframe stress.** Reflect on a recent stressful moment. Be critical about it and reflect on how stress was helpful or harmful. Remember, how you view stress can really nudge you down a negative path if you let it.
- **Stress dump.** Some stress is inevitable, but you can keep your response manageable by time-boxing it into a specific slot in your day. During that time, write down what is worrying you. Then review and ask yourself: can I turn this into a problem I can solve? Then think of a plan to tackle actionable worries and acknowledge and let go of the others.
- **Talk it over.** Talk things through with someone who can help you reframe problems and figure out how to deal with stressful situations.
- **Non-meditation meditation.** Try guided imagery, taking a short pause in your day to imagine yourself in your 'happy place'. Take five minutes to practise some slow, deep-breathing exercises to activate the neurons that signal to the vagus nerve, leading to activation of the parasympathetic nervous system. Do a body scan, progressively tensing and relaxing muscle by muscle, starting in your feet and working up your body.
- **Try ecotherapy.** Ecotherapy is the umbrella term for the many benefits of spending time in nature. Humans have a deep connection to the environment – in particular green

spaces – and failing to nurture this takes a toll on many aspects of wellbeing, particularly the immune system. Ecotherapy has been shown to improve mood, reduce feelings of stress and fortify the immune response.

- **Give your brain a rest.** Often, the working week can feel like scaling a mental mountain against the glare of a computer screen. Even for those of us who have jobs we enjoy, there is often a sense of so much coming at us at once, so much to process, that we just can't deal with it all. We endure a kind of base level of mental tension and busyness that never totally dissipates. Your brain needs a rest. Rest is not an indulgence or a vice; it is about replenishment The default mode network (DMN) is the term given to the brain systems that come to life when you daydream, and it links aspects of immune function to psychological and behavioural states. The DMN can moderate inflammation, and inflammation can disrupt the DMN.[21] To let your mind drift and activate the DMN, you need to do activities where you are not processing information. Watching TV, scrolling social media or reading a book might all feel restful, but are not brain rest in the sense of letting your mind wander. To really engage in this, you have to do a lot less, perhaps sitting and staring into space, or try a mindless, repetitive task, such as vacuuming.

Hormetic stress tools

Hormesis is a fancy word for 'what doesn't kill you, makes you stronger'. The devil is in the detail, however, because for stress to have a beneficial effect, you have to control the timing and dose to assist your body in adapting, and encourage your own innate capacity to manage challenges when they come.[22] This works via numerous molecular mechanisms, including activating the vagus nerve, boosting your relaxation response and strengthening the nervous system against stress, as well as increasing antioxidants and molecules associated with cellular resilience.[23] Classic examples include exercise, fasting, phytonutrients and extreme temperature exposures (such as a sauna or plunging into ice-cold water), all of which act as acute stressors, stimulating you to adapt and rejuvenate your body systems in a positive way (provided your stress container is not already overflowing). You may have heard of Wim Hof, also known as the Iceman, who is famous for being able to withstand extremely cold temperatures and has used cold (and breathing) to completely stop immune-system inflammation.

Hormetic responses have been demonstrated to help you live longer, reduce oxidative stress, and improve your immune system and your mood. This is why I routinely do things that are mildly uncomfortable, such as sea swimming or, occasionally, forms of challenging high-intensity exercise.

YOUR MENTAL-HEALTH BLUEPRINT

Start with a weekly check-in. Take a few moments to note down two or three points for each of the following questions:

- How do I feel physically? Mentally? (Notice and admit what you are feeling. Try to name the feeling.)
- How's my thinking today? Am I having unhelpful thoughts? How are my thoughts making me feel? (Consider how you talk to yourself and the choices you make in your day-to-day life to support your mental wellbeing. Remember, busy is the enemy of clarity. It is important to manage how you think, feel and behave in a solution-

focused way. If you are stuck in a stress rut, it might feel permanent, but it can be reversible; nudge: this is where self-compassion comes in useful.)

- How is my social health? Do I have strategies in place to get the connection I need? What one thing can I try this week?
- When have I felt resilience? (Reflect on that experience.)

Take fifteen minutes

Can't take a day for yourself? That's ok. Find an hour. Or even just fifteen minutes – did you know that's only 1 per cent of your day?

- Choose five things to explore this week for your emotional and social wellbeing. For example, can you introduce a self-compassion break into your day? Can you increase the time you spend in nature across your week?
- Take fifteen minutes out of your day to focus on one of these. What's one small thing you can do for yourself during this time? For example, how would your day look if you just took this moment to be gentler with yourself and invite in some self-compassion? Or reconnect with a personal activity that you love? Or learn something new? And it doesn't need to be fifteen minutes – it can be more or less, but once you start to make time, use it wisely (no scrolling social media)!
- If you find yourself worrying about something, remember to pause and ask yourself – will this problem matter in

ten minutes, one day, one week, six months . . .? The answer might be that it will matter in a year or more from now, but it's helpful to triage your worries in this way.

Goal setting

Time to set some goals. Refer back to p. 64 to recap on how to set SMART goals, remembering to focus on *your* why, and no one else's. Goals are successful when they are based on our values. This will help you to kickstart and maintain positive changes. Remember also, making changes isn't easy, especially against the tide of stresses in our environment.

Reflect on your weekly check-in (opposite) and use what you have learned in this chapter. Focus on the process, not the outcome, and prioritise sustaining new behaviour changes to get you there. Anchor your goals to automatic behaviours you have in your life and keep it positive. Choose a convenient period to start, avoiding stressful times at work or busy social weeks. Share your goals with those close to you, or find like-minded individuals who share similar ones. Social support creates accountability, making you more likely to stick to your goals.

Be honest with yourself. But also, be kind. See this process not as the path to achievement, but as an important step to focus your attention on the things that support your emotional and social wellbeing, providing key elements of a healthy, balanced life, as well as strengthening the resilience needed to buffer against the stresses of daily living.

Short-term goals What would you like to achieve over the next 2–4 weeks?	**Medium-term goals** What would you like to achieve over the next 2–4 months?	**Long-term goals** What would you like to achieve over the next 6–12 months?
1. 2. 3.	1. 2. 3.	1. 2. 3.
Start date:	Start date:	Start date:

What will you need to do to accomplish your goals?		
In the short term...	In the medium term...	In the long term...

Consider what has gone well: notice your wins, no matter how small. Pick out the positives and note down what you enjoyed.

What has not gone so well? Take stock; note what you disliked most. Identify barriers so you can work towards overcoming them.

Keep reflecting on your immunobiography: what do you want its next chapter to look like?

Front-load your day

Your prefrontal cortex – the thinking, plotting, planning, conscious part of your brain – fatigues with use. So as the day wears on, your thinking wears down. Front-loading is a simple technique that builds momentum and fuels motivation. If you want to get your day off to a positive start, try front-loading by planning so that a large proportion of activities, such as exercise, happen early in your day. By making time for your emotional and social wellbeing early, you set the tone for the rest of the day, knowing that you did something positive for your mental wellbeing before surrendering your best-laid plans to the reality of work/family/kids/friends/life.

Turning obstacles into superpowers

Limiting factors are the things that stand in the way of you achieving your goals. We deal with limiting factors almost every day, but sadly, some problems just won't go away or get fixed easily. When this happens, they can really take their toll on our mental wellbeing. This means problem solving is a really important skill to develop

Turn your biggest obstacles into superpowers with the IF → THEN approach:

- If I feel overwhelmed by a situation → then I'll pause and pay attention to my feelings.

When you pay attention to these feelings, you often recognise the problems sooner. For example, feeling angry whenever you talk to your boss may be a sign that there is a problem at work. But you can't solve the problem until you identify what the issue is.

Try not to get caught up with finding the 'right' solution. Sometimes there is no right answer, but it's easier to find a *good* solution when you feel calm and are not being self-critical. It can also be helpful to brainstorm a lot of solutions to choose from. Consciously work on emptying your stress tank and cultivating an inner circle of supportive friends, family or professionals who can help you brainstorm. And if at any stage you are really struggling, refresh your knowledge by refamiliarising yourself with the details in this chapter.

Cutting-edge scientific insights confirm the importance of the two-way street between the immune system and the brain. By acknowledging the real impact of the intricate mind–body connection on our health, we gain a clearer understanding of the links between our own personal lived experiences, our personalities and their health effects. And by implementing the tools outlined in this chapter, we can support both brain and body better.

CHAPTER 9:

Sustainable Movement

Since Hippocrates first advised us more than 2000 years ago that exercise (though not too much of it) was good for health, the science supporting the importance of physical activity has developed apace.

We know conclusively that being physically active keeps us more resilient to infections and reduces their duration.[1] And without doubt, an active lifestyle can alleviate many of the chronic inflammatory disease challenges we face today. In fact, physical inactivity contributes to 40 per cent of long-term inflammatory health conditions, causing as many deaths in the UK as smoking[2] and being considered the biggest public health problem of the twenty-first century.[3] Not only does physical inactivity impact on our body composition and cardiovascular health, it is also a key contributor to immune ageing, increasing the risk of infections, cancer and chronic inflammation-related poor health.[4]

THE PROBLEM WITH 'EXERCISE'

I'm sure everyone reading this wants to harness the immune-strengthening, metabolism-boosting benefits of exercise. Then why are so many of us not doing enough of it? And why are most public-health interventions aimed at raising our activity levels such a tough sell?

Hippocrates' advice aside, humans haven't evolved to exercise. It's a very modern thing. Our ancestors moved enough to do what they needed and find adequate food. It would have been very rare to have a surplus of food and little need to move. But modern life is structured in a way that means we do not have to move to fulfil fundamental needs, such as finding food, shelter and water. It's just too easy to avoid movement.

So how do we do something very ancient in a modern way?

By definition, exercise is a contrived experience with connotations of looking better or losing weight. It's a modern-day proxy for the lack of movement in our daily lives, a very deliberate way for a very deliberate outcome. Let's start by reframing exercise as 'movement'. Irrespective of our personal fitness goals, focusing on more movement opportunities throughout the day is foundational, because all movement counts. It's also more achievable (going back to what you learned about goal setting earlier – see p. 63) and more inclusive. Then you can supplement with exercise, as required or as you desire.

Next, is our affective response. Knowledge and belief in the health benefits motivate initial involvement and return to activity following relapse, but feelings of enjoyment and pleasure have been scientifically shown to be stronger motives for continued participation.[5]

Exercise in the conventional gym-going sense is fine, but it's important to remember that movement is fundamentally human and crucial to our wellbeing. So let's start to think of it less as being confined to a gym and more as movement, strength and play. A life where moving and living are one and the same thing, not separate entities, is the ultimate goal. Developing a body that moves well is the ticket to a place where we feel we can live better. Ultimately, how well – and how much – we move determines how well we engage with the world and establishes our larger purpose in life.

Future-proofing our fitness outside the gym is a key learning from the COVID-19 pandemic. COVID has shown us that we can't rely on the gym as the only place to get our movement in. Building gym-free movement opportunities into our daily routines is the only way to secure consistent good health for the long term. In fact, non-exercise activity thermogenesis (NEAT) is the energy expended for everything that is not sleeping, eating or sport-like exercise, and includes walking to work, performing household tasks and even fidgeting.

MORE MOVEMENT, MORE OFTEN, MORE WAYS

You might want to beat your marathon time or squat your personal best, but those specific goals may not be supporting your health in the ways that matter. Don't overcomplicate it. Just as you need diversity, abundance and variety with key nutrients in your diet, so the optimal way to move your body throughout your day is with diversity and abundance and variety. This will look different for everyone and depend on your starting point, personal goals and other factors, such as lifestyle or underlying health conditions. In fact, the least active individuals stand to gain the most from a small increase in physical activity. For example, we know that if you are sedentary, some exercise is better than nothing to offset some risks. A meta-analysis (a large and robust way of evaluating lots of different studies) suggests that while higher sedentary time is associated with increased risk of death, the risk can be partially offset by thirty to forty minutes of moderate-to-vigorous physical activity per day.[6, 7] Regular movement can also positively impact your immune system in a relatively short space of time[8] – and it's never too late to start. Plus, it doesn't need to be long, intense or unpleasant to be effective.

Think of the immune effect of exercise as having a housekeeper. If you have really let things go, it will look a lot better on their first visit than if they had never come. But the more frequently they come back, the better and cleaner the house will look. Exercise is essentially a housekeeping activity that helps the immune system to patrol the body and detect and evade bacteria and viruses, manage oxidative stress and lower unnecessary inflammation. You can't necessarily exercise once in a while and expect to have an illness-clearing immune system. But come back for more movement on a regular basis and your immune system will be better prepared for anything life throws at it.

START WITH MOBILITY

Whatever your athletic goals are, your ability to move well will directly affect what you can do and how well you can do it. Mobility is often overlooked, yet it is an essential part of physical movement, minimising injuries and opening up opportunities, making it the gateway to being able to take full advantage of the benefits of the other physical activities you enjoy.

One of the misconceptions about being mobile is that you have to be very flexible. Flexibility is only a fraction of the equation. Being able to move well is a combination of flexibility, strength and motor control. The human body should be able to co-ordinate bending, rotating, shifting, stabilising, squatting, lunging, crawling, running and climbing from multiple angles and planes. As use-it-or-lose-it organisms, we can re-educate and rehabilitate our joints towards a healthier range of movement by practising and playing with our full range of motion. This keeps us moving, which keeps us healthy.

Ten-minute morning mobility ritual

Working on mobility can take many forms, from static and dynamic stretching and foam-rolling massage to working with a physiotherapist or movement coach. This can all feel quite confusing and overwhelming. More important than specific mobility 'tools' or exercises is how consistently you move, breaking up those static postures and giving your body the 'medicine' it needs for improving mobility. If you spend most of your time sitting, you'll become very good and efficient at sitting. Spend more of your time moving in lots of different ways and you may well become good at that, too! However you move, try to make time to do so within your full range of motion. This might mean taking time to regularly open your hips through stretching or do some full shoulder rolls.

As a big advocate of front-loading my day with intentional behaviours (see p. 213), I do mobility work early – because the time up until the moment I have to leave the house for the school run/work is possibly the only point at which I have a modicum of control over the things I want to do for myself. This way, on days when my schedule expands into catastrophic mayhem, I still feel like I've engaged in some movement/physical practice. With that in mind, here is your ten-minute morning mobility ritual to help you dip your toe into mobility for better movement and a better-functioning body:

First work through your body:

- Neck – how does it feel? Tight on one side?
- Overhead reach – can you comfortably lift your arms overhead? Do your ribs flare up (where the lower part at the front of your rib cage protrudes forwards and out)? Are your arms at the same height?

- Toe touch – how close or far away from your toes are you? Do you feel a stretch in your hamstrings or your lower back?
- Squat – can you easily sit in a squat? Or is it an uncomfortable position for you? Do your ankles roll, knees cave or upper back round? Are your arms both at the same height?

Now slowly work through the following moves. As you do so, remember to breathe deeply and fully, relaxing your body and letting go of tension. Always work within your own range of ability.

Cat-cow

Cat-cow is a gentle flow between two positions that warm the body and bring flexibility to the spine.

- Start on your hands and knees with your wrists directly under your shoulders, hands pointing in front of you and your knees under your hips.
- Move into cow pose, dropping your belly towards the ground. Lift your chin and gaze. If you have neck issues, keep your chin in line with your torso. Try to feel the distance between your shoulders; broaden and draw your shoulders away from your ears.
- Now move into cat pose by drawing your belly to your spine and rounding your back towards the ceiling, like a cat stretching.
- Repeat the sequence as many times as you like, aiming for at least 5–10, taking a pause to enjoy each cat and cow.

The resting-squat sit

A resting squat is a posture where you squat down fully, lowering your hips towards the ground, with your weight equally distributed.

- Start barefoot, spreading your feet hip-width apart and pointing your toes straight ahead.
- Now squat, going as low as you can. Try not to raise your heels off the floor or slump forwards. If this feels very difficult, hold onto something, such as a doorframe, as you squat. You can also try putting a cushion under your heels.
- Aim to do 3 squat sits, staying in each one for at least 30 seconds. then start to build towards staying longer in them.

Spiderman lunge to thoracic rotation

This move is great to open your hips and chest. It can be performed as part of a warm-up, or you can hold the position for a deeper stretch.

- Place your hands directly under your shoulders in the push-up starting position; turn the inside of your elbows forwards.
- Step your right leg forwards and place to the outside of your right hand.
- Take your right hand and first reach through underneath your body, before taking that arm up to the sky. Lower your hand, return the leg to the starting point and repeat on the other side.

Overhead shoulder mobility

Improve your shoulder mobility with the help of a stick – for example, a broom handle.

- Grab the stick in front of you with both hands, starting with a pretty wide grip.
- Keep your elbows straight and lift the stick up and over your head.

- Bring it as far back as you can, while keeping your elbows straight. Try not to let your ribcage flare.
- Repeat, aiming for 5–10 times.
- Once you are comfortable with the width of your grip, start to move your hands a little closer. Don't rush it.

Downward dog

This is particularly beneficial for creating length throughout the entire body, from your feet all the way to your back. It also develops strength in the wrists, shoulders and back muscles.

- Start off on all fours and make sure your knees are slightly behind your hips. Your hands should be shoulder-width apart and your fingers spread out wide.
- Press your hands into the mat, gently tuck your toes under and take a deep inhale.
- Keeping your hands pressed into the mat, exhale deeply, lifting your knees off the floor and straightening your legs as much as you can. Take a few breaths in this position, paddle out the feet and enjoy the stretch to the back of the legs. Try to keep your belly drawn in, heels rooting towards the floor, shoulders actively drawn away from your ears and fingers spread wide and active.
- Come back to all fours, then repeat. See if you can increase the number of deep breaths you take in this position.

MUSCLE

From those who do no physical activity to those for whom fitness means racking up steps on their pedometer or maxing out on cardio, strength training is perhaps the best thing for immunity.

For all of us, no matter our age, strength training can add healthy years to our lives. And no steps needed!

Sadly, muscle power has long played second fiddle to cardio, with 75 per cent of the UK population failing to get enough strength exercise. Sometimes referred to as resistance training, strength training refers to conditioning the strength and function of your muscles by adding some resistance to them, triggering your muscles to grow and adapt. You don't need to lift weights or even join a gym. Resistance can be picking up a heavy object, such as a child, carrying shopping bags or moving logs, rocks or anything with mass. The World Health Organization recommends at least two strength sessions per week. This is a good baseline to aim for. Muscles will respond to load or force regardless of age, so there are benefits for everyone to include strength and resistance movement, whatever their starting point. A twenty-year-old is in a good place to build their muscle bank account (and I don't mean body-building style) to buffer some of the inevitable sarcopenic losses that come with age, while research shows that one bout of resistance exercise leads to muscle growth in ninety-year-olds.[9] So it's never too late – or too early – to initiate a resistance-work programme. And as I said, it's about diversity and abundance – trying different things and finding activities you enjoy. Search online for variations of body-weight exercises, such as push-ups, keep a resistance band next to your desk, do Pilates or a yoga class . . .

MOMENTUM

The momentum pillar refers to aerobic activity, often called 'cardio' exercise – the kind of activity that gets your heart beating faster. This is the most beneficial type of exercise for your cardiovascular system (your heart, lungs and blood vessels) and is when your body is using 'aerobic metabolism' to produce energy from fat and glycogen (the stored form of sugar) in the presence of oxygen.

In order to benefit your health and longevity, you need to be doing *some* cardio. But before you shout 'I hate cardio', remember we are reframing exercise.

Build your aerobic base

The intensity of cardio can be split into 'training zones', which reflect your level of exertion based on a percentage of your maximum heart rate. These zones range from zone 0 (at rest) up to zones 5–6 (nearing maximum intensity or all-out effort). Moving in what we call your aerobic base, or zone-2 training, generally involves exercising at a constant moderate level of intensity for a specified duration (usually for a minimum of thirty minutes). This is paced at a level that makes you breathe faster and feel warmer, but where you can still hold a conversation (so you don't have to torture yourself, turn purple and collapse in a pool of your own sweat at the end of it). Typical activities include walking, jogging, cycling, swimming, skipping, stair climbing and rowing. But this also includes activities of daily living, such as walking to the shops, gardening and cleaning.

For most people, this will mean experiencing an increased heart rate and breathing rate during the activity to a point where their heart rate is between 60 and 70 per cent of their maximum, but it will vary according to existing fitness levels. If you have a heart-rate monitor, a quick way to calculate this is 180 minus your age. And for those who like numbers, this is about 100 steps per minute when walking (i.e. 1500 steps in 15 minutes, or 3000 steps in 30 minutes) or walking a fifteen-minute mile.

Regularly engaging in zone 2 by simply walking at a brisk pace will provide this immediate benefit to your immune system, and the benefits add up. In fact, walking five or more days of the week lowers the number of upper-respiratory tract infections (such as the common cold) by more than 40 per cent.[10]

There is no 'best' cardio, but I can't emphasise enough the value of zone 2 activities, such as brisk walking. Being consistent is key here, so the goal is to explore and share training methods and habits that are sustainable. Simple brisk daily walking will lead to important physiological adaptations that will help you perform better in all forms of movement with a much lower risk for injury. Walking might not burn as many calories as running, but it produces the same risk reduction for inflammatory disease, while taking less of a physiological toll on your body as compared to higher-intensity cardio. All of which makes it more accessible and a great place to start if you are currently not moving much at all, yet easy to build up to as much as four to six times per week. It is also less demanding on your central nervous system. If you're stressed out on life and juggling a heavy life load, zone 2 facilitates a parasympathetic response in the body, think 'flow state'.

However, training indefinitely in just one cardio zone with one type of activity is like training just one muscle in your body. To get the most out of moving, aim for progression, variation and challenge to encourage beneficial adaptations that add up over time. Try to switch up the type of activities, the frequency, duration and intensity.

We can build our aerobic base by spending time in zone 2, topped up with small amounts of higher-intensity training. You can track intensity using a heart-rate monitor and work towards incorporating activities that target all zones in some capacity.

RECOVERY

Recovery is our secret superpower. It's perhaps the most underused, chemical-free, safe and effective therapy available to us. If only we were better at it, though.

Do you ever find it hard to rest enough to feel really recovered and ready to go? Do you go to the gym, even though your body (or brain) is not up to it? Ever taken on extra responsibilities, even when feeling fatigued? While many of us might find it hard to shake the 'no-pain-no-gain' mantra, recovery is crucial. Very few things in life, the body included, can keep going without taking time for recovery. In fact, recovery is defined as purposely doing things to help our bodies return to a better state. As such, it is vital in helping our bodies to perform at their best and allowing us to engage fully in life.

How important recovery is to you as an individual will depend on the type, frequency and duration of physical activity that you engage in, as well as any body-composition goals and personal preferences.

Keep it simple by following the five Rs of recovery[11] to ensure that you are fully prepared and keeping your immune system strong:

Rehydrate

Rehydrate soon after finishing your session. Get into the habit of drinking adequate fluids to ensure you will be hydrated both during and after exercise.

Refuel

Refuelling with dietary carbohydrates will replenish the muscle and liver fuel stores (called glycogen) that you have burned through exercise. But this is also important to ensure you have enough energy in your body to support your daily activities, including your energy-intensive immune system. The timing and amount of carbohydrates you will need after exercise needs to be fine-tuned, depending on how much energy you are expending across the day, how your energy levels are and how long before your next exercise session.

Generally speaking, post-workout refuelling is something to consider following longer sessions of forty-five minutes or more. The body is most effective at replacing carbohydrate and promoting muscle repair and growth in the first sixty to ninety minutes after exercise; however, this will continue for another twelve to twenty-four hours, which means that it's ok to wait until your next meal to refuel. Just remember that in the post-exercise period, it takes about four hours for carbohydrates to be digested and absorbed into muscle and liver tissues to be incorporated as glycogen.

Rebuild

This is perhaps the most important way you can support your body physically through nutrition. Protein ingestion gives you the building blocks necessary to synthesise muscle protein. Along with resistance training, this is important for preventing muscle loss, especially as you age. A good amount to aim for, in particular for elderly or very active people, is 25–30g protein per meal.[12]

Not all protein sources are created equal in terms of their amino-acid (building-block) composition, though. Historically, animal proteins were considered superior when it came to supporting muscle-protein synthesis. A closer look tells us that this is due to animal sources generally being higher in the amino acid leucine, but this is also found in plant-based sources, though in more variable amounts. So try to be judicious with plant-based protein, diversifying your sources to ensure you meet your leucine needs (2–3g per meal). (See p. 118 for high-leucine foods.)

Restore

Restoring micronutrients (vitamins and minerals) is important for recovery, too.[13,14] Micronutrients support energy production and the mitochondria that help us to move. They also provide antioxidant functions, which is particularly significant if you exercise regularly, and they are important for the immune system, so make sure you consume enough of them.

Rest

Rest is also part of your overall recovery strategy. Your body needs rest to recover and get stronger from hard workouts. A rest day is one that doesn't involve exercise at all, but where you plan to relax and do light movement, such as errands and housework instead. Active recovery is slightly different. This is where you include low-impact activities at an easy intensity to keep blood flow and movement in your muscles and joints and complement the demands of higher-intensity activities. This might include stretching, gentle yoga, walking. Both rest and active recovery are tools you can use to achieve your fitness goals.

MAINTAINING MOVEMENT

Some might say exercise is medicine, in which case, of course, it's possible to over- or underdose. Exercise adherence is generally the place where most of us stumble. Many people are unwilling to exercise due to lack of time and motivation. And for those who are older or have chronic diseases, exercise can also cause pain, which limits it further, for obvious reasons. Even for someone like me who loves to move, it isn't always enjoyable, and sometimes I am just too tired and mentally drained after a day of work to even contemplate going out for a walk (even if I've spent my whole day sitting at a desk). We also know that the rigorous regimes of elite athletes can lead to overtraining syndrome, a constellation of problems, including reduced immunity. Perhaps you have been conditioned to think more is better, or you are pursuing a specific training goal, putting that before your body's health needs. Severe overtraining is about moving too much without proper fuel and recovery, leading to immune-system fatigue, and potentially leaving you open to infection and illness.

The best approach is to find a way to stay active that feels good and tickles your reward centre, because the best dose of exercise is the one that gets you coming back for more. Do what you feel your body needs and what you enjoy. Move with compassion. Each day will present the inevitable challenges to moving your body, which means it can be tough mentally: skipping workouts, cutting them short or deviating from your regimen in other ways usually leads to feelings of guilt, disappointment, self-doubt and lack of motivation. And negative self-talk is not the best way to get back on track.

The first step to establishing a sustainable workout routine is to wipe out any destructive feelings, such as guilt and frustration, with a heavy dose of self-compassion. 'Exercise snacking' refers to small, even tiny, morsels of physical activity (such as standing for a few minutes after sitting for a while), and is supported by scientific research as an effective way to improve your health.[15] The activity does not need to be lengthy, tiring or involve formal exercise, although it can be vigorous if you choose to make it so. 'Exercise snacking' is a powerful way to reframe our collective mindset about exercise, allowing us to view it as a treat, rather than a chore. When we break down a task like this, it requires less mental willpower to achieve it, thus challenging the 'all-or-nothing' mindset that is so pervasive when it comes to fitness.

YOUR MOVEMENT BLUEPRINT

Choose a convenient period to start to introduce changes to your physical activity. Avoid stressful times at work or busy social weeks. Remember that vague, unrealistic or uninspiring goals (or none at all) set you up to quit at the first (inevitable) hurdle. Rather than search out the next quick fix or complain about how situations and circumstances 'made' you fall off the wagon, you need to start out in a way that will protect you against hurdles. That requires a little planning, taking into account incidental movement during your day and engineering your environment and schedule in a way that breaks up sedentary behaviour.

If you are movement deficient . . .

. . . but committed to a physical activity programme and setting goals for yourself, it's helpful to first identify your personal barriers. By troubleshooting and developing tactics in advance, you'll have better success in overcoming them. (See pp. 233–4 for some of the most common barriers.)

If you're an exercise misuser and abuser . . .

. . . here are some questions to ask yourself when healthy movement becomes an obsession:

- Do you feel a high level of anxiety or guilt if you miss a workout?
- Do you exercise even though you have an injury or are unwell?
- Do you miss social events with friends and family so you can exercise?
- Are you afraid of gaining weight if you can't exercise?
- Is your primary motivator for exercise burning calories?

If you have answered yes to most of these questions, then it might be a good idea to pause and consider your relationship to exercise, acknowledging that you may have an unhealthy pattern of physical activity. While we know moderate physical activity benefits your immune system, pushing yourself too hard can impair it.

Dialling down your weekly exercise can be challenging, but several athletic organisations, including the International Olympic Committee, provide recommendations that are worth keeping in mind to guide your training plan if you're ramping up for a competitive event (or other reasons) in order to reduce your odds of getting sick.

- Develop an individualised training plan that suits *your* lifestyle and goals, but also allows you to achieve balance.

- Increase intensity in small increments.
- Include enough rest days to allow your body's immune system to recover. If you are feeling run down or have other symptoms of overtraining syndrome (such as increased resting heart rate, slow heart-rate recovery after training, mood changes and fatigue), you may need to tone down your workouts accordingly.

Goal setting

Time to set some goals. Refer back to p. 64 for a recap on SMART goals, and remember to focus on *your* why, no one else's. This will help you to kickstart and maintain positive changes. Remember also, making changes to help you move in a healthy and sustainable way isn't easy, especially in our modern environment, with computer-based jobs.

Find a way to stay active that feels good both physically and mentally. As I've said, the best dose of exercise is the one that gets you coming back for more.

Choose a convenient period to start, avoiding stressful times at work or busy social weeks. Share your goals with those close to you or find like-minded individuals who share similar ones. Social support creates accountability, making you more likely to stick to your goals.

- What's the one small thing you can do today/this week to improve how you move your body?
- Could you add more walks into your week?
- Keep reflecting on your immunobiography: what do you want its next chapter to look like?

Short-term goals What would you like to achieve over the next 2–4 weeks?	**Medium-term goals** What would you like to achieve over the next 2–4 months?	**Long-term goals** What would you like to achieve over the next 6–12 months?
1. 2. 3.	1. 2. 3.	1. 2. 3.
Start date:	Start date:	Start date:

What will you need to do to accomplish your goals?		
In the short term...	In the medium term...	In the long term...

Breaking down barriers

Even a switch to working from home means that any exercise you might have had during the day – whether cycling to work or walking to get lunch – may no longer exist. But while the way you work has changed, that doesn't mean you can't easily find ways to be more active during the working day. If you're committed to a physical activity programme and setting goals for yourself, it's helpful to first identify your personal barriers. By troubleshooting and developing tactics in advance, you'll have better success in overcoming them.

Some of the most common barriers are listed overleaf:

Lack of time	Monitor your activity levels for 1 week and identify at least 3 x 30-minute slots that you could use to move more. Then select activities that you can easily fit in (e.g. without requiring a trip to a gym).
Lack of accountability	Share your movement goals with friends and family, or join an online community to find people with similar goals who can offer a support network.
Lack of motivation/energy	Plan ahead and enjoy the satisfaction of checking exercise off your to-do list. Monitor for a few weeks and discover the times you feel most energised or adapt the type of movement to your energy levels on a given day.
Lack of resources	Turn everyday activities into movement opportunities: playing with your kids, housework, dancing in your kitchen . . . Or use the plethora of free classes available online, which require no special equipment.

Taking those first steps

The next step is to consider ways to intentionally break up sedentary periods. What easy or enjoyable ways can you think of to fit more opportunities to move into your daily life? It's sometimes helpful to look across four areas: home, how you travel or commute, work and play. Here are some examples:

- Set time limits on how long you sit before getting up.
- Give yourself reasons to get up and walk around frequently.

- Design your environment to help – for example, try standing instead of sitting at your desk. This has been shown to improve blood-sugar regulation and other markers of metabolic health in the long term.
- Get creative with your day: walk instead of using transport, take exercise snacks (see p. 230). The most recent evidence suggests that activity of any duration is good for health.[16]
- Ensure you factor in some movement when planning out your daily or weekly schedule, taking into account your work pattern.

The most up-to-date scientific recommendation is for those who work sitting at a desk to aim for at least two hours a day standing or moving around during work hours, building up to four hours, if possible.[17] Starting out, try adding at least thirty to sixty minutes of standing into your work day, perhaps by alternating between fifteen minutes standing followed by fifteen minutes sitting. Or perhaps try taking all your calls or meetings while standing.

CHAPTER 10:

Sleep and the Science of Rest

There's nothing like a good night's sleep to help you feel refreshed. Your body cannot keep up with the daily demands put on it when you are consistently not getting enough sleep, so it only makes sense that less sleep equals poorer health. Yet sleep is the one lifestyle lever most of us choose not to use. In fact, humans are the only species that deliberately choose not to sleep in favour of, say, watching TV, even though they are tired. Somehow, sleep falls down the priority list, or we forget to shift down through the gears in the evening, which means our brains are still in overdrive when we get into bed, falling into a less-than-restful sleep. But while we rest and recharge for the morning ahead, the immune system switches gears, embarking on a series of biological processes that restore and rejuvenate. Sleep gives our immune system a chance to recalibrate and rebuild, performing lots of housekeeping tasks – because during sleep there is less risk of us encountering an infection (as opposed to when we are out and about during the day). Plus, sleep is critical for all sorts of essential physiological processes, as well as our mental health. When we are well slept, we are more likely to engage in positive health behaviours that indirectly support our immune system.[1]

If you're consistently not sleeping enough or only getting poor quality sleep, this is something to be taken seriously, and you should always talk to your doctor if you are concerned. But with a few simple strategies, you can get the high-quality, restful sleep your immune system deserves.

HEAL YOUR SLEEP

Sleep itself is part of a twenty-four-hour process known as our circadian rhythm, or internal body clock. Think of sleep as something that begins the moment you wake up. In other words, what you do during the day will affect what happens at night.

Circadian rhythm is all synchronised by a master clock in the brain. This clock is directly influenced by environmental cues, especially morning light, which is why the cycle is tied to that of day and night. When properly aligned, a circadian rhythm can promote consistent and restorative sleep by helping to make sure that the body's processes are optimised at various points during a given twenty-four-hour period. For example, the cells of your immune system and their functions are also anchored to your circadian rhythm. Circadian oscillations coincide with different tasks needed by your immune defences at different times of the day, which is why when your sleep is off – i.e. insufficient or of poor quality – your immune system will be a bit off, too.[2]

Melatonin is one of the key hormones responsible for orchestrating our circadian rhythm. Its secretion from the pineal gland in the brain changes according to daylight time and night length and with the seasons. A wide range of factors can suppress melatonin,[3] including night-time exposure to light, ageing and even some medications. Natural morning sunlight is at the blue side of the light spectrum, signalling the body to suppress the production of sleepy melatonin and alert the body to wakefulness. We then experience a surge of the stress hormone cortisol, which turns our brains and bodies on, helping us to feel alert and ready for the day. Decent exposure to morning sunlight helps to maximise the effect of this morning cortisol release, giving the body a little kickstart to get the circadian rhythm normalised and improve evening melatonin.

Wake-up action plan

There is no hard-and-fast rule, but most of us need seven to nine hours' sleep (maybe more for those with a heavy life load). The first step to fulfilling your sleep requirement is to work out how much you need:.

- Write down your 'why'. Appreciating the value of sleep for your wellbeing is key.
- What time do you need to (or can you) consistently wake up? If you want to reprogramme your sleep pattern, this question is crucial. Your biology is on a schedule, and if you want it to work properly, then you should be, too.
- When you wake, the first thing to do is to embrace daylight. Maybe you think the lights in your bedroom are bright, or that you can just look out of the window, but it's worth going outside for morning light exposure rather than relying on the light coming in your windows. The reality is that even on a cloudy day, the intensity of light outside is substantially (two to three times) higher than it is indoors. Don't believe me? Try a lux meter app on your smartphone. Bright light through your eyes during the day is not only good for your sleep but also supports neurotransmitters and brain health.
- Keep a consistent wake time. When your get-up time is consistent, your internal clock will recognise that as the time to start producing circadian alerting signals.

- Now consider bedtime. What time will you need to go to bed to give yourself enough time to sleep before your ideal wake time?
- Like an aeroplane preparing to land, getting ready for sleep each evening takes time – use the bedtime action plan below.

Bedtime action plan

- Go to bed at the same time every day – your body thrives on routine.
- Keep the temperature in your bedroom cool; no more than 18°C, if possible.
- Keep the bedroom completely dark so that you're not disturbed by light, which your brain detects even when your eyes are closed. Eye masks can be useful.
- Take some gentle exercise every day. There is evidence that regular exercise, including stretching and aerobic exercise, improves restful sleep. Taking it outdoors can also tick the box of sunlight exposure.
- Rest and digest, leaving plenty of time between your last meal and going to bed.
- Make an effort to relax for at least an hour and a half before going to bed – try a warm bath, massage, meditation. Write down your thoughts to encourage your mind to let go of the worries and stresses that might get in the way of sleepiness.
- Follow nature's lead and soften the lights.
- Consider getting a traditional alarm clock so that your smartphone can stay out of the bedroom.

Once you have sorted your wake–sleep schedule using the guides on pp. 238–9, aim to stick to it six or seven nights a week.

TACKLING TIREDNESS

We all get tired from time to time. Late nights, long working hours or the kids keeping you up at night can all leave you feeling temporarily worn out. Then there will be periods when life has challenged you – perhaps when you have overdone things or are recovering from illness. At these times, you will need extra rest.

Fatigue differs from tiredness, which can usually be relieved by sleep and rest. Fatigue is overwhelming and accompanied by an unpleasant physical, cognitive and emotional symptom described as tiredness, but which isn't relieved by sleep and rest.[4] It's not a diagnosis in itself, but a symptom of something else – often, underlying inflammation – but it can also be associated with stress, anaemia, poor sleep, thyroid issues, underlying disease, ongoing infection, certain medications and even mental ill health. Relationship issues, financial worries and anything that is consuming a lot of mental energy, not just physical, can be involved.

When you are experiencing extreme tiredness or fatigue, it's important that you seek support from your healthcare provider and work together to identify the underlying cause (or causes). The good news is that if no medical conditions are identified, you are likely to be healthy. The not-so-good news is that, as with so many other things we've talked about, there is no one-size-fits-all approach to fatigue because the elements that cause it are likely to be multifactorial, including diet, lifestyle, environment and mental wellbeing. Your starting point is to examine all areas of your life using the results of the self-assessment we did earlier (see pp. 41–53) to start to unpick what needs to change if you genuinely want to get your energy back.

There are steps you can take in tackling fatigue, but your specific approach to getting and keeping energy levels running optimally is likely to be unique to you. As a general guide, I recommend the following:

- **Time management** An out-of-control to-do list takes its toll on your mental energy, as well as physical. Activities should be achievable and manageable, in line with how you are feeling. I like to use the four Ds for this:
  - **D**o what you need to do.
  - **D**elay what you can.
  - **D**elegate – i.e. ask for help!
  - **D**ump any unnecessary tasks.

- **Rhythms and routines** Our bodies naturally operate and thrive on rhythms. Make sure your circadian biology is in sync (see p. 237) and schedule certain activities for points in the day when you generally feel most energised.
- **Ultradian rhythms** These are like mini versions of circadian rhythms and normally take place over a cycle of 90–120 minutes. Divide up tasks into short ultradian chunks, then take a break to rest and recharge.
- **Movement** It may seem ironic, but there is some evidence for exercise being effective for fatigue in certain groups of sufferers. There's no easy answer to whether exercise will help or hurt you. The answer may, in fact, be both, depending on how you approach exercise. I would recommend you discuss with your doctor to understand if exercise might be of benefit in the context of your situation.[5] Longer sitting times are associated with more feelings of fatigue, so even if exercise isn't available to you, it's good to try and break up that sedentary time. Remember to start slowly and get moving but don't do more that you feel you can.
- **Mindset** Fatigue can become a self-fulfilling prophecy. Focusing on how badly the fatigue is affecting you may actually make it persist.
- **Address nutritional shortfalls** It should go without saying

that you need to be fuelling your body properly as part of dealing with fatigue, cutting out poor diet habits that are not serving you well, such as heavy reliance on caffeine or alcohol. Avoid undereating calories and address any micronutrient deficiencies.

YOUR SLEEP BLUEPRINT

Life today seems to move faster than ever. Every hour is consumed with so many tasks that we never really rest, except when we collapse at the end of the day and stay up watching Netflix rather than going to bed, just so we feel like we have had a bit of time to unwind. Then, even though we know we should go to sleep, we cannot seem to get mind and body into the relaxed state needed to fall into the restful sleep we require.

But as you now know, there are lots of effective solutions to the problem of poor sleep, the key being to work towards setting up strong morning and evening rituals that you can consistently sustain without feelings of frustration and defeat.

Goal setting

Time to set some goals. Refer back to p. 64 to recap on SMART goal setting. And remember to focus on *your* why, no one else's. This will help you to kickstart and maintain positive changes. Remember also, making changes isn't easy, especially against the never-ending to-do list and busyness of today's 24/7 world.

Reflect on what you have learned in this chapter. Focus on the process, not the outcome, and prioritise sustaining new behaviour changes to get you where you wish to be. Anchor your goals to automatic behaviours you have in your life and keep it positive. Choose a convenient period to start, avoiding stressful times at work or busy social weeks. Share your goals with those close to you, or find like-minded individuals who share similar ones. Remember, social support creates accountability, making you more likely to stick to your goals.

- What's the one small thing you can do today/this week to improve your sleep and get more rest?
- What strategies can you employ to work on your tiredness and fatigue?
- Can you alter your bedroom environment to make it more supportive of good sleep?
- Keep reflecting on your immunobiography: what do you want its next chapter to look like?

Short-term goals What would you like to achieve over the next 2–4 weeks?	**Medium-term goals** What would you like to achieve over the next 2–4 months?	**Long-term goals** What would you like to achieve over the next 6–12 months?
1. 2. 3.	1. 2. 3.	1. 2. 3.
Start date:	Start date:	Start date:

What will you need to do to accomplish your goals?		
In the short term...	In the medium term...	In the long term...

- Consider what has gone well: notice your wins, no matter how small. Pick out the positives and note down what you enjoyed.
- What has not gone so well? Take stock, note what you disliked most. Identify barriers to help you work towards overcoming them.

Turning obstacles into superpowers

Identify your limiting factors and use them to formulate possible next actions. This might mean adjusting a goal to make it more achievable, for example, or minimising any barriers highlighted. Then turn your biggest obstacles into superpowers with the IF → THEN approach:

- If I work late on my computer → then I'll adjust my screen and use blue-light blockers to reduce exposure to sleep-disturbing light.
- If I have trouble falling asleep → then I'll try to get out for some morning sunlight to help set my circadian rhythm.

Finding ways to make your goals more achievable involves problem solving and experimenting. And if at any stage you are really struggling, refresh your knowledge by refamiliarising yourself with the details in this chapter, always keeping in mind how much your health stands to gain – from strong immunity and mental clarity to better physical performance and reduced risk of a whole host of diseases.

CHAPTER 11:

Outside-In Immune Support – Curating a Healthy Environment

Since earliest times, humans have needed to be sensitive to their surroundings to survive. We have an innate awareness of our environments and have evolved the ability to seek out spaces that not only do no harm, but also have certain health-promoting qualities. You could say our health is the sum of our relationship with both ourselves and our environments.

We humans have been evolving for well over 4.5 million years, but it's only in the last hundred or so that we have lived with a cacophony of noises, pollution, artificial lights and household and personal-care products teeming with potential chemical, physical and psychological stressors and irritants with the capacity to set off a cascade of unwanted inflammation and aberrant immune responses. And just as our environments have changed dramatically and become more out of balance, so too have our immune systems.

I use the term 'environment' to encompass all the things we breathe, absorb, put on and in our bodies, and feel and interact with, from within our homes to the places we frequent. Our environments are very much part of our exposomes: a measure of all the exposures of an individual in a lifetime and how they relate to health to form our immunobiographies (see p. 32). Our bodies are constantly exposed to a plethora of challenges from the environment – not only infections, but all sorts of toxins, stresses and other insults, particularly from the air we breathe,

the food and drink we consume, the surfaces we touch, and the people and animals we come into contact with. To help us adapt to this ongoing environmental challenge, our immune systems have evolved a remarkable system of barriers to protect us as early as possible following exposure. To help optimise immunity, it is imperative that we nourish the immune system from the outside in. And thankfully, there is much we can do to support this.

The immune system is enriched at the barriers to the body where it is in constant contact with the environment – for example, the skin and lungs. This not only helps to protect these physical barriers, which may be vulnerable to infection, but also plays a key role in immunoregulation of the whole-body immune system, relaying signals and instructions as to what it should tolerate and what it should react to. And even though science has proven the strong link, we have been slow to catch up, leaving the role of the environment in our health neglected for too long. Whether or not we are conscious of it, however, the environment is a modifiable factor that can help us make important health-supporting changes that give us sustainable results. Even the best diet in the world isn't going to make us feel better if our environments aren't serving us well, too. So in this chapter, I want to change how you think about your environment and its impact on your health. Consider it the 'where' of your wellbeing.

GET INTO HEALTHY OUTDOOR SPACES

By the time you reach the age of eighty, you will have spent seventy-two years of your life indoors. Shocking, I know. Humans have become largely an indoor species, but much of our biology was shaped in the 4.5 million years before this happened. And because of this genetic hardwiring, we still crave being outdoors in nature. This is known as the biophilia hypothesis – the urge to affiliate with nature[1] – and a quite substantial and robust body of research clearly tells us that nature exposure is not only good for us, but essential.

As we saw on p. 201, one area in which this is strongly connected to our wellbeing is our stress response.[2] Natural environments decrease stress. Cortisol levels of people living in neighbourhoods with more green space were lower than in people in areas with little green space. In fact, as the percentage of green space in neighbourhoods increased, reported levels of stress decreased. Exposure to nature for thirty minutes over the course of a week reduced blood pressure, and ninety minutes of walking in nature, compared to a walk in an urban environment, reduced activity in brain areas involved with sadness and negative emotions. There is a trickle-down effect of having safe and accessible green space: people are likely to make use of it to move, exercise and play if it is well maintained and easy to access. Being able to walk to shops and facilities can reduce social isolation. And feeling safe in your home can help act as a buffer against the stresses and strains of the outside world.

There are some specific immunity benefits, too. Chemicals called phytoncides, released by trees and plants, improve the virus- and cancer-fighting cells of the immune system. This is why one of the best things I can prescribe for your immune system, no matter where you are at with your health, is a daily dose of nature. Nature-based health interventions (NBIs), such as 'green prescribing', can include therapeutic horticulture, biodiversity conservation pursuits or activities such as exercise in green spaces. Some researchers are looking at whether green infrastructure, such as urban parks and community allotments, could be designed and managed to generate microbiome-associated health benefits. Others are examining the possibility of 'rewilding' environmental microbiomes by restoring urban ecosystems and their microbial communities to a state that benefits human health.

Each environment has its own distinct microbiome, and our microbes are enriched by exposure to these.[3] The best environments for supporting your microbes are green and natural ones. Increasing the biodiversity of kids' playground environments, while encouraging them to play in the soil and with plants, improves microbial diversity and kids' immune systems after only twenty-eight days.[4] Sure, hygiene is important to prevent infection, but grubbing around in dirt and being in nature nurtures immunity, too.

CURATE HEALTHY INDOOR SPACES

There are many aspects about the outdoor places we frequent that we cannot change. But what about our homes and workspaces? Healthy buildings support healthy bodies (and brains) and can promote healing. As home features increasingly more in our evolving lifestyles, we have an incredible opportunity to curate our indoor spaces, too.

Less chaos

If you are an aesthete like me, creating a home with less chaos and more pleasant diversions is key to improving how you feel and, therefore, your mood, mindset, productivity and overall sense of wellbeing. Research repeatedly shows that a cluttered home is a stressful home, and it can have a knock-on effect to your immune system.

Cluttered spaces can operate like a toddler screaming for attention, distracting us and making it more difficult to process information. They can make us feel irritable, frustrated and stressed, draining and exhausting our mental focus.[5] Studies show that people who describe their homes using words such as 'messy', 'cluttered' and 'disorganised' have higher levels of cortisol – the hormone associated with stress. So if your home environment is untidy or filled with stuff in a way that seems out of control (and this doesn't just need to be physical stuff – it can also be a never-ending to-do list, an overflowing inbox or an unmanageable number of social media channels to check), this could be a strong signal that your environment is stressing you out more than you realise. Decluttering might even help you to sleep better; in fact, hoarders have been scientifically shown to have more trouble sleeping.[6]

It's often hard to find the motivation or a good reason for a proper clear-out, but it can help you feel better about your home and happier in yourself. Tidy up one room or section of a room today and see how it makes you feel.

More control

'We spend money that we do not have on things that we do not need to satisfy pacifying wants that further distract us from what we fundamentally need.' I'm not sure who first said this, but I've often heard it quoted, and perhaps in our world of massive consumerism, we all need reminding of it now and again.

We need to make a conscious effort to acquire less. Less clutter and less stress (and less debt) = better mental health and stronger immune systems that don't have to fight with immunosuppressive cortisol.[7]

Simplifying and decluttering our living spaces creates not only peace of mind, but has other benefits for health-promoting behaviours, too: less cleaning and a more organised household (stress-reducing in itself) mean extra time and energy for self-care, exercise, focusing on relationships and making space for hobbies, all of which are essential for personal wellbeing.[8] Eating (see box, below) and exercise are also influenced by the forces of environment, with studies showing that people with cleaner homes tended to be healthier and more physically active.[9]

Clutter, chaos and food

One of the most easily cluttered areas in our homes is the kitchen. But did you know that the state of your kitchen can influence your eating behaviour – and not in a good way? Studies show that people in a chaotic kitchen had more out-of-control mindsets. They also ate significantly more treats, such as cookies, than those in an organised space. So a chaotic kitchen can make us more susceptible to unhealthy food choices.[10]

Simplify your environment for better health

The queen of clean, Marie Kondo, advocates letting go of items that don't bring you joy, and while there will always be things you do need but that don't necessarily make you happy (a saucepan, for example), this can be a useful measure for getting rid of clutter.

Here are a few tips to get you started:

- **Choose quality.** Invest in a few quality stand-out pieces.
- **Find joy.** Decorate with meaningful items that give you a sense of joy.
- **Be selective with your clothing.** Apply a quality-over-quantity mindset to your wardrobe.
- **Downsize.** This doesn't necessarily mean moving into a

smaller home, but owning fewer objects is a great way to simplify your life.

- **Purge regularly.** Make time to donate bags and boxes of clutter on a regular basis.
- **Adopt a hands-off approach.** If you have an 'over-attachment' to personal items that make it difficult to part with them, have someone else help you.
- **Control the scroll.** Consider unfollowing toxic social media that's cluttering up your brain.
- **Curate your energy.** Start to observe your energy in different places you frequent. Notice where you feel depleted and where your energy feels restored. Now curate where you spend your time as much as possible.

There are so many ways to simplify your life, and the list above is certainly not exhaustive. Whether you begin with your kitchen cupboards or by taking a digital break, you'll start feeling happier and healthier by eliminating excess stuff, and stress, from your life.

Create pleasant diversions

Another tip is to create pleasant diversions inside your home.

Take noise exposure, for example. Dealing with noise pollution can be challenging and multifactorial, depending on where you live and the type of work and activities you do. Evidence shows that the stress of a noisy, confusing hospital room resulted in patients not only feeling worried, sad or helpless, but also experiencing higher blood pressure and heart rate, muscle tension, poor wound healing and delayed recovery. Consider noise-cancelling technologies if you are exposed to a particularly noisy environment for prolonged periods of time. Or add pleasant sounds. Most of us know intuitively that music's good for us, but there is also evidence for immunity benefits. Listening to music disrupts the stress chemistry of the sympathetic nervous system. Singing, listening to the sounds of nature or looking at a nature picture reduced sympathetic nervous system activity more quickly than non-natural sounds and pictures, and even increased pain threshold.

You might not have access to green spaces but keeping plants in your home environment can contribute to the benefits of biophilia (see p. 246). Just providing nursing-home residents with a plant to take care of led to a significant increase in lifespan. Over an eighteen-month follow up, those who weren't given a plant to care for (the control group) were twice as likely to die as those who were.[11] Plants have a stress-calming and anxiety-reducing effect and are known to boost mood;[12] they can also help to reduce background noise and provide a pleasant distraction, enhancing concentration and facilitating healing.[13,14,15] Finally, they are non-invasive and inexpensive; caring for them can give a sense of purpose without the bigger responsibility of, say, a pet or a child. Rest assured, I'll remain a passionate plant mama.

ADDRESS YOUR BODY BURDEN

If all the above is not convincing enough, there is an additional reason to clean up your home environment; I'm talking about toxins – an overlooked threat to our immune systems.

Immunotoxicology is the study of adverse effects on the immune system resulting from exposure to harmful agents. Broadly speaking, immunotoxicity can manifest as a reduction in immune competence, either as reduced function (immunosuppression and increased vulnerability to infection) or overzealous and inappropriate, upregulated immune responses (such as allergy and autoimmunity).[16, 17]

Can you sweat out toxins?

While I love a soothing sauna and its many immune-nourishing benefits, a regular sauna isn't the simple solution to a complex problem such as xenobiotics. A sauna itself does not directly participate in the detoxification processes mentioned later in this chapter. Sweat is primarily a reaction to cool ourselves. It is made up mostly of water and minerals, but environmental pollutants have also been found in sweat. BPA (bisphenol A, an industrial chemical), for example, has been scientifically shown to be effectively secreted through the skin in sweat. Nevertheless, to be clear, it is the liver that is the main detox organ in the body.

TALKING TOXINS

A quick look at some confusing terminology

Before we get stuck in with toxins and our environments, let's start by clearing up some confusing terminology:

- The word 'chemical' can feel alarming – but please remember, everything is a chemical.

- The word 'toxin' is a tricky one because it is misused in many contexts. The term toxin actually refers to dangerous compounds naturally found in nature, such as snake venom.
- 'Toxicants' refer to man-made chemicals that pose a threat to health. **Note:** I will use the term 'toxins' to encapsulate all environmental chemicals, both man-made and naturally occuring, that have the potential to compromise health, as it's more familiar than 'toxicants'.
- Pollutants are chemicals that are toxic in our environments and pose a risk to our health and ecosystems.
- Xenobiotic is the term used for chemical substances from natural or synthetic sources that are not naturally produced or expected to be found in animals. It can also cover substances that are present in much higher concentrations than are usual.
- 'Body burden' is the term used to describe the collective strain on our bodies from all the xenobiotics within each of us.

Don't be afraid of the terminology. And remember, chemicals have positive uses, too. It's just that we need to develop an awareness of what's in products and then make informed choices and changes accordingly.

Modern life is based around the use of thousands of potentially toxic chemicals. Even the healthiest of us are exposed to these both inside and outside of our homes each day. Might they be making us sick or contributing to poor health? How worried should we be?

Before you decide the only solution is to pack up your life and go to live on a mountain (far away from pesticide-spraying farms), don't panic. First, you can't completely eliminate toxic substances because, as I said earlier, some of them are in our environment in ways we can't control. We also need to consider the mental-health burden of developing a preoccupied concern around toxic exposure. Many things require extensive scientific examination and regulatory action from government. Sadly, regulation has not always been effective and science is not always able to keep up with the plethora of chemicals we are exposed to.

So while we can't deal with all possible toxin exposures, we can take a precautionary 'health-first' mindset that errs on the side of caution. This should not be an additional burden to our already busy lives, nor should it cause fearmongering. It's not about being perfect, but about making empowered and informed choices as consumers – what we buy, what we have in our homes and what we put into (and onto) our bodies. If each of us uses our individual power to make better choices, encouraging government and manufacturers to meet better safety standards (and care about people over profits), our combined efforts will make a big difference.

How much is too much?

People often try to defend the low levels of chemicals in consumer products, suggesting that they are so low as not to be harmful. We've all heard someone say dismissively, 'Even water can kill you if you have too much. It's the dose that makes the poison!' But is it?

Environmental factors contribute to more than 25 per cent of all global disease.[18] Toxic agents ranked fifth in underlying causes of US deaths in 2000.[19] And the number of registered chemicals has grown more than 30 per cent since 1979. Yet this is rarely talked about and the effects of exposure to toxins and the underlying biological mechanisms are not well understood.

It's true that just because you are exposed to something that is harmful doesn't mean it will necessarily harm you. And more chemicals don't always mean more disease. But there certainly is a high chance that it might. For example, if you are exposed to a cancer-causing agent, it doesn't necessarily *cause* cancer, but it does add to your body burden, increasing your chances of getting the disease.

We each have unique immunobiographies. This means not all people are equally sensitive to chemicals and potentially toxic substances. And we don't know *all* the effects of exposure to *every* chemical.

Serious effects of toxins can take years to realise, and almost none of us can test ourselves to see our own complete body burdens. Plus, there are so many new chemicals being introduced that the necessary scientific studies just can't keep up, and few look at the possible combined effects of different compounds. However, the good news is that the effects of environmental toxins – both indoor and outdoor – are, for the most part, cumulative; so a small exposure here or there is something a healthy body can deal with. This is a helpful way to think of it because we will never be able to fully avoid exposure to harmful chemicals in our environments.

TOP TOXINS – WHERE THEY ARE FOUND AND HOW TO REDUCE EXPOSURE

Toxins include much more than just the obvious toxic offenders, such as cigarette smoke and lead. In fact, the past fifty years have seen tens of thousands of new synthetic compounds introduced into the environment, and the list is ever growing.

Culprits include environmental exposure or exogenous sources – in the air we breathe, the food we eat, the water we drink and medications – and endogenous sources, such as hormones or the products of alcohol when it is metabolised within the body.

Hundreds of environmental substances have been found in the blood of humans, including flame retardants, chemicals from plastics, heavy metals, exhaust fumes, herbicides and those found in personal-care products, among others. These are pervasive in our modern environments, particularly our homes. A simple look at a person's morning routine shows the potential for being exposed to chemical compounds in deodorant, shampoo and make-up, not to mention artificial substances and heavy metals ingested through food, or chemicals inhaled through air-sanitising products or air pollutants.

Some have the potential to disrupt reproductive, developmental and neurological processes. Others are known to have carcinogenic, epigenetic or hormone-disrupting properties. Some have the capacity to directly impact the function of our immune cells and organs or cause inflammation, while others have indirect immune effects via an unwanted impact on metabolism or microbiome, or by causing elevated oxidative stress. Some appear to have a biological effect at minuscule levels, and certain chemical compounds are persistent and bioaccumulate within the human body. Individually, some chemicals might have little effect, but mixtures can heighten toxicity.

So let's look at some practical steps for non-toxic living, focusing on what we eat and what is inside our homes – because this, for the majority of us, is where our exposure comes from.

Dietary hazards

According to the World Health Organization (WHO), about 20 per cent of cancers are attributable to food toxins. Food toxins also increase the risk of dementia, autoimmune disease and allergies. Found naturally in foods, added during production or generated by cooking methods, they tend to be harmful either by causing oxidative stress, DNA damage or inflammation. These are the top toxic shockers to look for in your diet:

- **Acrylamides** are a by-product when foods with high sugar or starch content are heated at high temperatures (for example, fried-potato products, biscuits and crackers or baked products that contain sugar). The European Food Safety Authority confirms that acrylamides in food have the potential to increase the risk of cancer for people of all ages.
- **Heterocyclic amines** and **polycyclic aromatic hydrocarbons** form when meat – fish or poultry – are cooked using high-temperature methods. They are linked to oxidative stress and risk of chronic diseases.[20]
- **Nitrosamines** in processed and cured meats induce oxidative stress, inflammation and DNA damage and are linked to cancer, neurodegenerative diseases and metabolic dysfunction. The WHO has issued warnings on processed meats.
- **Plastics** used in food packaging have unclear impacts on our health but are associated with an exponential rise in plastic contamination of seas, rivers and lakes. Try to purchase fruit and vegetables that are not wrapped in plastics, opt for glass containers, look for plastic-free refilling

shops in your area and/or paper boxes composed of 100 per cent recycled paperboard.

- **Pesticides, herbicides, fungicides and bactericides** are used to prevent damage to crops. The risk is thought to be small here, but the evidence is mixed, so it's worth considering reducing your intake by washing fresh produce and choosing organic where possible.
- **Metallic compounds such as mercury** in seafood can be avoided by choosing smaller fish, such as sardines, which have lower levels.

Indoor hazards

The health of our planet is interconnected with our own. If you are one of the many millions of people living in a city, breathing more pollution than is healthy, then you may also be at greater risk of catching an infection or having poor health. The reasons are twofold. First, air pollution can cause or aggravate respiratory illnesses such as asthma or chronic obstructive pulmonary disease. And those illnesses can make you more susceptible to the worst effects of lung infections. Second, increased pollution increases susceptibility to infection, regardless of underlying health conditions. Polluted air from outside your home can get trapped indoors, adding to contaminants emitted from consumer products.

Most conversations around air pollution focus on outdoor rather than indoor air quality. But indoor air pollution is often eight times higher than that outdoors, even in cities (and this is the air you are breathing 90 per cent of the time). Why? Well, it's the cumulative result of many things, including keeping your windows closed, cooking, heating your home, the volume of consumer products used (cleaning, laundry, air fresheners and personal-care), cigarette smoke and certain building materials, such as flame retardants. The people most exposed to indoor pollutants tend to be those most vulnerable to their effects: the young, the elderly or those with compromised health who may already be struggling with other areas of supporting their health.

Given that we all spend a fair amount of time indoors these days, it's critical to be aware of the top indoor hazards:

- **Volatile organic compounds (VOCs)** are compounds emitted from a large range of sources, including furniture, carpets, building materials and personal-care products, and are present in just about all indoor air. Although more rigorous research is needed, a decline in lung function has been observed in people who are regularly exposed to products high in VOCs.[21]
- **Persistent organic pollutants (POPs)** are also known as 'forever chemicals' and are organic compounds that break down slowly and can get into our food chain. One of the most common is a perfluorinated chemical (PFC) called perfluorooctane sulfonate (PFOS), which in 2009 was added to the list of chemicals banned under an international environmental treaty called the Stockholm Convention on Persistent Organic Pollutants.[22]
- **Phthalates** are in everything from household cleaners to food packaging, fragrances, cosmetics and other personal-care products, as well as dust! Phthalates have been shown to increase the production of inflammatory proteins that can weaken our immune response to pathogens and cause immune dysregulation. In addition, phthalates may reduce gut bacteria diversity, thus negatively affecting the immune system.[23, 24, 25, 26]

My top tips to reduce exposure:

- **Let buildings breathe.** The simple act of opening a window, even for just five minutes a day, can reduce indoor pollution. Portable air purifiers can also be effective – just make sure they are the right size for the room and look for ones with carbon-based filters for VOCs.
- **Tackle dust and make your home a shoe-free zone.** People ingest approximately 45mg of dust each day. As well as potentially being a respiratory allergen, dust is a vector for several chemical hazards, such as phthalates. Make sure to do periodic wet cleaning of any surface where dust might settle, take your shoes off at the door as you enter your home and vacuum regularly.
- **Upcycle and repurpose furniture.** There's been a surge of interest in upcycling, but there is often also a health benefit that comes with used furniture. Off-gassing of VOCs from new furniture is often most prominent in the first few years of the product's life. This risk will be reduced in second-hand furniture – and it's good for the environment and more cost-efficient, too.
- **Create a love list and lose list.** Consider the wide range of household products used every day in your home. Then divide into those that you cannot live without, and ditch the others or swap out for less toxic versions. An added bonus is that fewer products equal less clutter, too.
- **Read product labels and trust your senses.** Read the labels on all the consumer products you use. Do your own research and trust your intuition. Even the best technology cannot match our own sensing ability.
- **Ditch the fragrance.** Generally, fragrances can be a source

of 200 or more different ingredients, many of which have not been fully explored. Choose products with low or no VOCs, which are also more environmentally friendly. For candles, for example, go for 100 per cent soy, beeswax or coconut wax with 100 per cent cotton wicks and scented with pure essential oils.

- **Clean up your cleaning supplies.** There are several eco-friendly, natural, 'green' cleaning brands on the market, which are clearly labelled and contain far lower levels of VOCs. Their packaging also tends to be biodegradable, which is a major plus in our plastic-saturated environment. Alternatively, you can make your own, using the many recipes available online.
- **Be precautious with plastics.** There are many chemicals in plastics, and it's not easy figuring out which are safe. Being precautious with plastics is not only beneficial for reducing exposure to potential xenobiotics, but also for the health of our planet. And we should all reduce single-use plastics where possible. Choose glass, stainless steel or ceramic containers to store food. I like to save glass food jars to store leftovers in the fridge.
- **Look out for damp.** This allows fungus and mould to grow, which can cause a wide range of conditions, from mild irritation of your airways to more serious infections if you have a lung condition, particularly in the UK where the weather can be damp.

HOUSE PLANTS AND AIR QUALITY

I love house plants and they're probably the one thing I'm happy to have too many of. Not only are they a cost-effective way to brighten up your environment, but they can also do wonders for your wellbeing (see p. 252). The internet is awash with claims that cohabiting with house plants will purify the air in your home. Nice idea, and as a house-plant aficionado I am keen to believe this. There is an oft-quoted NASA study[27] nearly as old as me that demonstrated that placing plants in a sealed chamber resulted in a significant improvement in air quality and reduced the presence of VOCs over a twenty-four-hour period. This has led to drastically overstated claims about the benefits of house plants on air quality – because it turns out you'd need an awful lot of plants to beat just opening the window.[28] But before you berate your home jungle for not doing its job, many subsequent controlled plant studies have shown improvements in VOCs over a very, very long time. In the meantime, however, remember to open your windows too!

Demystifying detox

While our priority should be to do our best to avoid toxins in the first place, we can also support our bodies' ability to remove them. Detox is a small word that has a lot of different meanings, and it triggers a variety of responses from people, depending on who you talk to – and possibly what they are selling.

Truth be told, detox is a natural biochemical process occurring in your body every single day without you even thinking about it. But there is some controversy over whether the body needs help flushing out unwanted matter, collectively known as xenobiotics (see box, p. 253), and which may be grouped as carcinogens, drugs, environmental pollutants, food additives, hydrocarbons and pesticides.

Let's look first at what the detox process entails when you encounter xenobiotics. There are several phases of detoxification metabolism taking place primarily in your liver cells, acting in concert to detoxify xenobiotics and remove them from cells. Although every biological tissue in the body has some ability to perform detoxification, the barrier cells of your gut, lungs and skin are all responsible for a localised level of this process.

Detoxification happens via three primary phases.

Phase I

This is all about transforming harmful substances into less harmful metabolites via enzymes, primarily those of the cytochrome p450 family (CYPs). Most pharmaceutical drugs, as well as our hormones and alcohol, are metabolised by phase I . This phase leads either to direct removal from the body via the stool or urine, or further detoxing is required via phase II.

Phase II

This is all about a process called 'conjugation', which takes the products from phase I out of your body via bile, urine and stool. There are various ways in which this occurs, all with fancy scientific names, such as glucuronidation and esterification. Phase II is considered the major pathway by which damaging environmental chemicals are removed from the body.

Phase III

This phase is all about transportation of phase-II conjugates, either to your kidneys for further filtration, then out of your body in your urine, or via the bile in your small intestine for elimination in your stool.

These stepwise processes of detoxification are largely influenced by genetics and environmental factors, including – but not limited to – diet. Other factors, such as advancing age, our microbiomes and lymphatic circulation, can impair these processes. The balance between phase-I and phase-II activity can be disrupted by certain toxic compounds, genetics and other lifestyle practices. This imbalance can then impair the removal of these compounds, leaving them free to wreak more damage.

How to support effective detox

Although our bodies are equipped with a system to eliminate the daily toxins we produce and are exposed to, we are becoming more and more overloaded, risking a significant body burden.

When it comes to what foods to eat to help our bodies alleviate any toxic burden, research is still is in its infancy, with most of the studies looking at the effect of foods and nutrients on detox being performed in animal models, while solid data in humans is still lacking. Some foods increase particular enzymes while decreasing others, so it's not as simple as recommending a specific food for detox. One key example is the furanocoumarins present in grapefruit juice, which inhibit specific CYP enzymes. The result is that the bioavailability of certain drugs is increased if taken after drinking grapefruit juice because they hang around the body longer. Therefore, some medications come with a grapefruit-juice warning.

It's complex: many foods, depending on their concentration or composition, appear to act as both inducers and inhibitors of the detox enzymes, but there are a few broad principles you can apply:

- **Phase-I detox** can generate oxidative stress. So it's crucial to eat a diet high in antioxidants like the polyphenols and flavonoids you met on p. 111.
- **Phase II** depends on B vitamins and the amino acid glycine (a building block of protein found in protein-rich foods

such as meat, dairy and legumes). Nuclear factor erythroid 2- related factor 2 (NRF2), the major genetic regulator of phase-II enzymes, is supported by the isothiocyanates and glucosinolates found in cruciferous vegetables and sulphur compounds in alliums such as garlic and onions. Curcumin in turmeric and flavonoids such as quercetin, ellagic acid and resveratrol also support phase II.

- **Phase III** requires adequate hydration for effective urine production and enough dietary fibre to support a proper functioning digestive system, so you can poo efficiently and frequently. Brown rice fibre is beneficial in eliminating toxins. And curcumin in turmeric shows promise in promoting excretion of toxins through bile flow.

YOUR ENVIRONMENT BLUEPRINT

My hope is that having read this chapter, you will no longer overlook your environment as a determinant of your health. Now it's time to start applying what you have learned through small changes to curate a healing home and turn your environment into a pillar of your overall wellness.

Write down your 'why'

What are your top personal reasons for improving your home environment? It might be that after reading this chapter you realise how important your environment is to your health, or because you now spend a lot of time working at home and want to improve your surroundings.

What matters is that you are able to articulate your own

reasons, which may not be directly health-related (although that would be a worthwhile bonus), because you are more likely to be able to change if you can align the 'pros' for doing so with real, specific and meaningful personal outcomes.

Goal setting

Start by reassessing your answers to the environmental questionnaire on p. 52. Now you have the knowledge and tools, take a moment to reflect on the key foundations of a healthy environment, and try to make this a weekly check-in.

Refer back to p. 64 to recap on SMART goals. And remember, focus not on the outcome you might have in mind, but the process, prioritising sustaining new behaviour changes to get you there. Progress is much more important than perfection, and it's important to prepare for setbacks, too – there is more than one path to any destination. To make your goals achievable and your actions sustainable, use problem solving and experimenting; the key is to work towards habits and rituals that you can use consistently for life without feelings of frustration and defeat.

- Adjust goals to make more achievable.
- Work on minimising any barriers identified.

Examples:

- What's one small thing you can do this week to simplify an area of your home?
- How can you engineer your week to make sure you spend more time in nature/green space?
- Can you audit your cleaning products?

Short-term goals What would you like to achieve over the next 2–4 weeks?	**Medium-term goals** What would you like to achieve over the next 2–4 months?	**Long-term goals** What would you like to achieve over the next 6–12 months?
1. 2. 3.	1. 2. 3.	1. 2. 3.
Start date:	Start date:	Start date:

What will you need to do to accomplish your goals?		
In the short term...	In the medium term...	In the long term...

- What has gone well? Notice your wins, no matter how small. Pick out the positives and note down what you enjoyed.
- What has not gone so well? Take stock, note what you disliked most. Identify barriers to help you work towards overcoming them.
- What can you do to make your goals more achievable? This involves problem solving and experimenting. Remember the key is to work towards small, sustainable changes without feelings of frustration and defeat.

PART 3

Supporting Specific Conditions

From mild infections to chronic disease, sometimes illness is unavoidable. As an immunologist, I often remind people that there are many aspects of the immune system that we cannot control, and because we are all immunologically unique, we will be susceptible to infection or developing illness in slightly different ways. Therefore, each of us needs to find our own individualised way to recover or manage illness when it strikes. In this final section, I'll share the knowledge and tools to help you do this.

Acceptance of a chronic long-term condition and a seemingly 'lesser' life can be a bitter pill to swallow. Let's face it, most of us struggle with self-acceptance even without chronic illness. We've already looked at the physical and mental benefits of self-compassion; well, self-acceptance and self-advocacy are also important, particularly when battling a health condition. When we accept illness, we can see it as an opportunity to acknowledge our situation and explore ways to help ourselves. Self-acceptance can help us to better communicate our needs, while self-advocacy can help on the journey to diagnosis – putting a stable support network in place and finding some time each day when we put ourselves first to work on recovery. This, in turn, strengthens our internal health-promoting forces and has a positive effect on objectively measured 'health'. Instead of letting a condition define us, we make it our goal to strive for living life to the fullest despite it.

You may receive a diagnosis that means a lifetime of prescription drugs, or you might want to go the natural route and shun conventional medicine. The two are often pitted against each other but are not mutually exclusive. Nutrition, lifestyle interventions and complementary health practices can influence your health, and many illnesses can be prevented, treated or even cured by them; but remember – others cannot. And it is critical to understand that, in many cases, these practices cannot *and should not* replace pharmaceutical drugs. Medicine was developed to save lives and treat disease. While it may be overprescribed or used as an easy fix for some problems, it's often invaluable.

This doesn't mean there isn't value in engaging in lifestyle changes, because these work with your immune system, not against it. There is a lot that you can do, because even if you are taking prescription drugs, better living through chemistry is always helped by better living. The use of medications is almost always going to be helped by building a strong core of general wellness. Laying the foundations to your wellbeing using the information in the previous section is more important than ever. We all know it isn't always easy to do the things that are needed to promote good health, but it's harder still when battling with poor health. Being unwell presents many more barriers to 'doing the right thing' for our health. And understanding those barriers is the first step in overcoming them.

It is important to be both cautious and realistic. In my view, if food really is medicine, then it can only be medicinal in the context of love, social connection, physical movement, good-quality sleep and everything you have learned about in the preceding pages. As you move through the forthcoming chapters, remember, there is no one-size-fits-all cure or protocol that I can offer - just suggestions grounded in scientific evidence. What benefits one person may not necessarily help another. You know yourself and your particular health challenge better than anyone.

CHAPTER 12:

The Battle Against Infection

Infections are caused by microscopic organisms known as pathogens – bacteria, viruses, fungi or parasites – that enter the body, multiply and interfere with normal function. They are still a leading cause of illness and death around the world.

We've all been there. A day of feeling inexplicably run down. A few days with a sniffle or perhaps a sharp pain in the back of the throat. Perhaps it's achiness in every joint of the body and, before you know it, you are down and out with the flu, struggling to sleep, exhausted and unable to accomplish a single thing. And chances are you'll get sick at the most inconvenient time.

Mostly, the immune system is preventing infection without us even knowing it. And living somewhere like the UK, where routine vaccinations and public health measures have dramatically reduced the risk of infectious disease, means that the threat we face from serious and deadly viruses, bacteria and parasites can perhaps seem remote. COVID-19 reminds us, however, that novel infectious microbes can strike when we least expect it.

As the scope of infection is broad, I will focus here on everyday minor infections. These illnesses may be common, but they comprise a significant majority of the acute illnesses that burden Western society, not only leaving us feeling unwell, but also carrying with them a high economic cost.

THE UNCOMFORTABLE TRUTH ABOUT INFECTIONS

The previous chapters have been concerned mostly with the health of our immune systems in the long term. But germs present a more immediate concern. Because there is a genetic component to how individual immune cells detect and recognise germs, there is quite a lot of variability in how people respond to infections. Some are prone to respiratory viruses, whereas others are more susceptible to gastrointestinal bacterial infections, for example. This is an uncomfortable truth about the immune system and has become an immunological talking point of the COVID pandemic: why do some people get minor symptoms, whereas for others, sadly, it's a trip to the ICU?

An underlying reason for this (in fact, one of several) is that germs consist of lots of different proteins. You might have heard about the coronavirus 'spike' protein, mentioned in reference to COVID-19. In a process akin to 'immunological roulette', different proteins are shown to our immune cells (see p. 16 on HLA molecules) and those that have a receptor that locks onto them are allowed to build themselves into an army producing highly specific antibodies and T-cell responses. This is normal and leads to what we call a polyclonal immune response. But the annoying thing is that only responses to a small number of proteins are helpful in clearing the infection. If your immune system targets the 'wrong' proteins, you might have a strong immune response but one that is of no help in protecting you from the invading germ. This has been seen in COVID-19: people developing a strong immune response but to the 'wrong' parts of the virus, so they struggle to eliminate the infection. This is independent of age and other factors, such as diet, lifestyle or co-morbidities (the presence of one or more additional conditions; these may add an extra barrier to an effective immune response).

We might not be able to avoid germs completely, and part of how our immune systems respond to them is beyond our control, but we can work on the things that *are* within our control, as outlined in the previous section of this book.

Immunodeficiency

Remember, germs are all around us, and it is perfectly normal to get the occasional infection; for adults, this can be up to six illness episodes per year. For certain people, however – particularly those with underlying illnesses, such as heart disease or cancer, or those who are taking medication that weakens the immune system – it's more difficult to avoid becoming ill with an infection.

Immunodeficiency disorders result in a full or partial impairment of the immune system, leaving you open to infection. Primary immunodeficiencies are the result of genetic defects, and secondary immunodeficiencies are secondary to other factors, such as HIV/AIDS, ageing or malnutrition. To discover if you have an immunodeficiency, testing will have to be done by your healthcare professional and should always be carried out within the context of a complete clinical history.

When you do get sick, a variety of approaches can be adopted for supporting your immune system and recovery during the short term. Whether it's a cough, cold or even COVID-19, my framework will set out what to do and how to get on the road to recovery.

Recommendations are based on the three phases of infection, because what is needed in one phase might not be appropriate for another. Each phase therefore requires its own focus.[1]

HEALING PHASE 1: AN OUNCE OF PREVENTION

Although no single method completely eliminates the risk of contracting an infection, there are several effective behaviours and nutritional and lifestyle factors that can limit your risk. Importantly, how you enter any infection can dictate how equipped your immune system is at handling it.

The germs that cause disease – pathogens – can be viruses, bacteria, fungi, protozoa or parasites. But before we talk about supporting your pathogen immune defences, your first line of defence is avoidance of germs in the first place. And understanding how infections are transmitted can help you to do this, limiting your chances of getting sick.

Pathogens enter through openings in the body – the respiratory, gastrointestinal and urogenital tracts – or breach the skin barrier. They can be transmitted through insect bites, touch, food and drink, fomites (non-living surfaces, such as metal, plastic or paper) or body fluids. To make us ill, pathogens have to reach their target site in the body and attach, multiply and avoid or survive attack by the immune system. Throughout human evolution, pathogens have been honing their skills to enter us and successfully evade our immune defences. Likewise, we are equipped with a breadth of different immune strategies to combat all sorts of pathogens.

Infection protection

COVID-19 has given us a timely reminder of the fundamentals of how not to spread your germs: situations involving people and shared space increase exposure. A lot of socio-cultural practices engaged in when people are together, and that we never really thought about pre-COVID-19 – shaking hands, embracing, kissing, hugging – play a part in the exchange of microbes.

Basic hygiene habits, such as handwashing and tissue etiquette, and the environments and spaces we frequent matter a lot when it comes to how likely we are to pick up an infection. This is why, unsurprisingly, we get sick after attending large events or travelling extensively on public transport. Or perhaps it's when the kids go back to school after the holidays, bringing home the germs transferred from close interaction with so many other children. Public health is everyone's responsibility, and our decisions are key to how infection spreads. And let's not forget our pre-COVID culture of presenteeism: people going in to work and continuing as normal while obviously contaminated with a lurgy. Not only are these people not fully functioning, they are also spreading pathogens to anyone they interact with throughout the day. Presenteeism is actually the costlier cousin of absenteeism. So if you're sick, and you know that you really need to rest, stay at home and do exactly that.

Risk factors for infection

Numerous factors (some of which are beyond our control) can leave you more susceptible to infection, including immunological age, gender, HLA (see p. 16) and other genes, levels of exposure to a pathogen and overall health status.

A co-morbidity may put you more at risk for a severe form of an infection or a longer duration to recover. Common co-morbidities that increase susceptibility to infection include metabolic diseases (type-2 diabetes, high blood pressure or heart disease), conditions with a raised baseline inflammation (this may be present even without a co-morbid diagnosis) or low micronutrient status (see p. 104 for key micronutrients in the immune system). Stress, overnutrition and inactivity could also be considered predisposing factors to infection.[2] Over the last few decades, numerous public-awareness campaigns have tried to get us to pay attention to the risks posed by chronic preventable conditions, such as diabetes, obesity, cardiovascular disease and hypertension. COVID-19 has put them all to shame, as we finally see clearly just how significant these co-morbidities are to our health.

Nutritional prevention of infections

Public-health practices, such as vaccinations and hygiene measures, mitigate risk very effectively but are not sufficient to support the immune system directly. A nutritionally poor diet pattern can lead to compromised immune reserves. Ensuring you are maintaining a healthy body composition with a calorie-appropriate diet and regular physical movement is also important. Prioritising protein and healthy omega-3 fats EPA and DHA can support our anti-microbial defences by providing the raw materials for infection fighting.[3] It is super-important to avoid deficiencies in any of the essential vitamins and minerals to ensure the best immune protection from infection. Even mild deficiencies in key essential micronutrients could jeopardise defences and increase the risk of infections.[4] When it comes to frequency of respiratory infections, such as colds and flu, vitamin D and A take centre stage.[5] Approximately one in five people has low vitamin D levels (defined as serum levels below 25 nmol/L). This is not so low as to cause rickets – a disease of overt vitamin D deficiency, visibly affecting the bones – but enough to reduce the effectiveness of the immune defences. Making sure you keep up with your vitamin D supplementation all year round is important, particularly if you are considered at higher risk of deficiency.

HEALING PHASE 2: INFECTION FIGHTING

There is no one-size-fits-all solution when you are sick, but your immune system does require two key things: proper resourcing and time.

Proper resourcing means consistently bringing together the different aspects of wellbeing outlined in Part 2 to collectively provide the foundations for a strong immune system. Then, when germs do manage to invade, your well-maintained immune system is normally pretty good at battling pathogens, alleviating symptoms and restoring you back to full health in a timely manner.

The second thing your immune system needs is time to do its job. The adaptive immune system, comprised of T cells and antibody-producing B cells, is slow and specific. It's estimated that human B cells generate about 10 billion different antibodies and approximately 100,000 different T cells in our bodies, each capable of binding to a different thing (antigen). Considering we have only 20,000 genes, the immune system has evolved a unique genetic process to provide us with this huge pool. When we become infected, the immune system searches in the

10-billion-strong pool of antibodies and 100,000 T cells to select those capable of binding to that specific virus. When a match is found, the B cell responsible for producing that antibody starts a factory to produce more. They also further refine the antibody so that it binds the germ even more effectively. Specific T cells that bind the germ are selected and expanded; they also develop specialised functions to deal with the nature of the threat. We also squirrel away a store of long-lived memory T and B cells that jump into action if the virus comes back.

Building armies of highly specific and specialised T cells and antibody-producing B cells can take several days or weeks; it even needs a few days to reactivate pre-existing immunity you might already have. This is also why symptoms start several days or even weeks after you have been infected (a side effect of the immune system doing its job, not the infection itself). If, however, you are worried that you are not getting better as quickly as you would expect, or you develop new or worsening symptoms as the infection progresses, it's always worth discussing with your doctor.

Fever is your friend

While your T and B cells from your adaptive immune system are busying themselves, your first line of defence is also working hard to kill the germs with inflammation. If you remember, one of the cardinal signs of inflammation is fever (see p. 21), also called pyrexia. Almost every animal on the plant can develop a fever. When we are healthy, our body temperature tends to gravitate around a constant 37°C (although there are fluctuations across a twenty-four-hour period). When we are fighting an infection, our temperature can rise up a degree or so (a mild fever) to about 39.5°C (high fever).

Fever is another example of why the immune system needs

a chance to do its work. It results from molecules produced by the immune system (known as pyrogens) triggering parts of the brain to adjust body temperature. This interferes with the ability of some germs to grow, but mainly it helps the immune system to do its job better by:

- increasing antibody production
- enhancing mobility of bacteria-killing immune cells
- reducing iron availability in the blood, sequestering it from germs (known as nutritional immunity)
- enhancing T-cell activity.

Although unpleasant, fever is a symptom of the immune system doing its job, not an illness in itself. It can feel distressing and taxing on your body as your resting metabolism increases by 13 per cent with each 1°C increase in body temperature. Uncomplicated, a physiological fever is harmless, beneficial and an important part of your immune response. (Note: environmental fevers, arising, for example, from heat stroke or exercise on a hot day, can be problematic due to the rapid rise in temperature.) It's helping you to get better quicker,[6] and this makes the question of when to treat a fever difficult.

In general, it is ok and safe to let a low-grade fever run its course, as it is likely to be short-lived. Often, the default is to use antipyretics (paracetamol, for example) to reduce fever, but recent evidence has called this into question, and it is now thought that antipyretics should be reserved for when the fever becomes too distressing, rather than with the sole aim of bringing it down. Studies even show that taking antipyretics before or at the time of receiving a vaccine may mildly decrease antibody production (but it stays within protective range). Remember, no matter how healthy and resilient we are, sometimes being sick is tough and it's always metabolically demanding, so occasionally, pharmaceutical interventions have their place.[7]

Set your self-care priorities: sleep, hydration and nutrition

Most minor infections resolve themselves or need just a little advice from a doctor or pharmacist. If you do find yourself sick, it can be hard to do anything other than not feel well. But you can also take measures to help yourself feel better with the basics of self-care. Nourishing and nurturing your body back to optimal health following illness involves allowing the time and energy for this to happen. If you're dealing with a cold, flu or worse, and you're not slowing down and acknowledging the symptoms, there is little that will help you to recover faster. Plus, there is plenty of evidence that having a cold impairs mood, alertness and working memory and that brain performance falls off, so there is no point trying to push on.[8] Being sick with an infection is a temporary state, but one in which it is more important than ever to invest in your wellbeing.

Sleep, rest, sleep, rest . . . repeat

Lack of sleep can, of course, leave you more vulnerable to infection in the first place, but fighting one, more often than not, requires more sleep. Infection-fighting immune cytokine interleukin 1b acts on neurons in the brain, signalling to increase sleep and inhibiting wake-promoting neurochemical pathways. Altered sleep during infection is a component of the acute inflammatory response and sickness behaviours designed to promote recovery by freeing up energy to support the metabolic demands of fever and the immune system.[9] As well as allowing the immune system to produce more infection-fighting cytokines, sleep also generates low levels of $G\alpha_s$-coupled receptor agonists, which favour the formation of immunological synapses needed to enhance T-cell responses.[10]

So sleep is more important than ever when fighting an infection. But it can be hard to achieve the quality of sleep you desire because infection is a known sleep disruptor. In fact, changes to your sleep pattern might be an early indicator of infection. The changes in sleep architecture that occur during infection include increasing the amount of time spent in deep sleep, which is helpful because it reduces the energy expenditure associated with competing activities, such as moving, and has additional: shivering is crucial to the generation of fever but does not occur during REM sleep.[11]

Key message? Rest really is the best medicine. Try to listen to your body: maximise night-time sleep and nap when you can until you are feeling fully recharged.

Hydrate and humidify

Good hydration keeps your mucus membranes soft and moist, helping the barrier to resist infection. It's also important for the flow of blood and lymph around the body, keeping tissues well oxygenated and allowing immune cells to perform their surveillance function.[12, 13] It's no surprise, then, that good hydration is associated with reduced infection, and not getting enough fluids might hinder your ability to recover.

To my knowledge, there are no clinical trials on how much hydration is right for recovery. Practise moderation: focus on maintaining your normal fluid intake and replacing any additional fluid loss (from sweating, vomiting or diarrhoea), but don't go overboard and drink multiple litres. Hot teas and soups should be your go-to, as they are also comforting and can ease nasal congestion, keep your respiratory system hydrated and thin out any mucus causing congestion.

Nutrition

Nutrition and infection interact with each other in a synergistic vicious cycle. Infectious episodes can result in hypermetabolism of nutrients and, in some cases, muscle breakdown can occur – the extent of which will depend on the type of infection and its duration. As we saw on p. 101, muscle is so important for the immune system that we don't want to lose it. Eating well before, during and after infection is, without doubt, the best course of action, but sometimes your immune system needs a little extra nutritional support when you are sick. But if you do get struck down with an infection, you may notice your appetite changes – one of many sickness behaviours. This could make it harder to consume the foods needed to shore up your immune system.

There are several nutrients, plant-based botanicals and supplements that can support these additional demands, counterbalance inflammation and oxidative stress, provide symptom relief and – possibly – shorten the duration of illness.

- **Protein** Providing the building blocks for infection-fighting immune cells and antibodies,[14] protein will also prevent muscle loss during times of prolonged infection or recovery. Aim for 1.5g/kg/day,[15] and focus on sources high in the amino acids glutamine and arginine, both of which are considered non-essential amino acids but become conditionally essential during an immune response. This is because they are used at a higher rate by the immune system during illness, helping to inhibit inflammatory responses in people recovering from surgery and serious illness.[16, 17] White meat is a rich source of both of these amino acids, which is one reason why chicken soup is considered an antidote to colds and flu. But they can also be found in nuts, beans and legumes.

- **Vitamin C and citrus bioflavonoids** When you are fighting an infection, your immune system uses much more vitamin C. Increasing consumption of vitamin-C-rich foods, such as citrus fruits and berries, or supplementing with up to 1g a day, can reduce the duration and severity of symptoms (although high doses can upset the digestive tract).[18] Be sure to maximise the benefits of vitamin C with citrus bioflavonoids, such as hesperetin, naringin, tangeretin and quercetin.[19] These compounds, often found in the pulp and the white core of fruits high in vitamin C, act synergistically with the vitamin to neutralise free radicals and support the immune response.[20]
- **Zinc and zinc-ionophores** Often regarded as the gatekeeper of infection protection, zinc is found in many foods, but is particularly high in meat, poultry, shellfish, nuts and seeds.[21] Supplements are unlikely to reduce your chances of getting a cold unless you are at risk of deficiency. But taking supplemental small doses of zinc repeatedly over the day (total daily dose of 10–40mg) can substantially reduce the duration of common colds.[22] (High doses cause unpleasant side effects, including nausea, diarrhoea and vomiting; ingestion of more than 1g in a single dose, or long-term supplementation with more than 100mg daily, can cause copper and iron deficiency.) Take the flavonoid quercetin when you supplement with zinc. It helps zinc to get inside your cells through its role as an 'ionophore', plus it has its own antiviral properties, too.
- **Selenium** Deficiency in selenium allows invading pathogens to mutate and infect for longer.[23] Brazil nuts, seafood and organ meats are the richest sources of selenium. The levels in plant-based sources will depend on the soil that the produce is grown in. Selenium is available as a supplement

and may be useful for those with insufficient dietary intakes, including the elderly and those with co-morbidities and high risk from infection. The selenomethionine form is the most bioavailable.

- **Polyphenol phytotherapy** The deep red and purple polyphenols found in berries are packed with antioxidants and anti-inflammatory compounds, but also show antiviral properties. This is one reason why elderberry supplements are popular for treating colds and flu, but it is not clear that these beneficial compounds survive processing. Opting for dark and colourful berries in your diet is probably just as effective.[24]

Never judge your mucus by its colour

A common misconception is that coughing up yellow/green mucus indicates bacterial involvement in the lungs and warrants antibiotics. Recent evidence, however, suggests that mucus colour does not indicate bacterial involvement and patients do not benefit from antibiotics. (Remember, antibiotics do not kill viral infections.) There may be points where antibiotics need to be considered (for example, where symptoms persist for more than ten days, a high fever isn't improving, or there is a thick, continuously white pus-like discharge), but each case will be different, so talk to your doctor if you are concerned.

NUTRITIONAL ANTIMICROBIALS

Too many visits to the doctor end with a prescription for antibiotics. There are perfectly valid, and often life-saving reasons for antibiotics, but they tend to knock out both good and bad bacteria, leaving a vacancy for harmful bacteria to move in, which can increase infection risk in the long term. Studies have shown that at least 20 per cent of antibiotics prescribed in primary care in England are inappropriate,[25] while nearly half of children with common colds are treated with them.[26] This not only damages our microbiomes, but adds to the growing issue of antimicrobial resistance. Stick to using antibiotics only when necessary – that is, to treat serious, confirmed bacterial infections and certain life-threatening diseases, and use them correctly, as recommended by your practitioner.

When you're dealing with minor infections, I recommend using Mother Nature's antibiotics, which can work just as effectively to reduce the harmful bacteria in your body, while also reducing inflammation and increasing the presence of good, protective bacteria:

- **Oregano oil** Contains carvacrol and thymol, two powerful antibacterial compounds.[27] Use only therapeutic grade oil or supplements, taking one to two drops daily and not for more than fourteen days.[28]
- **Honey** Showing antiviral actions in test tubes and with a lack of side effects, honey is deemed a better alternative to over-the-counter medicines for helping with sore throats and coughs.[29] A small serving of 2.5ml daily will suffice for the duration of the illness; combine with lemon and ginger for a soothing elixir. Manuka honey is an extremely rich source of antimicrobials, with growing scientific evidence

of its effectiveness on the skin for healing wounds.[30] Honey should not be given to children under one year of age.

- **Garlic** Containing chemical compounds, such as allicin, which have proven antimicrobial activity, garlic shows promise in human studies for the treatment and prevention of upper-respiratory viruses.[31] One study showed a single clove of raw crushed garlic activates multiple genes related to immune function.[32] If you don't fancy munching raw garlic (who does?), it's estimated that we need three times as much cooked garlic because some of the magic phytonutrients in garlic reduce with cooking.[33]

  Try the hack-and-hold method to optimise the immune-nourishing benefits of garlic:

  - Chop or crush the garlic.
  - Leave to sit for a few minutes to let the chemical reaction that generates allicin to take place.

  Add an extra clove the next time you are cooking with garlic. And grate a raw clove or two into dips, such as hummus and salsa, or salad dressings.

- **Turmeric and the curcuminoids** The curcuminoids in turmeric have antiviral and antibacterial activity.[34] It's also delicious and gives food a vibrant colour. Ideally, pair turmeric with a dash of black pepper, which can boost its absorption in the body by up to 2000 per cent.[35] Turmeric supplements can also help supply a more concentrated dosage of curcumin and can be taken in doses of 500mg twice daily to reduce pain and inflammation.[36]
- **N-Acetylcysteine** NAC is required for the production of

glutathione, our bodies' most powerful antioxidant. NAC also interferes with viral replication in the body and helps to thin mucous secretions, so the body can more easily clear them; 600mg NAC twice daily is effective in reducing respiratory viral symptoms.[37]

- **Quorum sensor inhibitors** 'Quorum sensing' refers to how germs 'talk' to each other using chemical messengers as they try to reach a critical threshold and spread their infection to other hosts.[38] Warming winter spices (ginger, cardamon, eucalyptus and clove) interfere with this process, alleviating pains and symptom-inducing inflammation, and are comforting ingredients to include when unwell.[39, 40]
- **Combining synergistic forces: β-glucans, lactoperoxidase and lactoferrin** Mushrooms and yeasts offer a plethora of antimicrobial properties, including immune-enhancing β-glucans. Try supplementing with β-glucans during periods of extra stress, infection risk or at the first sign of a cold or other minor infection. Your β-glucan-enhanced immune cells use various antimicrobial tools to do their job, including the immune enzyme lactoperoxidase (LPO) and lactoferrin. Regular supplementation with lactoferrin (between 600mg and 2g per day) has been shown to prevent incidence of colds and cold-related symptoms.[41, 42] LPO is a ferro-protein, which means it requires iron to function. It also requires cyanogens, which are phytonutrients found in brassica vegetables, such as broccoli, cabbage and Brussels sprouts.
- **Anti-adhesins** Fucoidans and funorans, which occur in edible seaweeds, have 'non-stick' properties that prevent disease-causing pathogens from adhering to our cells. They are particularly useful for infections of the oral cavity, protecting against gum disease. The sugar D-mannose has

shown encouraging results in displacing pathogens, such as *e. coli* from the urinary tract.[43, 44]

Probiotics for infection immunity

Whether you're fit and healthy (and aiming to stay that way) or already experiencing symptoms of infection and need some TLC, probiotics can be a great addition to your daily health regime.

There is a lot of interest in how probiotics can regulate immune defences against infections. They work in strain-specific ways, so it's important to pick the right strains that have been shown to be effective for your particular needs. Just remember that we are all different, and what has been shown to work in the scientific studies might not work for you.

The following are some probiotic strains shown to reduce the likelihood of catching common colds and flu, and to reduce their duration and severity: *Lactobacillus rhamnosus* GG, *Bifidobacterium lactis* BB-12, *Lactobacillus paracasei* CASEI 431®, *Lactobacillus acidophilus*-LBG80.

Note: When considering taking a probiotic, it's worth keeping in mind that even when there is supporting scientific evidence, it still doesn't guarantee that it will work for you. And remember, a consistently healthy diet, including a plethora of plant power, is more important than one or two bacterial species in a probiotic.

HEALING PHASE 3: PRO-RESOLUTION AND THE ROAD BACK TO HEALTH

When an acute infection starts to shift down a gear and resolve, the focus of care needs to shift with it, from an emphasis on supporting antimicrobial immunity to a downregulation of excessive inflammation and corresponding upregulation of pro-resolving to complete the cycle. You may be starting to feel better gradually, but in some cases, it can take several months, and sometimes a year or more, to feel fully recovered, and some people never return to normal completely due to long-term post-viral fatigue.

R & R: rest and repair your mind *and* body

Fatigue is a common symptom of many different infections, but it can linger long after you have recovered from the initial acute infection. Post-viral fatigue affects children, young people and adults of all ages alike. And the severity and length of time that someone experiences fatigue doesn't always reflect the severity of the initial infection or their previous fitness levels. Infections can affect people to different degrees, so give yourself the time you need to recover. Do not rush or push yourself.

Rest needs to be your priority. This frees energy for your body to finish off dealing with the infection and support resolution. And that means resting the body *and* the mind, because stress and worry use energy, too. Engage in quality rest, which might mean simply reducing your sensory input – such as putting down your phone – and incorporate relaxation techniques to help reset a stressed immune system (see p. 210 for ideas). It's important to spend more time on activities you enjoy and that leave you feeling restored, such as meditation or simply being in nature or deep breathing – anything low-energy that you gain pleasure from and that can be done with regular rests. This can shift your brain out of survival mode, which is crucial when you're healing.

Get plenty of restorative sleep, too. Poor-quality sleep is no joke. When we are tired, we're more irritable and depressed, our hormones are a wreck, we can't lose weight, we can't concentrate, our digestion is a mess, we get more spots, we get sick more often – and our immune systems don't have time to repair and rebuild. Try to reshuffle your priorities with the four Ds: **d**o, **d**elay, **d**elegate, **d**ump (see p. 241).

Post-viral fatigue can be difficult to describe and is often referred to as 'an invisible symptom'. It can start to interfere with every aspect of day-to-day life, so learning how to cope with it and feeling confident with helpful strategies may assist in reducing its impact (see also p. 240). If possible, get up and move around slowly and gently a few times each day to keep your body moving and to aid circulation of lymph, which guides the removal of inflammation. If you are too unwell for this, try to move around in bed a little – stretching out, moving all your joints and tensing and relaxing your muscles. When you start to feel better, aim to build up your daily walk gradually. Build up to your pre-illness level of activity super-slowly and do not push yourself too much. Overexertion could potentially knock you back energy-wise.

Nutritionally support a return to homeostasis

For recovery, nothing beats a balanced whole-food diet rich in plant diversity, protein and healthy fats (see Chapter 7). But any inflammatory response will result in a degree of oxidative stress, and you might be nutrient depleted from the extra demands of your immune system. You can help your body back to health by providing targeted nutritional antioxidant and anti-inflammatory support.

Omega-3s

DHA and EPA Omega-3s are my top choice for promoting a return to normal. This is down to their ability to form specialised pro-resolving mediators (SPMs), which orchestrate the resolution of the inflammatory phase before it gets out of hand and starts to damage cells.[45] You can find them in supplements from marine sources (or, if you are vegan, opt for an algae version). DHA and EPA omega-3s are also found in oily fish. (See also, p. 278.)

Bromelain

Bromelain is a complex mixture of protease extracted from the fruit or stem of the pineapple plant. It's been used in traditional medicine since ancient times to promote healing and soothe inflammation. Although the complete molecular mechanism of bromelain has not been entirely identified, it's considered safe and studies show clinical benefit in injuries, infections and respiratory-tract diseases.[46]

Plant power

Many plant phytonutrients support resolution of inflammation after infection. In particular, sulforaphane, resveratrol and curcumin have been shown to promote the genetic switch AMP-k, which shuts off inflammation and helps promote resolution.[47, 48] (See also, pp. 154 and 288.)

CHAPTER 13:

Supporting Immunity When You Suffer From Allergies

From a seasonal pollen allergy, known as hay fever, to perennial dust mite allergies to eczema, asthma and life-threatening food allergies, allergic reactions are among the leading causes of emergency hospitalisations in the UK. In fact, according to data published by the NHS, the number of children admitted with severe allergic reactions was up 72 per cent over the five-year period between 2013 and 2019. Eczema, allergies and asthma are known as the atopic triad because they so often occur together. Up to 80 per cent of children with eczema also have asthma or allergies to pollen, dust mites, pet dander, mould or certain foods.

To learn how to handle allergies and support your immune system, it is important to know what an allergy actually is. An allergic reaction is caused when the body's immune system reacts disproportionately to something called an allergen – a substance in the environment that is usually considered harmless. We hear about different allergens including pollen, mould, animal dander, peanuts and insect stings, causing allergies, but the reality is that, no matter the allergen, all allergies result from an underlying immunological issue.

There is currently no definitive cure for allergic conditions, but in this chapter, you will learn how to look upstream to identify root causes and your personal triggers. I will teach you how to create a downstream impact that will support your overall immune balance, putting you on track to defeat the symptoms, manage your condition and dramatically improve how you live with your allergy. I will provide particular focus on atopic rhinitis (also known as hay fever) and atopic dermatitis (eczema), and you can customise my recommendations, depending on your allergy and symptoms. It is also important to know that people can grow into allergies and out of them, and no one really knows why. It's also true that if you are unlucky enough to have one allergy, you are more likely to develop others. Getting the immune system under control is critical to reducing the likelihood of this happening. The good thing is that many of the approaches described in this chapter to control symptoms are also part of the prevention process.

WHY ARE ALLERGIES MORE COMMON TODAY?

Allergies of all kinds have become more common in recent decades. What's behind this epidemic? Increased awareness could be part of it, but that's not the whole story. We do know some people are genetically more susceptible than others, so one of the culprits is our genes.

The role of our genes

A family history of allergic diseases – known as atopy or atopic diseases – is the strongest risk factor for developing allergic symptoms. If you have a close family member who suffers from hay fever, or any other atopic conditions (such as asthma, eczema or food allergies), you're already at higher risk for developing a form of allergy due to genetics.

To date there is no single gene linked to all atopic diseases.

The genetic causes of allergies consist of a complex network of interacting genes; it's not just down to a few disease-causing mutations.[1] This means that your risk of developing asthma or another atopic disease depends on the interaction of all these genetic factors with a variety of environmental ones, which we'll discuss.

This network of allergy-related genes can impact things such as how easily we make IgE antibodies to allergens and how well they bind to mast cells (histamine containing immune cells), as well as how effectively our bodies metabolise and inactivate histamine using the diamine Oxidase (DAO) enzyme and histamine N-methyltransferase enzymes (HNMT). The unique constellation of genes underlying your allergy might be different from someone else with the same allergic condition.

The atopic march refers to the typical progression of related allergic diseases that often begin early in life, starting with atopic dermatitis (eczema), followed by allergic rhinitis (hay fever) and then atopic asthma.[2] Although not all children with eczema will develop the related conditions, almost 80 per cent will go on to develop asthma and/or allergic rhinitis and/or other food allergies. The more severe the eczema, the higher the risk for developing a food allergy later in life.

Rather than thinking of allergies as the result of a singular event or trigger, it's more helpful to consider them as the result of a complex series of internal and environmental inputs interacting with our genetics.

The role of environment

Allergic conditions are primarily the result of a generalised loss of immune tolerance for benign and harmless substances in our environments. The T helper 2 cell branch of our adaptive immune system becomes overactive and there are not enough regulatory cells to keep it in check. Consider it a warning sign that the immune system is highly vulnerable to the modern world in which we all now live.

Reduced biodiversity theory

'Good bugs' are the first stop after genetics when it comes to dissecting what's behind the pandemic of hay fever and other allergies. Every mucosal surface on your body, including your gut, lungs and nasal passages, is colonised by distinct communities of microbes, collectively known as a microbiota (see earlier chapter). Far from causing harm, these microbes teach your immune system to tolerate harmless environmental substances like dietary proteins and allergens, such as pollen.

For a long time, the 'hygiene hypothesis' was the leading explanation for the increase in allergies.[3] It's based on early studies conducted by epidemiologist David Strachan in the 1980s, which suggested that the immune systems of people who grow up in 'clean' environments, where they are exposed to fewer infection-causing bacteria, do not develop normally, causing them to pick fights with harmless allergens. But the hygiene hypothesis is an incomplete and now outdated explanation. I also find the use of the word 'hygiene' problematic. Basic hygiene matters for public health, and increasing the number of infections your child gets does not necessarily 'strengthen' the immune response to prevent allergies.

The 'old friends hypothesis', also known as the 'reduced biodiversity theory', has pretty much overthrown the hygiene hypothesis. This suggests that reduced contact with 'good' germs in natural environments (not the infection-causing germs or the number of infections) is key to educating our immune systems and preventing allergies.[4]

When it comes down to what microbial communities we need living on and in our bodies, the waters are still very muddy. Gut microbes are the best-studied, but we have communities of microbes all over our bodies, including in our lungs and skin. Though it's still early days in understanding the microbes that make up the 'lung microbiota', this is an important frontier in allergic airway diseases.[5,6]

Generally speaking, allergies are associated with changes to the balance of our gut microbiota.[7] Since the gut is home to 70 per cent of the immune system, shifts in microbes can alter immune regulation generally, throughout the body.

People with allergies tend to show signs of gut microbial dysbiosis (see p. 130), with more unhelpful microbe species in their gut and significantly fewer helpful ones compared to healthy people. One group of bacteria called *Acinetobacter* is notable because it seems to encourage immune cells to produce an anti-inflammatory substance called IL-10, which helps to regulate against unwanted immune responses, such as allergies.[8] Children growing up in homes that are surrounded by forest and agricultural land tend to have more of these actinobacteria and lower rates of allergy. The DAO enzyme, which breaks down histamine, is produced mainly in the gut, so gastrointestinal damage may lead to a reduction in the enzyme activity. (See p. 322 for my probiotic suggestions to help with hay fever.)

Other environmental risk factors and allergy aggravators

Passive tobacco smoke exposure after birth and even during the gestational period has been demonstrated as one of the stronger risk factors causally related to the development of asthma in children.[9] Children of mothers who smoked up to the end of pregnancy and continued to smoke after birth also turned out to have a significantly increased risk for allergic sensitisation to food proteins from hen's eggs and cow's milk.

Air pollution can physically modify allergens to increase their potency and damage our delicate body barriers which makes our immune cells more likely to respond inappropriately.[10]

A recent study found that birch pollen collected from trees in Munich, Germany, was more likely to provoke an immune reaction than pollen from trees in rural areas.[11] Pollution also attacks the delicate membranes in the respiratory tract, making people more susceptible to pollen. Many people who have never had hay fever before start experiencing it after moving to built-up areas. There is even data to suggest that babies who are exposed to pollution both before they are born and during their first year of life have a higher risk of developing allergies.[12]

The prevalence of both obesity and allergy has been increasing throughout the world, leading to the hypothesis that the two are linked. In a large study investigating the contributory effect of increasing body mass on the development and incidence of various atopic diseases,[13] obesity was found to clearly affect asthma and was associated with eczema, too. An increased risk of severe asthma in adolescents and children was also associated with consuming fast food three or more times per week,[14] while being overweight or obese is associated with an increased prevalence of allergic eczema.[15]

A lack of sleep can also affect things. People who slept at least seven hours a night suffered significantly milder symptoms than those who slept no more than five. Mast cells, that cause many allergy symptoms, are under circadian control,[16] which might be why our symptoms differ depending on the time of day. Allergic conditions such as asthma or allergic rhinitis have historically shown severity of symptoms to be exacerbated between midnight and morning.[17]

HAY FEVER (ALLERGIC RHINITIS)

Allergic rhinitis is an inflammatory condition that affects the inside of your nose and is caused by an allergen. Normally, the immune system is educated to tolerate these, but in the case of allergic rhinitis, it reacts inappropriately with an inflammatory response.

Allergic rhinitis is on the rise in adults and children, and was estimated to affect around one in every five people in the UK in 2013, compared with one in eight in the 1980s.[18] But a study in 2021 by Allergy UK suggests this may be an underestimate.[19] If you have a close family member with allergic rhinitis, you have a greater than 50 per cent chance of developing an allergy yourself. Not only do allergies have an inherited component, they are also gender-related. Studies show mothers are more likely to pass allergies to their daughters, and fathers to their sons.[20]

Allergic rhinitis can be seasonal or perennial (occurring all year round). In perennial allergic rhinitis, the symptoms usually relate to indoor allergens, such as house-dust mites, pets (including birds) or moulds. Hay fever is what we call seasonal allergic rhinitis, which occurs as a reaction to pollen from grass, trees and some weeds during the early spring and summer months. In general, it's the pollen of wind- not insect-pollinated plants.

The role of pollen

The distribution and abundance of allergy-inducing pollen is changing. This is thought to be due to climate change influencing weather patterns, altering how and when plants release pollen and how long it stays in the air.[21, 22]

Strangely enough, even though many of us consider pollen only an irritating allergen, it is antiviral, helping to remove viruses and activate the immune response against them. Pollen bioaerosols have been shown to deactivate aerosol viral particles, and thus lowering the spread of flu. This suggests it's one of several reasons why flu is a seasonal infection. (Others include weather-related changes, such as the amount of UV light, humidity and air temperature.) Pollen counts have even been explored as a predictor of flu epidemics.

It has also been suggested that hay-fever symptoms make it more challenging for SARS-CoV-2 viruses to get into our lungs, and that hay-fever medications, such as antihistamines, suppress COVID-19 symptoms. None of this has been properly worked out yet, but it makes for interesting discussion. It could be that social distancing and preventative behaviours are less relevant during pollen season, making pollen a protector against COVID-19 in spring.

What are the symptoms of hay fever?

Far from just a runny nose, the raft of symptoms can be hugely debilitating, drastically impacting quality of life and lasting for several months in the case of seasonal allergies or even all year round in perennial ones. Although symptoms somewhat resemble those of the common cold, allergies tend to last longer and typically do not include a fever. Any combination of the following symptoms is most common:

- Itchy eyes/ throat
- Sneezing, blocked/runny nose
- Watering, red eyes (allergic conjunctivitis)

- Headaches, blocked sinuses
- Shortness of breath
- Tiredness
- 'Post-nasal drip' – the sensation of mucus running down the back of the throat

There are also some less well-known symptoms:

- Itchy and sensitive skin, caused by direct contact with pollen; some hay-fever sufferers who experience eczema find their eczema gets worse when pollen is high
- Loss of smell caused by lack of air reaching the smell receptors located high in the nose, which can, in turn, lead to loss of taste
- Facial pain caused by blocked sinuses
- Feeling a 'little off' because the inflammation hay fever causes can interact with metabolism and stress chemistry

These symptoms become more severe when the pollen count is high or when you are exposed to your specific allergic trigger. Remember, it doesn't take much to trigger a reaction. Symptoms typically kick in once the pollen count reaches 50 (which means there are 50 grains of pollen per cubic metre of air).

Note: it's not just pollen that you might find yourself allergic to. Allergic antibodies can also cross-react to similar-looking parts of foods. This is called oral allergy syndrome. For example, a birch pollen allergen called Bet v 1 shares similarities with proteins in some fruits and nuts, so people with hay fever may occasionally notice swelling and itching in their mouths when they eat uncooked fruits, such as apples, peaches and kiwi. Hazelnuts, almonds or even soya milk can trigger it, too. It is usually harmless – but not always. One study found that oral allergy symptoms spread to other areas of the body in nearly 9 per cent of people with the condition, progressing to anaphylactic shock in 1.7 per cent of them.

Sensitisation

The first time an allergic individual encounters an allergen, the immune system misidentifies a harmless substance (pollen, for example) as a threat when it enters the body. This is known as 'sensitisation', and is a very important step in developing an allergy.

Antigen-presenting cells (immune cells that line our bodies' barriers) capture the incoming substances and present them to other immune cells, such as T and B cells. If the cells identify the substance as a threat, a cascade of immune responses is initiated. The B cells will produce a specific type of antibody called immunoglobulin E (IgE). T cells are instructed to become T helper 2 cells (Th2) and produce molecules called cytokines, such as interleukin-4 (IL-4), that encourage the production of these IgE antibodies.

Once released into the blood, IgE binds to mast cells (the major allergy immune cell), as well as other immune cells, such as basophils. You are now sensitised to this substance and your body considers it an allergen. Sensitisation can take place years before you first experience allergic symptoms, and when it happens you won't be aware of it.

Once sensitisation has taken place, some people will develop an allergic reaction when they're re-exposed to the allergen – the allergen will bind to the IgE on the mast cells and initiate an aggressive and immediate immune response. But you can go your whole life carrying allergen-specific IgE-bound mast cells without ever experiencing an allergic reaction or even being aware of the allergy.

The allergic reaction

Mast cells are huge granular cells, meaning they store many granules containing things such as histamine. When the granules are activated, they release their contents. This is known as degranulation. In the case of a pollen allergy, when pollen binds to IgE-coated mast cells in your nasal cavity, it causes the granules to rapidly release their contents. When this happens, mast cells release a whole host of toxic compounds. It's like a grenade going off in your nose!

Histamine is probably the best-known granule component, as it's targeted by anti-histamine drugs, which anyone with hay fever will be familiar with. But there are over 200 of these toxic mediators stored within the granules of mast cells, including enzymes that can damage our delicate tissues and cause scarring after a prolonged time, and prostaglandins and leukotrienes, which activate inflammation.

This release of histamine and other granule contents within seconds of exposure to an allergen causes sneezing, localised inflammation and the suite of symptoms associated with hay fever. There are also mast cells in the lining of the eyelids, which helps explain the inflamed and itchy eyes. This reaction is exacerbated by something called the naso-ocular reflex: when the nerves linking the lining of the nose to the outer surface of the eye are irritated, you get reddening and itching of the eyes, too. Mast cells line all of our bodies' barriers, and their degranulation is responsible for all other forms of IgE-related allergic reactions, such as allergic asthma (lungs), atopic dermatitis, aka allergic eczema (skin) and even anaphylaxis (blood vessels). As well as this immediate response, several symptoms can occur hours after exposure to the allergen and can last for weeks. These late-phase reactions can result in similar symptoms, but they can also cause tissue to be destroyed through a vicious cycle of damage and repair, where immune cells are continually recruited to the area and perpetuate inflammation.

Despite all this, histamine isn't 'bad'. The mast-cell granule contents actually evolved to aid with expelling parasitic worms and bacteria.[23] Their strategic positioning along our bodies' barriers – at the interface between our bodies and our environments (near blood, lymphatic vessels, nerve fibres and a range of immune cells, including epithelial and dendritic cells) – allows them to respond rapidly to invading microbes and any change in environment by communicating with different immune cells. They've been described as sentinels, ready to deal with whatever comes their way. Unfortunately, these normal components of our immune defences produce some unpleasant effects when released inappropriately by benign triggers such as pollen.

Histamine starts to become an issue when our bodies can't break it down fast enough, or we make too much. Some people don't break down histamine very well due to genetics and the composition of their microbiota (see 'The role of microbes', below). Histamine intolerance (HI) results if there's an imbalance between the build-up and breakdown of histamine. If this happens, histamine can start to affect normal body functions and we develop conditions such as hay fever.

How can I find out what allergens trigger my symptoms?

It may be useful to test which allergen you're allergic to as this can help with managing your symptoms. Diagnosing your allergy is typically based on your symptoms and history in combination with a skin-prick test. However, these can give false positives as the allergens are given under the skin where the immune response may be different from that inside the nose.

Another diagnostic testing option is blood tests for allergen-specific immunoglobulin E (IgE) antibodies, which your immune system produces in response to the allergen.

There is also a test called the component resolved diagnostics (CRD). This is a diagnostic blood test for IgE-mediated allergy, which will check your blood for IgE antibodies for a huge number of potential allergens. It's basically a more advanced lab technique for the diagnosis of allergies as it provides more detailed and accurate information.

Any allergy test *must* be combined with a thorough allergy-focused patient history to form an accurate diagnosis. In cases where patient history and IgE tests do not match, a doctor may consider an allergy provocation challenge test under specialist supervision, with gradually increasing amounts of the suspected allergen. This is particularly useful to rule out false-positive results, which can be a barrier in allergy diagnosis.

If you have hay fever and narrow down that you're allergic to birch tree pollen, be aware that allergies can change to encompass other pollens, too.

ECZEMA (ALLERGIC DERMATITIS)

Atopic dermatitis, commonly known as eczema, is a chronic inflammatory skin condition. Eczema in Greek means to boil over, which I am sure makes sense to anyone who suffers with this incredibly itchy, dry- and cracked-skin condition. Skin without eczema provides an effective barrier that protects the body from infection and irritation; it also forms a vital part of whole-body immune regulation. If you think of the skin as a brick wall, the outer cells are the bricks, while fats and oils are the mortar, holding everything together and acting as a seal. The cells attract and keep water inside, and the fats and oils also help to keep moisture in.

What are the symptoms of eczema?

The main symptom of eczema is itchy, dry, rough, flaky, inflamed and irritated skin. It can flare up, subside and then flare up again. Eczema can occur anywhere, but most commonly affects the arms, inner elbows, backs of the knees or head (particularly the cheeks and the scalp). It's not contagious and, in some cases, it becomes less severe with age.

Other symptoms include:

- intense itching (which scratching further inflames)
- red or brownish-gray patches
- small, raised bumps that ooze fluid when scratched
- crusty patches of dried yellowish ooze, which can signal infection
- thickened, scaly skin.

Eczema often begins in childhood but can occur at any age. If you develop eczema at an early age, your skin is likely to remain sensitive, even if there is no recurrence of eczema. Eczema can vary in appearance from person to person, and each individual may be affected in completely different areas. In paler skin tones it will look like patches of angry red skin, while in darker skin tones, it can look purple or grey.

Vulnerable skin barrier

In the case of eczema, we know that a 'loss-of-function' mutation in the filaggrin gene impairs how skin cells mature to form the

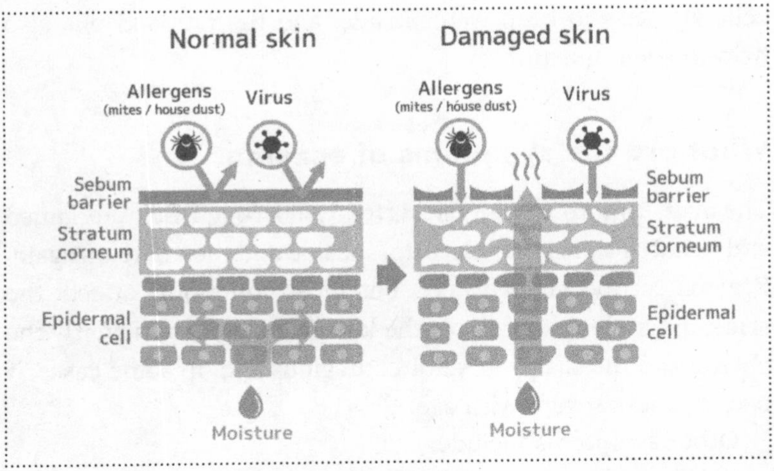

Figure 11 The skin barrier in eczema

outermost protective layer of our skin. Around one in ten of the UK population has reduced amounts of filaggrin in their skin because they have inherited a faulty copy of the gene for making it. Some people with a filaggrin deficiency will have normal or just slightly dry skin, while others may have quite markedly dry skin and a high risk of developing atopic eczema.[24] This is also linked to developing other allergic diseases, such as asthma and food allergies.[25]

How is eczema diagnosed?

There's no specific test that can be used to diagnose eczema, but a doctor may be able to recognise it by looking at the symptoms. A patch test can pinpoint certain allergens that trigger symptoms, such as skin allergies associated with contact dermatitis (a type of eczema). During this test, an allergen is applied to a patch that's placed on the skin. If you're allergic to that allergen, your skin will become inflamed and irritated.

Eczema flares: getting one step ahead of your triggers

The severity of eczema tends to come and go in 'flares'. There are many complex reasons why eczema may get worse, and the factors that can make this happen are called triggers. Triggers vary from person to person. They tend to be things you come into contact with in your environment, but even physical and emotional changes can cause a flare. Skin becomes inflamed, red and sometimes weepy, and the damaged delicate skin barrier can then be an entry point for infection. Eczema sufferers will know that it's incredibly difficult to get it back under control once something has set it off. This is why you need a flare plan.

Unfortunately, there is little clinical evidence to confirm what commonly suspected triggers really do produce flares of eczema. Some reactions happen straight away, but some can take a few days to manifest, so a symptom diary can be a great way to spot any patterns. Research has shown that 60 per cent of people with eczema who recorded skin appearance, treatments and triggers noticed an improvement in their skin. There are a variety of free eczema trackers online which can be helpful, and you can also consult the National Eczema Association's Eczema Product Directory.

Get into the habit of reading labels, especially before spending money on a product that might end up aggravating your condition (the dizzying abundance of products on the market can quickly lead to a money pit); look out for products labelled 'natural' or 'organic' – these are misleading terms.

The following are some of the most common eczema triggers:

- Personal-care and cleaning products, especially fragranced ones and also airborne room fragrances; double-rinse laundry to remove any detergent residues.
- Clothing – wool and synthetic materials can be

uncomfortable; 100 per cent cotton, bamboo or silk garments are ideal.

- Temperature – being too hot or too cold, or going from one temperature to another can trigger itching.
- Humidity – your efforts to protect your skin might need to double or even triple during periods of cold, dry air, as in the winter.
- House-dust mites – they are present in all homes and it's impossible to get rid of them, but their droppings can exacerbate eczema; washing clothing and bedding at 60°C kills them in these places.
- Animal dander, saliva and fur can be irritants for some people; clean all rooms regularly and ensure hands are washed after stroking or handling animals.
- Pollen and other airborne allergens; if affected by pollen, follow the tips on pp. 300 and 315.
- Damp and mould – spores from rotting vegetation and mould in buildings can cause a reaction in some children with eczema.
- Sleep – the circadian clock drives mast-cell function in allergies, so ensuring your sleep–wake rhythms are aligned is especially important.
- Stress – a known trigger of the allergic Th2 cells; stress-management techniques (see previous chapter) will need to be a part of your routine.

Eczema is notoriously unpredictable, and triggers can change over time. Flares can occur at any point, despite your best efforts. Self-compassion, as we've discussed (see p. 199), is one of the most anti-inflammatory acts you can do for yourself.

Your eczema plan of action

To get control when a flare occurs, you need a plan of action – an all-out mobilisation of tools against eczema to help relieve the symptoms, reduce the flare and limit its impact on day-to-day life. Your skin may be even more irritated and itchy than ever, leading to more scratching and damage. You may lose sleep at night, making you tired and less able to cope.

Short-term tools, such as topical corticosteroids (a type of cream that contains anti-inflammatory steroid ingredients), can be an important part of your flare care. Many people want to go all natural when it comes to their eczema, but sometimes natural products can't help repair the broken skin. Prescribed topical agents like steroids might be needed in some cases to help repair the broken skin so reducing risk of infection, clearing a flare and protecting your skin barrier. Importantly, when the skin barrier is 'leaky', there is a higher risk of food allergens entering the skin and sensitising the immune system, leading to food allergy. This has clearly been shown in eczema sufferers with peanut allergy. There are some risks associated with topical steroid use for eczema, so only used as prescribed by your healthcare practitioner.

Keep control with a good daily self-care routine

- **Moisturise, moisturise, moisturise!** Keeping your skin's moisture intact is one of the most important things you can do to help get control over an eczema flare. It's important to understand how and when to moisturise properly and which products are best to use when you have eczema. There is good evidence that less topical steroid cream is needed if skin is regularly moisturised. Even when the skin looks normal, there can still be immune activity there, so develop a daily skincare routine of moisturising, even when the skin looks good.

- **Curate your own selection of eczema-friendly self-care products.** Aim for fragrance-free products designed for eczema-prone skin. Finding ones that works can be a challenge, and what works for one person may not work for another. Also, as the condition of your skin changes, so can the effectiveness of a product. A manufacturer may also change the formulation of a product from one year to the next. And remember, it can take a month of consistent use before you see any improvement. Spot-checking is a must when trying out a new product. Just apply a little on a trouble spot, wait a couple of days and see whether you have a reaction. Never try more than one new product at a time.
- **Watch the temperature when you're washing.** Wash with water that isn't too hot and add to it an eczema-friendly emollient to stop skin drying out. You can also apply an eczema-friendly skin emollient directly to your body before getting into the bath if you find the water very aggravating. Do not spend too long in the bath (up to twenty minutes). Do not use soaps and other non-eczema friendly washing products (particularly those that contain sodium lauryl sulphate – SLS), as these can potentially irritate and dry the skin. In several population studies in the United Kingdom, the hardness of water has been documented as a factor that may drive eczema. Consider adding a small amount of water softener to bathwater.
- **For cracked, bleeding or weeping areas of skin,** you may need additional short-term tools, such as bandages and wraps or antimicrobials to deal with an infection. Eczema is most often infected by a bacterium called *Staphylococcus aureus*, which is found in greater numbers on the skin of people with eczema than in the general population.

Infected skin looks red and 'angry' and it is usually wet with small yellow spots and sometimes yellow crusts. Talk to your doctor if you think your skin is infected. Correct diagnosis is vital for appropriate treatment.

Skin microbiome

The skin microbiome is different from that in the gut, both in composition and function. Research about it is in its infancy, but in skin conditions such as eczema, sufferers have different amounts of certain bacteria, which can lead to flare-ups, so better understanding this balance could lead to potential treatments.

Some people first experience psoriasis after streptococcus throat infections, suggesting that our immune systems do have an effect on skin diseases. We are just beginning to explore this link, and more research is needed in this area.

Eczema habit-reversal therapy

Stress can increase the desire to scratch; and sometimes, scratching (which can be pleasurable) may occur as a subconscious behaviour and become a habit that makes eczema worse. Some people have benefited from habit-reversal therapy: for one week, keep a daily tally of bouts of scratching. Try to identify when and how you scratch, what you scratch with and how your skin looks and feels afterwards. When you feel like scratching, clench your fist gently instead, or grasp something (a small ball, for example) for thirty seconds.

TAKING ACTION AGAINST ALLERGIES

If you suffer from an allergy or eczema, I am sure you are desperately looking for practical tips to make it more bearable.

From the start, I think it's important to accept that, as yet, we do not have a complete cure and there isn't sufficient evidence to support a single diet, nutrient or supplement protocol that will work for everyone. There are many things about your condition and the reasons you developed it that you cannot control. But it can be your responsibility to live in a way that will allow you to thrive nonetheless. It might be just that little bit harder and require a little more focus and attention to your health.

Fortunately, there are some simple tips to help you reduce the effects of allergens on your body. Both natural and pharmaceutical, they can minimise symptoms to almost undetectable levels and give you back your quality of life. I also think it's important to reiterate that allergies can come on abruptly and can resolve by themselves.

As a starting point, I'd suggest practising self-compassion (it's well-known to be anti-inflammatory – see p. 199), and make sure you have an understanding network of people and healthcare providers around you to provide support.

Allergen avoidance

To control your allergy, you might be relying on antihistamine and other pharmaceutical interventions, going all natural or using a combination of both approaches. But whatever you choose, make sure you also avoid allergens where possible. Here are some tips for doing this:

- Monitor pollen counts in your area to help you decide when to go outside.
- During peak pollen times (this will vary depending on your location, weather conditions and the type of pollen you are allergic to, but tends to be morning, until around midday) try to stay indoors and keep windows closed or wear a mask when outdoors (the latter is now more socially acceptable due to COVID-19).[26] Plan outdoor activities when pollen is lowest.
- Light rain helps to clear pollen, but heavy rain seems to whip more up into the air, especially if it's windy as well as rainy.[27]
- Aim to keep indoor humidity between 40 and 60 per cent. Dust mites flourish in environments with more than 60 per cent humidity, and a warm, humid environment also promotes the growth of mould – another allergen that can also trigger asthma flares and lung infections. Below 40 per cent can irritate the skin and lung body barriers, making them more vulnerable.
- Wash your face/take a shower and blow your nose frequently when the pollen count is high.
- Use large-coverage sunglasses when you're outside.
- Get tested or learn to understand your personal allergen triggers.
- Wash your clothes and clean your home regularly to remove settled pollen. A regular cleaning schedule is essential in combating most household allergens. Wash bed sheets frequently for fewer dust mites.
- Use a balm, such as Vaseline, around the inside of your nose to form a barrier, and a saline nasal spray to irrigate and soothe inflammation in nasal passages.
- Remove mouldy soil and dead leaves from your pot plants if you have perennial allergies.

- Create allergen-free zones in your home (keeping windows closed against pollen, or spring cleaning to remove dust mites, dander and other household pollens).

Having an allergy doesn't need to be an obstacle or reason not to enjoy life. It just might mean that you need to work a bit harder to make things more bearable. You can't know how your body will react to new things unless you try them, so living a full life involves a certain amount of calculated risk to find the right balance between being fearful and cautious.

Antihistamines

Antihistamines are probably the best-known type of allergy medication, and most are readily available from a pharmacy without prescription. Typically, they start to work within thirty minutes.

There are several different types of antihistamine; some have been used for many years and have a reputation for making people drowsy. Modern antihistamines, such as acrivastine, cetirizine, desloratadine, fexofenadine, levocetirizine and loratadine, are less likely to have that side effect.

In general, antihistamines are all similarly effective in reducing the symptoms of hay fever. Non-drowsy ones are often preferred during the day, while drowsy ones may help you sleep at night if your symptoms keep you awake. Oral antihistamine pills can be used on their own, but relief is often better when combined with a nasal spray and eye drops, which provide more targeted relief. If you are using antihistamines, make sure you do so correctly: start ahead of the allergy season and use them consistently, as they can prevent as well as treat the symptoms of allergies. Discuss with your doctor which types you should try and the best time to take them and why.

Antihistamines don't usually cause severe side effects, and

any possible ones should be listed on the medication leaflet. Check with your pharmacist for any contraindications with other medications you may be taking, or other conditions (for example, pregnancy, as pregnant women are not normally included in trials to develop these medications). Alcohol interacts with antihistamines (and can cause histamine release), so best avoid it if you're suffering badly from hay fever.

Antihistamines are still widely prescribed for eczema, despite lack of evidence of their effectiveness. Results of double-blind, randomised trials have found that oral antihistamines do not effectively treat the itch associated with eczema. American Academy of Dermatology guidelines state that intermittent short-term use of sedating antihistamines may help insomnia secondary to itch but should not be used directly for management of eczema.

DIET, GUT HEALTH AND NATURAL REMEDIES

Although there's encouraging evidence that diet, supplements and natural products may be able to help with allergic conditions, it's important to acknowledge there is either no evidence for some claims, or the evidence is of low quality or limited.

Allergies are a sign of inflammation and generalised immune dysregulation. Ensuring good gut health and following an anti-inflammatory diet pattern are fundamental. Accepting that you may have to double down on your efforts is a huge step but an important part of the process. This includes limiting foods associated with a pro-inflammatory diet pattern (see p. 81) and focusing on a diet rich in plants with an emphasis on fruit and veggies and a diversity of plant fibre. Where possible avoid key factors known to disrupt gut health and ensure exposure to natural green environments, which can nurture our own microbiomes. Studies suggest that dietary fibre and the metabolites produced when your gut microbes break down that fibre can regulate mast-cell function.[28] Including fibre-rich foods made from beans and pulses supports immune balance via fertilising the gut microbiome (see p. 322 for my probiotic suggestions).

Foods rich in vitamin C, flavonoids and carotenoids are beneficial because of the anti-inflammatory, antioxidant and anti-allergy properties of these compounds.[29] It's also important to ensure that you don't have deficiencies in any of the essential micronutrients (vitamins and minerals) that support proper immune function. Research shows that people with allergies often suffer from nutritional deficiencies and may need enrichment with protective factors, such as selenium, magnesium, vitamins C and D and omega-3 fats. In particular, the histamine-clearing DAO enzyme is dependent on vitamins B6, B12, iron, zinc, copper and vitamin C.

Notable foods and supplements with evidence for alleviating allergic symptoms of hay fever and histamine are listed below.

Quercetin and the flavonoids

The flavonoid quercetin is a polyphenol known to inhibit mast cells, helping to prevent histamine release.[30] It's considered one of the best food-based anti-allergy agents. It also counters the oxidative load of an inflammatory condition. Foods containing quercetin include onions, capers, peppers, apples, leafy greens and berries; it's also found in many other foods, although levels vary depending on how the food is grown. A typical Western diet provides approximately 0–30mg of quercetin per day, but with a diet rich in flavonoid-packed foods, we can provide our bodies with much more.[31] Quercetin as a supplement is generally recognised as safe, and no side effects have been noted for doses of a few grams a day. The anti-allergy effects of quercetin are typically seen in doses of 1000mg twice a day. The appropriate dose for you will depend on your age, gender and medical history. Speak to your healthcare provider to get personalised advice if you choose to take this supplement.

Foods that contain vitamin C typically contain quercetin and each helps with the absorption of the other. Other flavonoids that have shown beneficial effects on allergies include fisetin, kaempferol, resveratrol, epigallocatechol-3-gallate (ECGC) and genistein and myricetin. The good news is that flavonoids are also anti-inflammatory, helping to promote an anti-inflammatory status in the body.

Pomegranate

A study using polyphenol-rich pomegranate juice demonstrated that bioactive compounds from the fruit have the potential to reduce IgE binding and allergy sensitivities.[32]

Chamomile

There's a small amount of evidence that chamomile extract has potent anti-allergenic effects and that these are linked to the ability of bioflavonoids, such as apigenin, to inhibit the release of histamine from mast cells.

A word of warning: chamomile has proteins similar to those found in ragweed and may therefore cause oral allergy syndrome (OAS) in some people who are allergic to ragweed pollen (a phenomenon known as ragweed-chamomile cross-reactivity). The associated oral allergy symptoms may include itching or swelling of the tongue, lips or roof of the mouth.

Nettle

Widely considered an antihistamine, nettle also contains compounds that beneficially modulate the immune response. Nettle may also inhibit tryptase, an enzyme released alongside histamine and promotes its effects. Nettle was reported to be beneficial at a dose of 300mg freeze-dried preparation each day.[33]

Bromelain

An enzyme from pineapple, bromelain been shown to relieve hay fever or sinusitis in several human clinical studies by working as a natural antihistamine, anti-inflammatory and decongestant. Its enzymatic activity can help with fibrosis (scarring) that often occurs in the nasal passages following constant cycles of allergic inflammation.

The therapeutic dose reported for hay fever ranges from 400 to 500mg of bromelain three times a day (with a potency of 1800–2000mcu). Bromelain is thought to enhance the beneficial effects of quercetin by improving its absorption.[34]

N-Acetylcysteine (NAC)

NAC is a natural sulphur-containing amino acid derivative that protects against oxidative stress. NAC has been documented as an effective mucolytic agent (supporting the clearance of mucus) in people with lung and sinus conditions where there's increased production of mucus. NAC helps reduce the viscosity of mucus so it can be more easily removed.[35] While specific research on the use of NAC for allergic rhinitis hasn't been conducted, its affinity for mucus membranes, both as an antioxidant and mucolytic, means it may have applications as part of a treatment protocol for hay fever. Recommended therapeutic dosages range from 500mg to 2g daily.

Omega fatty acids

The omega-3 long-chain polyunsaturated fatty acids eicosapentaenoic acid (EPA) and docosahexaenoic acid (DHA) inhibit mast-cell activation and help settle allergic inflammation.[36] Studies in skin models suggest that DHA can increase filaggrin expression, helping to repair this protein, which is commonly defective in eczema, and attenuat skin inflammation.[37] EPA has been shown in animal studies to improve the skin barrier via an effect on ceramides in skin.[38] Evening primrose oil and borage oil, which are rich in the omega-6 fat called gamma-linolenic acid (GLA), also show some promise in enhancing barrier function of the skin.[39]

Supporting your liver

Supporting the health of your liver before the hay-fever season starts is also worth considering. Increasing cruciferous vegetables (such as broccoli, cauliflower, cabbage and radishes) in your diet, as well as including the diverse antioxidant phytonutrients found in colourful produce (in particular, berries, soy, garlic and even spices such as turmeric) have been noted to support liver detoxification processes.[40]

A spoonful of honey . . . or pollen?

Honey has long been recommended by some as a hay-fever preventative, but does it actually work? Very little research has been done to find out. In a small study conducted in the US, people were given one of three substances to take: pasteurised honey, unpasteurised honey or a corn syrup artificially flavoured to taste like honey. Participants didn't know which they had been given and were told to take a tablespoon a day, alongside any usual treatment they took to ease their hay fever. Neither type of honey made a difference to the severity of their symptoms.[41] While we know that bee pollen does have some health benefits, there isn't a great deal of firm evidence to support this. If you like honey, then go ahead, but I wouldn't expect a dramatic improvement from this alone.

Probiotics

Caring for your gut health through diet and lifestyle is foundational, but there is some interesting research coming out on the preventative and therapeutic role that probiotics can play, too.

The following probiotic strains have been shown to have immune-regulatory properties that may help in the prevention and treatment of allergies: *Lactobacillus paracasei* LP-33,[42] *Lactobacillus rhamnosus* HN001,[43] and *Lactobacillus acidophilus* NCFM®.[44] But see also 'Note' on p. 290.

Some microbes are histamine producers, using an enzyme called histidine decarboxylase to convert the histidine present in various proteins into histamine, even if the food is not a histamine-rich one. In healthy people this is not problematic, and these microbes do perform lots of beneficial tasks. Based on the very limited research so far, the following are considered potential producers of histamine: *Streptococcus thermophilus*, *Lactobacillus casei*, *Lactobacillus bulgaricus* TISTR 895, *Lactobacillus helveticus*, *Bifidobacterium longum*, *Lactobacillus plantarum* D-1033. If you have a probiotic supplement that is a blend of bacteria, pay attention to the inclusion of these species; they may not necessarily be problematic, but they could aggravate your symptoms.

The bottom line is, supporting gut health is the top priority in managing histamine intolerance. Rebalancing the gut microflora and improving gut integrity is a key step to doing this.

Low-histamine or other exclusion diet?

A low-histamine diet is one that is designed to exclude foods and drinks that are either histamine-containing or histamine-triggering in the body, as they may aggravate allergy-associated histamine symptoms. But be aware that when searching online for histamine-releasing foods you may be confronted with a *huge* list that includes many healthy items, such as fermented foods, fish and even some fruits and vegetables. I'd suggest you work with a qualified practitioner before attempting to cut out long lists of foods – because unless you have a specific mast-cell disorder, the evidence is limited.

The best way to figure out if food could be helping or hurting your allergy is by keeping a food diary. Note down what you eat, when you eat it and how your symptoms are for two to three weeks, then look for correlations. Remember, it can take three to four days for food to leave your system, so symptoms may not appear immediately after you eat them. And again, you should not remove food (an exclusion diet) without the supervision of your healthcare professional, who can advise on the best way to approach this and ensure that you replace any missing foods with others of similar nutritional value.

BIOPSYCHOSOCIAL SUPPORT

There are many psychological and emotional factors that can affect such as eczema and hay fever. It's been suggested that hundreds of extra decisions need to be made on a daily basis, which is exhausting in itself and certainly increases the life load you must carry. You may find your symptoms get worse when you are under stress (indeed, having an allergy can itself be a source of stress) because the stress chemistry upregulates the immune Th2 response that drives IgE antibodies that stick on mast cells. While it's important to avoid stress as much as possible, it's also important to cultivate an awareness of your levels (see Chapter 8) and prioritise emptying your stress cup. A lack of sleep can also adversely affect things. One study showed that people who slept at least seven hours a night suffered significantly milder symptoms than those who slept no more than five hours each night.

A recent survey by the British Skin Foundation revealed that nine out of ten dermatologists agree that not enough importance is placed on the psychological effects resulting from skin conditions such as eczema, and that sufferers do not have adequate access to psychological support. Although specialist psychological services for people with skin conditions are in short supply, it's definitely worth checking your local area as some do exist. Talk to your GP, dermatologist or dermatology nurse who will be able help. Even if there is no skin-disease-specific wellbeing service in your area, talking-based therapies are readily available and can greatly reduce feelings of low mood or anxiety. Look online for charities, support groups, forums and relevant self-help websites.

CHAPTER 14:

Thriving with an Autoimmune Disease

When the immune system is working as intended, it is balanced and resilient, defending against germs and tolerating the daily challenges in our environments. But sometimes it can start to lose its protective function and attack normal, healthy cells. When this happens, there is a loss of tolerance to the self that results in inflammation, antibodies and immune-cell attack on our own bodies, damaging our tissues and organs. The result? Autoimmune disease (AD).

In this chapter, I will share the wealth of knowledge I have accumulated on how to support yourself successfully, thrive and enjoy your life, even with an AD.

WHAT IS AUTOIMMUNITY?

Psoriasis, rheumatoid arthritis and lupus are all examples of AD, but there are some hundred different clinical syndromes collectively called ADs, and they all have one thing in common: a body-wide breakdown in all the checks and balances that regulate and balance the immune system. The body starts trying to fix a problem that isn't there, using the weaponry normally reserved for infection fighting to attack its own cells and tissues. Elevated inflammation, oxidative stress and premature immunolgocial ageing ensue and, over time, you end up with a disease diagnosis. This means that autoimmunity involves more than the area that is obviously affected by the condition (for example, it's not only the joints that are impacted for those with rheumatoid arthritis). As well as chronic pain, you might experience a lack of energy, failing body parts and a host of other physical symptoms that ultimately reduce overall quality of life. And often, these are only one part of the problem. For many AD sufferers, the mental and social side effects are worse, taking a toll on overall mental wellbeing: worrying about what to eat at a restaurant with friends when you fear the whole menu, extra measures (such as medication or special footwear), that you need to put in place for days out or holidays scheduling recovery time and forgoing activities that could leave you too exhausted. On top of all the ordinary demands of everyday life, this can be a recipe for mental exhaustion.

It is estimated that 5–8 per cent of the population have a diagnosed AD. In the UK, AD has been in the top ten leading causes of death in all age groups under seventy-five – a startling figure that some consider a huge underestimation. ADs need careful diagnosis and management, otherwise you could be setting yourself up for worse problems down the road. An unmanaged autoimmune disorder means an out-of-control immune system. This significantly raises your risk of developing more than one autoimmune disease (polyautoimmunity – defined as the presence of more than one autoimmune disease in a single patient; or multiple autoimmune syndrome – MAS – when three or more autoimmune diseases coexist) due to the intermix of susceptibility factors and a state of perpetual inflammation and immune dysregulation. ADs are also associated with a host of other unpleasant symptoms and conditions, including sleep disorders (such as sleep apnoea and insomnia), heart disease and cancer.

AD symptoms can be misleading or fly under the radar for a long period of time. Sadly, many people present with symptoms only after their disease has been wreaking havoc for many years and much damage has been done. This means getting a diagnosis can be challenging. It's estimated to take an average of four and a half years for a diagnosis, and during that period a patient typically has seen four doctors. Getting a correct diagnosis can be made even more complicated because symptoms can flare on and off and vary from one person to another with the same disease.

WHAT CAUSES AUTOIMMUNITY?

Before we can look at how to help your AD, we need to understand the causes. Your AD isn't the result of one thing – although it may have been triggered by one. It is the product of a perfect storm of multiple broad and varied factors known as the 'mosaic of autoimmunity' (see figure 11), which represents an interplay between your unique mix of genetics and several other factors, with many contributors still unknown.[1] In fact, the onset of at least 50 per cent of autoimmune disorders has been attributed to 'unknown trigger factors'.

Understanding the breadth of factors that contribute to the mosaic of autoimmunity gives us greater insight into how to approach the management of your condition. Within the mosaic, there are three broad elements that drive AD:

- An underlying genetic susceptibility
- Exposure to certain environmental influences
- Poor gut microbiome and gut-barrier health

Genetics

Most autoimmune diseases are polygenic, which means there is no single autoimmune gene responsible, but rather a combination. Most of the predisposing AD genes that have been identified are linked to the immune system in some way. Our immune system HLA genes play a significant genetic role. In fact, the way the HLA genes work means we all have some potential for autoimmunity – a side effect of the evolution of this beautifully complex system crafted to protect us. Autoimmunity may be a price we pay for producing immune cells that can detect a huge range of pathogens' molecular codes. Sounds weird, right?

Having a set of HLA genes that predispose you to autoimmunity might also protect you from certain infections. It's our collective diversity that stops us from being wiped out as a species.

You might think that you can't change your genetics, but epigenetics (see p. 34) – that is the turning on and off of the genes we have inherited – does contribute.[2] Diet, lifestyle and environment can all impact which genes our bodies turn on and off.

Environment

Environmental factors play a central role in triggering autoimmunity. Even if you have the predisposing genetics, there is normally an environmentally driven triggering event (or events) that provokes the start of autoimmune processes in the body. Environmental triggers can be sudden or subtle events way upstream of signs and symptoms, making them hard to pinpoint.

Toxins

As you saw in Chapter 11, health is the sum of our relationship with the environment and the many potentially toxic substances we are exposed to in our everyday lives. There is a well-established link between tobacco smoking and disease onset, for example.[3] But for other potentially toxic environmental exposures, the role in autoimmunity is less clear and very little has been studied of the body burden (see p. 252) that we individually accumulate over a lifetime.

Infections

Infections have long been known to play a role in triggering autoimmune disease.[4] Epstein-Barr virus (EBV), cytomegalovirus (CMV), some herpes viruses, rubella, hepatitis A and C have all been implicated in the initiation of autoimmunity. But how do infections cause our immune systems to turn on us? Here are a few possibilities:

- **Molecular mimicry:** some parts of an infectious germ show a sufficient molecular similarity to molecules in our own cells that a cross-reaction occurs.
- **Bystander activation:** the infection leads to activation of the self-reactive immune cells we may all harbour.
- **Epitope spreading:** the infection causes sufficient damage to trigger a self-reaction from the immune system. That means, in essence, that a primary inflammatory process – to an infection, for example – may cause tissue damage in such a manner that certain components of our bodies that are normally immunologically 'hidden' from the immune system become 'revealed' and evoke a secondary auto-immune response.

- **Presentation of cryptic antigens:** antigens are the molecules our immune cells recognise when they are triggered. Cryptic antigens are molecular parts of us that normally go unnoticed by the immune system but are accidentally unleashed during infection.

Stress

Stress is now considered a significant contributor to the onset of autoimmunity.[5, 6] Indeed 80 per cent of people diagnosed with an AD report stressful events prior to disease onset, while a higher incidence has been seen among people who were previously diagnosed with stress-related disorders. **Note:** a stress-related disorder is slightly different from just being stressed, as it is a well-defined condition or disease that develops following a specific and intensely stressful event. A dramatic example is post-traumatic stress disorder (PTSD), in which a serious physical or psychological injury leads to a host of problems, including dysregulation of the immune system and stress axis.[7, 8]

Unfortunately, not only is stress a potential factor in triggering an AD, it can also exacerbate symptoms. Plus, a diagnosis of an autoimmune disease can in itself cause considerable stress, creating a vicious cycle, shrinking your stress container and contributing significantly to the exhaustion and pain of living with autoimmune disease.

It has even been proposed that there is an 'autoimmune personality', whereby certain tendencies confer a significant risk for AD. These include over-giving empathy for others while ignoring your own needs, trouble with being your authentic self, suppression of so-called negative emotions, being a people pleaser/perfectionist, and consistent overachieving without sufficient boundaries – i.e. that person who cannot say no.

Diet

Numerous foods have been studied as potential factors in triggering or fuelling the storm of autoimmunity but, disappointingly, the results from the majority of studies have been equivocal. That's not to say that diet doesn't play a role. While studying individual foods hasn't got us very far, the overall pattern of your diet matters more.

It's no surprise that studies show that AD patients tend to have a poorer diet pattern (as defined by the Healthy Eating Index – HEI-2010) with lower than the recommended intake of fruits, vegetables and fibre, and higher than recommended refined and ultra-processed foods.[9] Regular consumption of sugar-sweetened beverages is associated with increased risk of AD,[10] as is the so-called 'Western diet', which is rich in high-calorie, nutrient-poor foods. Eating this way appears to act as an environmental trigger in genetically susceptible individuals through enhancing the systemic immune-inflammatory response and by compromising antioxidant status.[11] This also indirectly impacts autoimmune risk through the associated co-morbid conditions that arise from a poor diet, such as poor blood-sugar control, obesity and metabolic dysregulation.[12] In fact, BMI is causally associated with an increased risk of AD.[13] Of course, BMI does not distinguish the composition of your muscle and fat mass, which will have specific influences on your immune system and inflammatory set point. We do know that sarcopenia (see p. 102) is prevalent in people with certain ADs, especially where there is a disease-associated disability, and this is directly correlated to fat.

Gut health

The gut is where much of your whole-body immune regulation is crafted. It's also a barrier to the outside world (see p. 125) – a huge site where genes, immune system and environmental exposures interact. A low diversity of microbes in the gut is associated not only with increased risk of developing an AD, but also poorer outcomes. Individuals with AD almost all have a dysbiosis (see p. 130) of their microbiome, both in the gut and oral cavity.[14] Dysbiosis impairs immune regulation and can contribute to chronic inflammation, both of which are contributors to the onset of autoimmunity in genetically susceptible individuals. ADs are also frequently associated with a leaky gut.[15] Zonulin is a protein made by the gut barrier and dictates its integrity. It is used as a biomarker of leaky gut and has been found to be raised in many autoimmune diseases.[16] This allows toxins, microbial endotoxins and incompletely digested molecules of food to access the bloodstream. And because these substances are unfamiliar to the immune system, it will be put on inflammatory red alert.

Gut dysbiosis and gut permeability are, of course, interlinked and not mutually exclusive. We don't know if gut dysbiosis and barrier permeability is a cause of AD or an effect of having one, but changes in the gut often occur upstream of AD development. But if the gut microbiome is balanced and the gut barrier isn't compromised, it may be possible to keep the development of autoimmunity in check, even when there is a strong genetic predisposition.

Putting it all together – your immunobiography

You may have a genetic predisposition, but this doesn't necessarily mean you will go on to develop autoimmunity symptoms. Over time, you may develop poor gut health as a result of a fast-paced life, taking antibiotics for minor illnesses and decreasing intake of fibre and plant diversity. This sets you up for autoimmunity, but it may take an additional environmental trigger, such as an infection or a stressful life event, to set in motion the process that ultimately leads to symptoms. But for others, the road to autoimmunity is long and littered with issues, each of which contributed to the autoimmune burden. Reflecting on your health journey can reveal some of the potential antecedents to your present-day condition.

HOW TO THRIVE WITH YOUR DISEASE

Where to start with this incredibly complex health puzzle? First, we have to confront the elephant in the room: can you cure your AD? There are few simple answers in immunology, but the straight answer to this question is: no, you can't cure an AD. But that doesn't mean autoimmunity needs to be an obstacle to a good life. Despite all the negatives of an AD diagnosis, you can still live well. It might be harder and require more focus, but it is possible.

So if you can't cure it, what can you do?

The focus of initial care with an AD is to put it into remission. Remission is when your symptoms disappear; but they can always return – hence it is not a cure. Remission can happen spontaneously, sometimes in pregnancy, or with combinations of medications, supplements, nutritional interventions and lifestyle changes (that we will discuss in this chapter). One of the most difficult parts of living with an autoimmune condition is the unknowns. How long will the remission last before another flare? But understanding that autoimmunity is variable and incurable and having realistic expectations can be a pivotal part of your health journey.

Following diagnosis, you may be offered medications and suggestions to counter symptoms and inch you towards remission. Many of these therapies comprise immunosuppressive and anti-inflammatory medications that globally dampen immune responses or new-generation monoclonal antibodies, which are more targeted in their disruption of immunity. These conventional therapies are often necessary, and you should follow the advice of your healthcare team. But they are an imperfect solution. They rarely attack only the disease-causing immune cells, do not reinstall the lost immune tolerance and can cause many unpleasant side effects and unintended consequences, such as increasing your risk of infection and long-term risk of malignancy. This often pushes sufferers to turn to food, supplements and lifestyle as a way to manage their disease, seeking out root causes, focusing on immune support and ways to reinstate immune control and improve T-regulatory function.

I like to think in terms of not an either/or approach, but a synergy of both. Healing isn't always an eradication of disease or even a complete remission of symptoms. Sometimes it means reaching a point of balance, whereby we curate our lives to be as full and healthy as we can within the constraints of our condition. Making the changes suggested in the following pages will aid in supporting your overall wellbeing but must be balanced with an acceptance that symptoms and flares can still occur.

Learn how to be a patient

Self-advocacy as a patient is so important. One of the first steps in both diagnosis and healing is to start to tell your story. Fit the puzzle pieces together and take charge of identifying your own unique mosaic of causes. That includes a family history, if you can. Write it down, compile your immunobiography and record all your symptoms to share with your doctor, even if they seem unrelated. This will help to trace your antecedent events (for example, trauma, infection, family history). It also helps you to see your health in big-picture format. Things start to feel like less of a mystery and you may find possibility where there was once devastation.

Please do emphasise to your doctor how your symptoms are impacting your quality of life, highlighting multiple issues if you have them. And don't be afraid to ask for reasons for and against a particular diagnosis, investigation or treatment. Explore whether your doctor's surgery has practitioners trained in or with a special interest in a particular area that relates to your condition. Take responsibility for your health 'admin' by calling, following up, asking for clarification or to see somebody else if you don't feel you are getting anywhere – there really is someone out there who can help you.

Self-advocacy is a process of asking questions and learning from your healthcare team. When you don't understand something about your disease, your medication or your symptoms, ask the question again. Following your diagnosis, you might feel motivated to become your own health detective, searching Dr Google and turning up protocols that claim to reverse, cure and eradicate your AD. But in my experience, this leaves people frustrated, confused and overwhelmed. Remember, even with the same autoimmune disease, no two people will have the same causes and triggers, which means there can be no one-size-fits-all 'protocol' for autoimmunity. Understand your condition; educate yourself about it as much as you can – but use credible sources, such as your healthcare team and websites such as NHS and AD charities.

Give yourself the gift of letting go

An AD diagnosis is life-changing and frightening, and you might find yourself confronted with a real mix of emotions: shock, as you process your new reality, and perhaps even some positive feelings, such as immense relief if it's taken years of unexplained symptoms to get answers. Learning how to live with the symptoms of autoimmune disease is a steep learning curve that can be hard and frustrating. You want to feel 'normal' again, so hold tight to the life experience you desire.

The fact that there is no cure does not equate to life being over. There are so many things that can help and allow you to thrive despite your condition. It will take a degree of readjustment and reframing your wellbeing. And the first step to doing that? Release and accept your new you.

Your attitude and how you look at things is absolutely everything. It's not your fault you developed an AD, but your outlook can make it more difficult to deal with; conversely, you are also part of a solution that can allow you to thrive daily. You can control your attitude to your diagnosis, accepting the loss of the life you once knew. Notice as you move through the different stages from denial to anger, sadness to acceptance.

Healthy boundaries and stress-management techniques

Using the tools described in Chapter 8, create your own toolkit to manage your stress axis. You are now your priority. Start checking in with yourself regularly – not to beat yourself up, but as a reminder that you need to nourish well and learn to recognise when you're not, making space to reprioritise.

We free up energy for healing when we establish and maintain healthy boundaries, so you might have to make diet and lifestyle changes that are socially unacceptable to some people in your life. But you can also control your attitude towards those around you. Your condition might be invisible to others, so try to accept that some might not understand your daily struggles. Don't pretend that everything is ok if it truly isn't, and aim to surround yourself with those who can show empathy, support and understanding.

ANTI-INFLAMMATORY EATING FOR LIFE

While prescription medications remain at the forefront in the battle against autoimmune disease, diet and lifestyle changes can improve quality of life. But where to start? Since everyone reading this will be at a different point in their journey, consider that all ADs have a common thread – inflammation. Consequently, an anti-inflammatory dietary and lifestyle foundation is the base upon which everything else stands. It's the ground-level support upon which you can personalise additional layers.

Take control of your inflammation through the blueprint in Part 2, because these foundations really are the same for everyone, irrespective of any disease diagnosis. But with an AD, keeping on top of the basics will be significantly more important. You might not have as much wiggle room as the person next to you who doesn't have an AD.

AD anti-inflammatory diet pattern

Up to 75 per cent of people with an AD believe that food plays an important role in their condition. This means patients are often looking for diet/supplement advice or sharing anecdotal experiences around nutrition and their condition. This can become a bit of a minefield, especially if you have just been diagnosed. Worryingly, more than 50 per cent of AD sufferers blindly undertake diet and supplement interventions on their own.

The good news is that diet *can* play an important role in how well you live, but perhaps not in the way you have been led to believe. To clarify: diet is not the sole cause of your AD, nor is a diet change or a supplement regimen a cure. It is just one of potentially many levers in the causal mosaic of your overall condition.[17] Following an anti-inflammatory diet pattern is a starting point to support your body in tackling the common denominators of all ADs:

- Inflammation
- Immune imbalances
- Inflamm-ageing
- Oxidative stress
- Gut-microbiome and gut-barrier issues

Data strongly supports an anti-inflammatory eating pattern (with powerful phytochemicals, healthy fats and fibre) like the Mediterranean diet to benefit chronic pain, improve inflammatory markers and complement existing drug therapies.[18] Importantly, diet can be part of the puzzle of getting back the quality of life you want. Your starting point is to apply the principles in Chapter 7.[19]

Specifically, the following are some of the most well-researched nutrients shown to benefit AD:

- **Powerful polyphenols** such as ellagic acid – these are found in dark-coloured berries[20] and fruits such as pomegranate (which is also an excellent prebiotic).[21]

- **Citrus flavanones** such as hesperidin, apigenin and naringin are found in lemons, limes, oranges, grapefruits, as well as peppermint, oregano and leeks.
- **Epigallocatechin-3-gallate** (EGCG) in green tea is shown to improve symptoms and reduce the damage in some animal models of AD.[22]
- **Curcumin,** an active phytonutrient ingredient in turmeric, has potent anti-inflammatory properties, blocking inflammatory cytokines and enzymes via the same pathway as the non-steroidal anti-inflammatory drugs prescribed to many AD patients.[23]
- **Sulforaphane** from cruciferous veggies helps buffer the burden of oxidative stress and excessive inflammation seen in AD.[24]
- **Ginger** contains more than forty different antioxidant compounds, including phenolic gingerols and shogaols, that can decrease AD by increasing immune regulation and Treg cells.[25]
- **Garlic** has anti-inflammatory properties and has been shown to provide benefits for AD inflammation and symptoms as an adjunct to medication.[26]
- **Vitamin D** levels can be lower in people with autoimmune diseases.[27]
- **Omega-3** fats show promise in reducing the inflammatory burden of autoimmunity;[28] there is no established upper limit and scientific studies tend to use very high doses, so consult your healthcare provider before supplementing.

Avoiding nutrient deficiencies

The disability associated with some ADs, as well as the mental load and side effects from treatment methods, medications and the disease itself, can impact appetite and the ability to nourish yourself.[29, 30] Plus, typical drugs used in the treatment of ADs can cause side effects, such as nausea, vomiting, stomach pains, mouth sores and decreased appetite. This means people with AD are also at higher risk of developing nutrient deficiencies. This, in combination with a poor overall diet pattern involving overconsumption of empty calories, added sugars, salt and saturated fats, will leave you feeling worse than you need to. Ensure you are supplementing daily with vitamin D (and omega-3, if you are not eating oily fish). If you are worried about the quality of your diet quality or have restricted lots of foods, talk to your healthcare practitioner about appropriate multivitamin supplements that may be a good option for you.

Gut support

Nourishing your gut is non-negotiable. Focus on plant-based diversity as it helps to fertilise your inner ecosystem, ensuring your microbes are happy factories of immune-regulating metabolites.

You may want to consider trialling a probiotic. A combination of *Lactobacillus casei* 01, *Lactobacillus acidophilus*, *Bifidobacterium bifidum* and *Lactobacillus fermentum* has been shown to provide some benefits when tested in randomised controlled trials (these are among the most robust scientific studies) in autoimmunity. But see also 'Note' on p. 290.

Note: taking live bacteria in the form of probiotics might not be a good idea if your gut barrier is damaged since these bugs could translocate into your blood and cause septicaemia. Always talk to your doctor before starting.

'Controversial' foods

All too often, I see people with an AD embarking on highly restrictive diets without guidance from a qualified nutrition professional. They quickly restrict large numbers of foods, and while they sometimes feel improvements in their symptoms, they can start to feel imprisoned by their diets. Diet can certainly become a source of confusion for a newly diagnosed patient. They have read online which foods 'cause' autoimmunity, or they see that someone else with the 'same' diagnosis is thriving on specific nutritional adjustments.

Several foods are demonised when it comes to AD symptoms and are therefore often excluded by AD patients. Let's take a look at some of them.

Gluten

Coeliac disease is an autoimmune condition caused specifically by proteins within gluten, a component of certain grains, causing inflammation in the gut.[31] Coeliac disease requires strict elimination of gluten-containing foods. But does gluten play a role in other AD, too?

Many susceptibility genes for coeliac disease are shared with those for other ADs. Fragments of gluten and other parts of gluten-containing plants have been shown to induce zonulin release (see p. 332), increasing leaky gut and potentially contributing to vague symptoms not restricted to the gut, such as 'brain fog', headache, fatigue, joint and muscle pain, leg or arm numbness.[32, 33] This happens even in people free of AD, but if the gut is healthy and balanced, it can deal with this insult without any adverse effects. For those with an AD, or AD susceptibility, however, it can be problematic. So far, the link in the scientific evidence is rather weak,[34, 35] so just remember, individual tolerance to gluten will depend on things such as your own gut microbiota (GM). Not everyone with an AD needs to exclude it, unless they have tested positive for coeliac disease or find a significant improvement in symptoms when excluding it. Cutting out gluten-containing foods risks cutting out lots of fibre and other essential micronutrients. It can even negatively alter the microbiome. Because of this, such interventions should only be done under the supervision of a specialist nutrition professional.

Dairy

Dairy gets a bad rap, yet not only is it *not* associated with worsening AD, but diets that include it are linked to better outcomes in AD, while diets that exclude it or promote low intakes should be discouraged.[36] Dairy foods are a rich source of nutrients, such as vitamin D, iodine, calcium and protein. So if you're considering cutting out dairy, the best approach is to use my elimination-diet framework (see p. 344) to discover the effects for yourself. And work with your healthcare team to ensure you are not missing out on key nutrients.

Sugar and salt

If sweet or salty is your thing, it might be worth trying to curb foods high in added sugar or salt. In experimental settings, both sugar and salt have individually been shown to make autoimmunity worse by activating inflammatory immune cells,[37, 38] while anecdotally, foods high in added sugar and salt are often reported to trigger autoimmune symptoms in sufferers. You might not need to cut these foods out entirely, but think about the proportion of UPFs (ultra-processed foods) you consume – are these taking away space from more healthful foods?

Nightshades

Nightshades are the edible parts of flowering plants from the Solanaceae family, and include tomatoes, peppers, potatoes and aubergine. These foods have a host of proven nutritive benefits, being rich in nutrients, such as vitamin C, and phytonutrients, such as lycopene and anthocyanins, as well as powerful antioxidants. It may seem odd, then, that they are considered in a negative light when it comes to AD, but concerns arise from their alkaloid content. Alkaloids are bitter-tasting substances that act as a natural insect repellent. In the case of nightshades, a particular alkaloid called solanine, concentrated in the stems and leaves rather than the actual fruit or vegetable, has been flagged as a cause of concern in worsening inflammatory AD. However, no data conclusively supports a connection between inflammatory conditions and alkaloids. In fact, studies show that anatabine – another alkaloid compound found in nightshades – has powerful anti-inflammatory effects in people who have joint pain and stiffness from autoimmune and inflammatory conditions.[39]

How to do an elimination diet successfully

Most food-intolerance tests on the market are of poor quality and unreliable. Rather than indiscriminately avoiding foods, performing an elimination diet is the gold standard to help you identify any dietary triggers or just foods that make you feel less well, irrespective of your AD. This requires a meticulously scientific approach, as essentially you become your own experiment. Done correctly, it can be a powerful tool, not only for helping to identify potentially triggering foods, but also by fostering a greater level of self-awareness, encouraging you to tune in and listen to the messages your body is sending. The more rigorous you are, the more you will learn about foods and your condition.

While it can be challenging, navigating an elimination diet doesn't have to be stressful. If you prepare and plan ahead, you can move through the weeks successfully and, before you notice, it will be time to begin expanding your diet again. Remember to challenge yourself to address emotional connections to foods or any beliefs about 'good' and 'bad' foods that may be difficult to unstick objectively.

Note: always talk to your doctor before starting any diet alteration or adding a new supplement to your regimen – and also whenever you feel out of your depth.

- Be methodical, starting with one specific food at a time.
- List all the places where this one food may be found (for example, gluten hides in many unobvious places, including supplements, sauces and meat substitutes), then plan your diet and prepare for the week.
- Aim to exclude the food for twenty-one days. This might be challenging, so try to do it when you have a quiet few weeks with plenty of time to cook at home, meal plan and food prep to ensure you have lots of options.
- Complete avoidance is very important to calm inflammation and get clear results.
- At the end of the exclusion period, try to reintroduce the food and eat a few generous portions that day.
- Observe to see if any symptoms arise. If they do, this could be a sign that the food is not agreeing with your system.
- Check in with your bowel habits. Did they improve during the three-week elimination?
- Wait four days before eliminating a different food.

You may not need to eliminate a food completely and perhaps not for ever. You might want to experiment with your own personal tolerance level. Eliminating an offending food in combination with working on your overall healing, gut health and microbiome can allow you to safely and slowly bring foods back into your diet, starting small and working up to tolerance. Remember, this is all about plant diversity and aiming to include, ultimately, as many powerful antioxidant, anti-inflammatory and gut-loving nutrients as you can.

The autoimmune diet protocol (AIP)

The AIP is a restrictive dietary approach developed specifically to reduce inflammation and other symptoms of autoimmune disorders. It pops up on Dr Google when you search for food-based solutions to your autoimmune condition.

The AIP involves an exclusion period with elimination of a wide range of foods, dietary additives, emulsifiers and Western dietary patterns, followed by phased reintroduction. AIP promotes the consumption of nutrient-dense whole foods, such as vegetables, fruits, mono- and polyunsaturated fatty acids and non-processed meats. So far, so healthy, right? But there are a few issues. There are currently only three studies looking at AIP in humans with autoimmune diseases; two observing patients with inflammatory bowel disease, which showed some improvements in symptoms and inflammation;[40, 41] and a very small pilot study in autoimmune Hashimoto's thyroiditis, which showed no statistically significant changes in relevant blood markers, although patients did share improvements in quality of life.[42] Currently, there are no large, well-designed, high-quality studies.

AIP is highly restrictive and hard to sustain. This could lead to nutrient deficiencies, unintended weight loss and erosion of a person's relationship with food. It's my view that in the near future we may step closer to specific diets for autoimmune disease, but probably only under the guidance of nutrition professionals, as an adjunct to other therapies and concomitant with lifestyle modifications.

CAN I USE FASTING TO HELP MY AD?

The concept of intermittent fasting has been trending for some time now and its relationship with autoimmunity is creeping into popular media. Fasting by consuming only water for a prolonged period (usually a minimum of twelve hours) produces a range of changes within the body, which can reduce oxidative stress (remember this occurs with the day-to-day running of our bodies) and inflammation. Fasting is also associated with a process called autophagy. Literally meaning 'self-eating', autophagy is the body's way of consuming and degrading old, worn out or damaged cells. Fasting can induce autophagy, which is, broadly speaking, the term used to refer to the clearing out of unwanted cells and cell debris, including autoimmune cells. Some scientific studies have shown clinical reductions in autoimmune symptoms using fasting regimes.[43] Fasting can also be a tool to induce beneficial alterations to the gut microbiome and gut barrier.

We still don't have a strong, effective protocol for how long a person must fast to experience these benefits, and this may, in any case, be different for everyone. When fasting, you may incur a calorie deficit, which can exaggerate muscle loss and nutrient deficiencies, which can already be an issue for those with AD.

There may be benefits to be had from daily time-restricted eating (TRE) – a pattern that focuses on when you eat, restricting food into a time window without limiting the amount of food over a twenty-four-hour period. Although there is little data on the benefits of TRE for AD, we do know it can improve gut-barrier function, blood sugar and metabolic health, as well as encouraging a calorie-appropriate diet.

The bottom line? The science is still so immature that I'd caution against doing any kind of fasting protocol without professional guidance.

Your nutritional goals

The overall aim should be to 'add in' as many beneficial whole, minimally processed foods as possible. If your body doesn't tolerate certain foods well, this is not always a sign that you need to exclude them, but more that you need to better support your gut microbes because they are doing most of the legwork to digest your food properly. If your gut is out of whack, food may be irritating your gut microbiome and gut barrier, thereby adding to your inflammatory load, and consequently aggravating your symptoms.

- Try to reduce ultra-processed foods and replace them with more whole foods.
- Aim for a portion of fibre-rich foods, a variety of fruits and vegetables, a protein source and healthy fats at each meal.
- Be careful with foods high in saturated fat, salt or sugar.
- Perform a well-controlled elimination diet on any suspect foods.
- Talk to your healthcare professional before embarking on any diet changes or supplement regimens.

EXERCISE SMART

When you have an AD, your body still needs to move and stay strong, mobile and healthy to reduce the risk of infections and chronic inflammatory conditions. Physical activity is proven safe and beneficial in people with a diagnosed AD and can reduce the side effects and symptoms significantly. Exercise, when done in the right way, is anti-inflammatory and can reduce fatigue and enhance mood and relieve stress as well as reducing the likelihood of frailty. We know that physically active AD patients tend to have a milder disease course and reduced risk of downstream consequences and co-morbidities, such as heart disease, as well as a better quality of life.[44, 45] On the flip side, exercise can aggravate AD symptoms if done in the wrong way.

Understandably, there can be a lot of fear and apprehension around exercising, not to mention a lack of information on the type you should or should not be doing. Physical activity with an AD first involves releasing preconceived notions of how we should exercise. You cannot exercise like everyone else because your AD body is not like everyone else's. And too much exercise *can* make your symptoms worse. A body with an AD needs to exercise for a body with an AD. You must be careful about how to exercise to ensure you get the benefits without the nasty side effects. It's a double-edged sword and it probably feels like you just can't win. But you *can* exercise, and a little bit goes a long way.

Symptom flare-ups, such as exhaustion, pain and the busyness of life, might mean you never feel ready. You'll tell yourself that you can't exercise until the flare-ups go away, until the exhaustion passes or until life gets less busy. But you don't need to feel better before you get moving. Instead, you can *use* movement to help you feel better. Living with a chronic inflammatory disease means you need the health benefits of exercise more than ever because it can help to decrease the exhaustion, pain and flare-ups. So don't put it off until you feel better. Instead, think about how you could incorporate just a teeny bit of exercise into your day to get those benefits.

Still confused or concerned? Let me take some of the guesswork out of it for you.

Striking a balance

As exercise can either power you up or drain you down, physical movement must be just right. Of course, this is very individualised and depends on how you feel, where you are at with your AD journey and your life load.

Ignore mainstream exercise messaging (for example, 'no pain, no gain') and the heavy focus on the aesthetic results of physical movement ('How to lose weight fast' and 'Six weeks to a six-pack'). These approaches are problematic in themselves, but completely inappropriate for people with AD, and can trigger added stress, force a flare and leave you disconnected from what your body is telling you. Respect those little signs that nudge you, telling you that you have done too much. And define your own goals.

A strong immune system needs strong muscles

Muscle is downright fundamental for healthy immune function and supporting metabolic health, both of which are out of whack in AD. It also reinforces a sense of enhanced quality of life and mental wellbeing, allowing you to be able to walk, bend, play, hike and engage in activities that bring you joy. Sadly, living with an AD can take its toll on your lean muscle mass due to years of living with pain, exhaustion, flare-ups and fear of movement.

Sarcopenia is also highly prevalent in people with AD and a known contributor to poor overall outcomes from living with a chronic disease.[46]

Living with AD means you still need to move and maintain muscle, but you need to be doing it differently. Your focus should be on rebuilding strength and maintaining lean muscle mass through gentle, restorative strength training and resistance exercises. How should you practise these? A teeny, tiny bit each and every day: slow and steady wins the race. If you flare, immediately reduce what you are doing. This is a signal that your body is not coping.

Try the following to work gently and slowly on building your foundations:

- Regular aerobic movement that raises your heart rate (this could be walking or light activities around the house, such as tidying). Daily is ideal, but frequency, duration and intensity will depend on your current health.
- Don't neglect muscle-strengthening exercises, as well as flexibility, mobility and balance two to three days per week.
- Include a daily tension-release routine that includes relaxation and stretching.
- Aim to complete several small routines across your week that, combined, include the whole body – even parts not normally seen in exercise programmes, such as feet, ankles and wrists.
- Work at your own pace, starting gently, with little intensity, and progressing in intensity over time.
- Keep a note of any movement that can be done without initiating a flare-up.
- Respect your limits and work within them.
- Make it fun! Find opportunities to move your body that also make you smile and max out on all the feelgood chem-

icals that can help with things such as pain. Find activities in places you enjoy and with people who make you feel supported, motivated and happy.

- Allow plenty of time to recover, replenish and rebuild. This may vary from person to person, depending on other things that are going on in your life, but look out for those messages that you need recovery time. These might be subtle, like finding yourself in a bad mood or being short with those around you. Or you may have prolonged body aches, joint pain and other such symptoms. Alternate active days with other days where you slow down and give your body time to recover.

AN INTEGRATED ANTI-INFLAMMATORY LIFESTYLE

For many people, diet is the largest lever in their autoimmune management. But although it plays a foundational role, it does not go the full distance. On any autoimmune journey it is imperative to use an anti-inflammatory diet pattern as part of an overall lifestyle approach.

Be sure to carve out space in your schedule for you and your condition. Self-care is a keystone part of managing your AD, alongside diet, exercise and medication. And the best part is that you can have fun with self-care. The goal is to enjoy and relax. It may take some experimentation, some trial and error, to fit your needs, but just get exploring. Carve out a slot of time just for you. Whatever you choose to do with your time, make it part of your routine every single day. Remember, this is non-negotiable.

Strong connections with the people around you will always

matter the most. There will be hard times, but with the right support you can weather the storms. Focus on bringing people into your life who can hold you up even when it gets hard. Unplug from negativity. This might include difficult relationships with loved ones or social media feeds. Ditch all the stuff that leaves you feeling drained and unsupported.

Now that you have a greater awareness of your body and how it is under constant physical stress from an AD, it might be easier to understand why living with a chronic illness can make you less able than others to handle additional outside sources of stress. Use Chapter 8 to help you consider your stress container. Think about the many additional types of stress outside your AD that you encounter every day. These everyday stressors can have a big impact on your ability to manage (or not manage) your AD. Explore the multitude of options for stress management. What works best is different for everyone, but as long as you arm yourself with some stress-management tools, you will benefit.

Self-care action plan

Which areas of your life require better balance? Is it sleep (see p. 237), stress (see p. 201) or your envrironment (see below)?

What can you do today to move towards better self-care?

Do an audit of relationships and activities in your life that feel draining and are not serving you.

Plan your day and week; keep a note of how much you can manage and adjust your load based on how you feel.

Environmental action plan

Although it can be impossible to know your true body burden or undo some of the exposures that you have experienced in the past, you can clean up your current environment and unburden your toxic load by avoiding some of the biggest environmental triggers listed on pp. 256–60. Being proactive, continuously supporting your body's own powerful detoxification systems, will alleviate any symptoms of your condition that may be related to toxicity.

PREPARE FOR A FLARE

If you suffer from an autoimmune disease, chances are you will be familiar with the sudden worsening of symptoms, known as a flare. A flare is a sign that your immune system isn't coping with both your AD and the demands of your life. It takes the form of an increase in symptoms specific to your condition (such as overwhelming fatigue, body aches and pains, a severe rash or stomach upset), but may also be accompanied by depression, anxiety, low mood, insomnia and brain fog. Sadly, this can last anywhere from weeks to months, substantially derailing your quality of life. It can knock you for six and make it even harder to pull back towards balance.

During a flare, your AD is active and your autoimmune processes are in the midst of attacking your own body. Autoimmune T cells are actively viewing parts of the body (such as tissues, an organ or even a group of organs) as foreign invaders and attacking them. Unfortunately, during an AD flare, regulatory T cells (Tregs), which are designed to control immune responses and maintain tolerance of the body's own antigens, are not functioning properly to prevent this immune-system attack. As you can imagine, this causes a lot of inflammation in the body and risks a process called 'epitope spreading' (see p. 329), causing a worsening of your condition and potentially predisposing you to development of more AD.

Know your triggers

Causal factors that initiated your autoimmunity are hard to pin down. But figuring out what is triggering a flare can feel even more challenging.

You might be thinking, 'But I'm healthy – why am I experiencing a flare?' It is important to look beyond the symptoms themselves to identify things that always make them worse. Whether that's alcohol, poor sleep or stress, exposure to certain products, infections or changes in the weather, when you tune into your own personal triggers, you can start to curate ways to apply preventative measures to contend with them.

Everyone's triggers will be different. For some, they might be hormonal. For example, we know that menstruation is accompanied by changes in immune function and that some conditions go into remission during pregnancy, yet return with a vengeance afterwards, whereas the opposite is true of other ADs.

Seasonal changes may also lead to flares. For example, the lack of vitamin D in winter correlates with increased disease activity in certain ADs. In the winter, there are also more infections that can be associated with flares, while spring pollens or leaf mould in the autumn may contribute, too.

Flare-ups are often most likely to arise when you are run down or as a result of lifestyle factors causing additional inflammation and oxidative stress. But they can also occur at random, without a clear trigger, seemingly caused by nothing that you can identify with any certainty. I personally think that flare-ups can be your body's expression of some form of physical, mental or emotional stress. This could be an infection, lack of sleep, nutritional deficiency, overexertion, grief or stress, and anxiety caused by traumatic life events. Paying close attention to your body and how circumstances may have changed right before a flare can help you to figure out the puzzle.

Take action

While it is hard – even impossible – to prevent an autoimmune flare-up, there are strategies to help manage the triggers that may be preventable.

- Keeping a log of your daily habits, meals and emotional health around the time of a flare-up can be an excellent tool for identifying triggers.
- If you know or suspect the trigger, then take action to avoid it.
- Slow down! Accept that you cannot continue in business-as-usual mode; a flare will take you out and require more from you. Ask for help and use the four Ds: **d**o what you can; **d**elay other tasks; **d**elegate where possible; and **d**ump everything else, so you can prioritise getting well.
- Try to identify ways to reduce the amount of stress in your life. For example, politely say 'No' to extra activities or additional responsibilities.
- When you have a flare-up, it's likely you won't want to exercise at all. You are probably already exhausted and may be suffering from severe joint and muscle pain. But gentle, low-impact exercises can help to improve fatigue and musculoskeletal pain, even in a flare-up.

- Make sleep and rest a high priority to help with recovery and repair of damaged tissues, replenishing energy stores and removing excess inflammation.
- Trust that this flare-up will pass and you will feel better. Flare-ups do not last for ever. Take care of yourself, try to keep perspective and think positive thoughts.

Improving your sense of wellbeing while living with your AD will be highly individual. Some people embarking on a lifestyle overhaul might experience a dramatic improvement, while for others it can be slower and more difficult. You won't know what to expect until you start and see how your body responds. The road to good health, especially if you have been sick for a long time or have a complex case, is never a straight line. It is often slower than you would like, and the most common trajectory is one step forwards and a few steps back. When you start to get better, suddenly there is hope. But the setbacks are hard. They are, however, a really important part of the process, teaching you many things – not least your relationship with your triggers.

Final Word

As clichéd as it might sound, your health really is your wealth. And it could have a larger impact on our future economic situation than many of us realise. The sudden arrival of COVID-19 might have moved this closer to the forefront of your mind, but knowing often isn't enough to drive us towards real lifestyle change.

So how do you acquire this elusive wealth? Well, for the minority it can be the privileges you are born with, genetic or otherwise. For the rest of us, living well means attending to every area of our lives: small, consistent investments across all elements take us in the direction of becoming self-made health millionaires.

Still, it can be challenging to know which route to follow or who to listen to. We have more access to health-related information than ever before, yet alarming statistics on the growing number of immune-related poor-health conditions. I'm not here to add to the background noise or to promise you a quick fix (I really wish I could). Rather, my hope is that this book will give you the science-based tools and knowledge that will empower you to take control of your health. But I also know that more information is not enough. Improving one's wellbeing is as much about psychology as it is immunology. Spending a day at a health spa is probably less beneficial than challenging our behaviours, changing our environments or making small improvements to our daily habits.

On any journey, we need to begin by becoming well orientated and well grounded in where we are and what we want to achieve. That is why this path will look different for each and every one of us. Rather than an X on the map where the trail ends, it's about doing our best to prepare for what might be around the next bend. Let this book guide you on how to personalise your approach and weave it all together with achievable goals and consistent habits. Like a mountain guide, I am not here to do the climbing *for* you, but to improve your chances of success by providing a good, solid rope to support you on your own personal path.

As science continues to unravel the perplexing questions around how and why our diets, lifestyles and environments make us ill, we can take action on what we already know works. Remember, you don't have to be perfect to be well. It's about incremental growth and travelling the path with heart. Self-compassion will empower you to embrace challenges and setbacks as part of the process and allow you to let go of anything unhelpful to which you have been holding fast. You are your own best asset. Make this a part of your identity: *this is what I do; this is who I am*. Your immunobiography has got you to this starting point – now let's embrace a healthier future without dragging the past behind. Start writing the next chapter today.

Acknowledgements

A book is rarely the work of just the author named on the front cover. This book is the result of hard work by a number of people. Firstly of course I have to thank my (long suffering) family, especially my children and husband for their patience and support as I juggled the writing on top of everything else. My parents, John and Margaret, as well as my in-laws, Lorraine and Tony, for their continued support of everything that I do.

Thanks to my 'inner circle' – those wonderful friends who know who they are. This period of my life was filled with many intense and stressful moments. My dear friends who continued to check in on me and were always there when I needed someone to laugh or cry with.

To Carly, I couldn't ask for a better, more supportive and compassionate manager. Without you the vague book concept in my head would never have made it into a book proposal, let alone a finished manuscript. You have been there guiding me through every step from idea to publication and I am both grateful and honoured to be able to work with you. And of course, to Holly and the rest of the Found Entertainment family for their continued efforts and encouragement to grow in this space in an authentic way.

Finally, to my publisher Yellow Kite. Carolyn, the editorial director, for giving me this opportunity, for believing in me and providing me with valuable support to get me to the end of the process. I never thought I'd get to write one book, let alone two. To Anne for her enduring patience during the editing process. And the fantastic Yellow Kite team for all your support and ideas to help me bring this book to life and to a wide audience.

References

INTRODUCTION

1 *Long Term Conditions Compendium of Information: Third Edition – GOV.UK*. (n.d.). Retrieved 26 October 2021 from https://www.gov.uk/government/publications/long-term-conditions-compendium-of-information-third-edition
2 Ayres, J. S. (2020). 'The Biology of Physiological Health.' *Cell 181*(2). https://doi.org/10.1016/j.cell.2020.03.036

CHAPTER 1

1 Choo, S. Y. (2007). 'The HLA System: Genetics, Immunology, Clinical Testing, and Clinical Implications.' *Yonsei Medical Journal*, *48*(1), 11. https://doi.org/10.3349/YMJ.2007.48.1.11
2 Fricke-Galindo, I. and Falfán-Valencia, R. (2021). 'Genetics Insight for COVID-19 Susceptibility and Severity: A Review.' *Frontiers in Immunology*, *12*. https://doi.org/10.3389/FIMMU.2021.622176

CHAPTER 2

1 Tracy, R. P. (2006). 'The Five Cardinal Signs of Inflammation: Calor, Dolor, Rubor, Tumor . . . and Penuria (Apologies to Aulus Cornelius Celsus, *De medicina*, c. A.D. 25).' *Journals of Gerontology: Series A*, *61*(10), 1051–1052. https://doi.org/10.1093/GERONA/61.10.1051
2 Nathan, C. and Ding, A. (2010). 'Nonresolving Inflammation.' *Cell* 140(2). https://doi.org/10.1016/j.cell.2010.02.029
3 Blanco-Melo, D., Nilsson-Payant, B. E., Liu, W. C., Uhl, S., Hoagland, D., Møller, R., Jordan, T. X., Oishi, K., Panis, M., Sachs, D., Wang, T. T., Schwartz, R. E., Lim, J. K., Albrecht, R. A. and tenOever, B. R. (2020). 'Imbalanced Host Response to SARS-CoV-2 Drives Development of COVID-19.' *Cell*, *181*(5). https://doi.org/10.1016/j.cell.2020.04.026
4 Baylis, D., Bartlett, D. B., Patel, H. P. and Roberts, H. C. (2013). 'Understanding how we age: insights into inflammaging.' *Longevity & Healthspan*, *2*(1). https://doi.org/10.1186/2046-2395-2-8
5 Hunter, P. (2012). 'The inflammation theory of disease: The growing realization that

chronic inflammation is crucial in many diseases opens new avenues for treatment.' *EMBO Reports*, *13*(11), 968. https://doi.org/10.1038/EMBOR.2012.142

6 Luthra-Guptasarma, M. and Guptasarma, P. (2021). 'Does chronic inflammation cause acute inflammation to spiral into hyper-inflammation in a manner modulated by diet and the gut microbiome, in severe Covid-19?' *BioEssays*, 2000211. https://doi.org/10.1002/BIES.202000211

7 Sayed, N., Huang, Y., Nguyen, K., Krejciova-Rajaniemi, Z., Grawe, A. P., Gao, T., Tibshirani, R., Hastie, T., Alpert, A., Cui, L., Kuznetsova, T., Rosenberg-Hasson, Y., Ostan, R., Monti, D., Lehallier, B., Shen-Orr, S. S., Maecker, H. T., Dekker, C. L., Wyss-Coray, T., . . . Furman, D. (2021). 'An inflammatory aging clock (iAge) based on deep learning tracks multimorbidity, immunosenescence, frailty and cardiovascular aging.' *Nature Aging*, *1*(7), 598–615. https://doi.org/10.1038/s43587-021-00082-y

8 Elliott, M. L., Caspi, A., Houts, R. M., Ambler, A., Broadbent, J. M., Hancox, R. J., Harrington, H., Hogan, S., Keenan, R., Knodt, A., Leung, J. H., Melzer, T. R., Purdy, S. C., Ramrakha, Sandhya, Richmond-Rakerd, L. S., Righarts, A., Sugden, K., Thomson, W. Murray, Thorne, P. R., Williams, B. S., Wilson, G., Hariri, A. R., Poulton, R., Moffitt, T. E. (2021). 'Disparities in the pace of biological aging among midlife adults of the same chronological age have implications for future frailty risk and policy.' *Nature Aging*, *1*(3), 295–308. https://doi.org/10.1038/S43587-021-00044-4

9 Akbar, A. N. and Gilroy, D. W. (2020). 'Aging immunity may exacerbate COVID-19.' *Science 369*(6501). https://doi.org/10.1126/science.abb0762

10 Oh, S.-J., Lee, J. K. and Shin, O. S. (2019). 'Aging and the immune system: the impact of immunosenescence on viral infection, immunity and vaccine immunogenicity.' *Immune Network*, *19*(6). https://doi.org/10.4110/IN.2019.19.E37

11 Lian, J., Yue, Y., Yu, W. and Zhang, Y. (2020). 'Immunosenescence: a key player in cancer development.' *Journal of Hematology & Oncology*, 13(1), 1–18. https://doi.org/10.1186/S13045-020-00986-Z

12 Aiello, A., Farzaneh, F., Candore, G., Caruso, C., Davinelli, S., Gambino, C. M., Ligotti, M. E., Zareian, N. and Accardi, G. (2019). 'Immunosenescence and its hallmarks: how to oppose aging strategically? A review of potential options for therapeutic intervention.' *Frontiers in Immunology*, 0(SEP), 2247. https://doi.org/10.3389/FIMMU.2019.02247

13 K, K. and K, G. (2021). 'The Impact of Sedentary Lifestyle, High-fat Diet, Tobacco Smoke, and Alcohol Intake on the Hematopoietic Stem Cell Niches.' *HemaSphere*, 5(8). https://doi.org/10.1097/HS9.0000000000000615

14 Mihaylova, M. M., Sabatini, D. M. and Yilmaz, Ö. H. (2014). 'Dietary and Metabolic Control of Stem Cell Function in Physiology and Cancer.' *Cell Stem Cell*, 14(3), 292. https://doi.org/10.1016/J.STEM.2014.02.008

15 Worley, J. R. and Parker, G. C. (2019). 'Effects of environmental stressors on stem cells.' *World Journal of Stem Cells*, *11*(9), 565. https://doi.org/10.4252/WJSC.V11.I9.565

16 Aiello, A., et al., op. cit.

17 Zhu, X., Chen, Z., Shen, W., Huang, G., Sedivy, J. M., Wang, H. and Ju, Z. (2021). 'Inflammation, epigenetics, and metabolism converge to cell senescence and ageing: the regulation and intervention.' *Signal Transduction and Targeted Therapy*, 6(1). https://doi.org/10.1038/S41392-021-00646-9

CHAPTER 3

1 Grignolio, A., Mishto, M., Caetano Faria, A. M., Garagnani, P., Franceschi1, C., Tieri, P. (2014). 'Towards a liquid self: how time, geography, and life experiences reshape the biological identity.' *Frontiers in Immunology*, *5*(Apr). https://doi.org/10.3389/FIMMU.2014.00153

2 Lijoi, A. F., Tovar, A. D. (2020). 'Narrative medicine: Re-engaging and re-energizing ourselves through story.' *International Journal of Psychiatry in Medicine*, *55*(5), 321–330. https://doi.org/10.1177/009121 7420951039

3 Renz, H., Holt, P. G., Inouye, M., Logan, A. C., Prescott, S. L. and Sly, P. D. (2017). 'An exposome perspective: Early-life events and immune development in a changing world.' *Journal of Allergy and Clinical Immunology*, 140(1), 24–40. https://doi.org/10.1016/J.JACI.2017.05.015

CHAPTER 4

1 Aeberli, I., Gerber, P. A., Hochuli, M., Kohler, S., Haile, S. R., Gouni-Berthold, I., Berthold, H. K., Spinas, G. A. and Berneis, K. (2011). 'Low to moderate sugar-sweetened beverage consumption impairs glucose and lipid metabolism and promotes inflammation in healthy young men: A randomized controlled trial.' *American Journal of Clinical Nutrition*, *94*(2), 479–485. https://doi.org/10.3945/ajcn.111.013540

2 Myles, I. A. (2014). 'Fast food fever: reviewing the impacts of the Western diet on immunity.' *Nutrition Journal* 13(1), 1–17. https://doi.org/10.1186/1475-2891-13-61

3 Sheeran, P., Maki, A., Montanaro, E., Avishai-Yitshak, A., Bryan, A., Klein, W. M., Miles, E., Rothman, A. J. (2016). 'The impact of changing attitudes, norms, and self-efficacy on health-related intentions and behavior: A meta-analysis.' *Health Psychology: Official Journal of the Division of Health Psychology, American Psychological Association*, *35*(11), 1178–1188. https://doi.org/10.1037/HEA0000387

4 Lally, P., van Jaarsveld, C. H. M., Potts, H. W. W. and Wardle, J. (2010). 'How are habits formed: Modelling habit formation in the real world.' *European Journal of Social Psychology*, 40(6), 998–1009. https://doi.org/10.1002/EJSP.674

5 Bovend'Eerdt, T. J., Botell, R. E., Wade, D. T. (2009). 'Writing SMART rehabilitation goals and achieving goal attainment scaling: a practical guide.' *Clinical Rehabilitation*, 23(4), 352–361. https://doi.org/10.1177/0269215508101741

CHAPTER 5

1 *The Eatwell Guide – NHS* (n.d.). Retrieved 27 October 2021 from https://www.nhs.uk/live-well/eat-well/the-eatwell-guide/

2 Ashton L. M., Hutchesson M. J., Rollo M. E., Morgan P. J., Collins C. E. (2017). 'Motivators and Barriers to Engaging in Healthy Eating and Physical Activity.' *American Journal of Men's Health*, *11*(2), 330–343. https://doi.org/10.1177/1557988316680936

3 Pacheco, A. F., Balam, G. C., Archibald, D., Grant, E. and Skafida, V. (2018) 'Exploring the relationship between local food environments and obesity in the UK, Ireland,

Australia and New Zealand: a systematic review protocol.' *BMJ Open*, 8(2), e018701. https://doi.org/10.1136/BMJOPEN-2017-018701
4. Monteiro, C. A. (2009). 'Nutrition and health. The issue is not food, nor nutrients, so much as processing.' *Public Health Nutrition*, 12(5), 729–731. https://doi.org/10.1017/S1368980009005291
5 Monteiro C. A., Cannon G., Moubarac J. C., Levy R. B., Louzada M. L. C., Jaime P. C. (2018). 'The UN Decade of Nutrition, the NOVA food classification and the trouble with ultra-processing.' *Public Health Nutrition*, 21(1), 5–17. https://doi.org/10.1017/S1368980017000234
6 Rauber, F., da Costa Louzada, M. L., Steele, E. M., Millett, C., Monteiro, C. A. and Levy, R. B. (2018). 'Ultra-Processed Food Consumption and Chronic Non-Communicable Diseases-Related Dietary Nutrient Profile in the UK (2008–2014).' *Nutrients*, 10(5). https://doi.org/10.3390/NU10050587
7 Rico-Campà, A., Martínez-González, M. A., Alvarez-Alvarez, I., de Deus Mendonça, R., de la Fuente-Arrillaga, C., Gómez-Donoso, C. and Bes-Rastrollo, M. (2019). 'Association between consumption of ultra-processed foods and all cause mortality: SUN prospective cohort study.' *BMJ*, 365. https://doi.org/10.1136/BMJ.L1949
8 Hall, K. D., Ayuketah, A., Brychta, R., Cai, H., Cassimatis, T., Chen, K. Y., Chung, S. T., Costa, E., Courville, A., Darcey, V., Fletcher, L. A., Forde, C. G., Gharib, A. M., Guo, J., Howard, R., Joseph, P. V., McGehee, S., Ouwerkerk, R., Raisinger, K., Zhou, M. (2019). 'Ultra-Processed Diets Cause Excess Calorie Intake and Weight Gain: An Inpatient Randomized Controlled Trial of Ad Libitum Food Intake.' *Cell Metabolism*, 30(1), 67-77.e3. https://doi.org/10.1016/J.CMET.2019.05.008
9 Zinöcker M. K., Lindseth I. A. (2018). 'The Western Diet-Microbiome-Host Interaction and Its Role in Metabolic Disease.' *Nutrients*, 10(3). https://doi.org/10.3390/NU10030365
10 Prescott, S. L. and Logan, A. C. (2017). 'Each meal matters in the exposome: Biological and community considerations in fast-food-socioeconomic associations.' *Economics & Human Biology*, 27, 328–335. https://doi.org/10.1016/J.EHB.2017.09.004
11 Cena H., Calder P. C. (2020). 'Defining a Healthy Diet: Evidence for the Role of Contemporary Dietary Patterns in Health and Disease.' *Nutrients*, 12(2). https://doi.org/10.3390/NU12020334
12 Steinberg, D., Bennett, G. G. and Svetkey, L. (2017). 'The DASH Diet, 20 Years Later.' *Journal of the American Medical Association* (JAMA) (317(15), 1529. https://doi.org/10.1001/JAMA.2017.1628
13 Davis C., Bryan J., Hodgson J., Murphy K. (2015). 'Definition of the Mediterranean Diet; a Literature Review.' *Nutrients*, 7(11), 9139–9153. https://doi.org/10.3390/NU7115459
14 Shan Z., Li Y., Baden M. Y. (2020). 'Association Between Healthy Eating Patterns and Risk of Cardiovascular Disease.' *JAMA Internal Medicine*, 180(8), 1090–1100. https://doi.org/10.1001/JAMAINTERNMED.2020.2176
15 Vajdi, M. and Farhangi, M. A. (2020). 'A systematic review of the association between dietary patterns and health-related quality of life.' *Health and Quality of Life Outcomes*, 18(1), 1–15. https://doi.org/10.1186/S12955-020-01581-Z

CHAPTER 6

1 Toft, P. and Stroem, T. (2018). 'Fever during septic shock, friend or foe?' *Journal of Emergency and Critical Care Medicine*, 2, 42–42. https://doi.org/10.21037/JECCM.2018.04.06

2 Makowski, L., Chaib, M., Rathmell, J. C. (2020). 'Immunometabolism: From basic mechanisms to translation.' *Immunological Reviews*, *295*(1), 5–14. https://doi.org/10.1111/IMR.12858

3 Araújo, Cai, and Stevens, (2019). 'Prevalence of Optimal Metabolic Health in American Adults: National Health and Nutrition Examination Survey 2009–2016.' *Https://Home.Liebertpub.Com/Met*, *17*(1), 46–52. https://doi.org/10.1089/MET.2018.0105

4 Andersen, C. J., Murphy, K. E. and Fernandez, M. L. (2016). 'Impact of Obesity and Metabolic Syndrome on Immunity.' *Advances in Nutrition*, *7*(1), 66–75. https://doi.org/10.3945/AN.115.010207

5 Wood, T. R. and Jóhannsson, G. F. (2020). 'Metabolic health and lifestyle medicine should be a cornerstone of future pandemic preparedness.' *Lifestyle Medicine*, *1*(1), e2. https://doi.org/10.1002/LIM2.2

6 Carroll S., Dudfield M. (2004). 'What is the relationship between exercise and metabolic abnormalities? A review of the metabolic syndrome.' *Sports Medicine (Auckland, N.Z.)*, *34*(6), 371–418. https://doi.org/10.2165/00007256-200434060-00004

7 Logette, E., Lorin, C., Favreau, C., Oshurko, E., Coggan, J. S., Casalegno, F., Sy, M. F., Monney, C., Bertschy, M., Delattre, E., Fonta, P.-A., Krepl, J., Schmidt, S., Keller, D., Kerrien, S., Scantamburlo, E., Kaufmann, A.-K. and Markram, H. (2021). 'A Machine-Generated View of the Role of Blood Glucose Levels in the Severity of COVID-19.' *Frontiers in Public Health*, 0, 1068. https://doi.org/10.3389/FPUBH.2021.695139

8 Berry, S. E., Valdes, A. M., Drew, D. A., Asnicar, F., Mazidi, M., Wolf, J., Capdevila, J., Hadjigeorgiou, G., Davies, R., Al Khatib, H., Bonnett, C., Ganesh, S., Bakker, E., Hart, D., Mangino, M., Merino, J., Linenberg, I., Wyatt, P., Ordovas, J. M. . . . Spector, T. D. (2020). 'Human postprandial responses to food and potential for precision nutrition.' *Nature Medicine*, *26*(6), 964–973. https://doi.org/10.1038/s41591-020-0934-0

9 DiPietro, L., Gribok, A., Stevens, M. S., Hamm, L. F. and Rumpler, W. (2013). 'Three 15-min Bouts of Moderate Postmeal Walking Significantly Improves 24-h Glycemic Control in Older People at Risk for Impaired Glucose Tolerance.' *Diabetes Care*, *36*(10), 3262–3268. https://doi.org/10.2337/DC13-0084

10 Burton H. M., Coyle E. F. (2021). 'Daily Step Count and Postprandial Fat Metabolism.' *Medicine and Science in Sports and Exercise*, *53*(2), 333–340. https://doi.org/10.1249/MSS.0000000000002486

11 Crosby, P., Hamnett, R., Putker, M., Hoyle, N. P., Reed, M., Karam, C. J., Maywood, E. S., Stangherlin, A., Chesham, J. E., Hayter, E. A., Rosenbrier-Ribeiro, L., Newham, P., Clevers, H., Bechtold, D. A. and O'Neill, J. S. (2019). 'Insulin/IGF-1 Drives PERIOD Synthesis to Entrain Circadian Rhythms with Feeding Time.' *Cell*, *177*(4), 896-909.e20. https://doi.org/10.1016/J.CELL.2019.02.017

12 Valdes D. S., So D., Gill P. A., Kellow N. J. (2021). 'Effect of Dietary Acetic Acid Supplementation on Plasma Glucose, Lipid Profiles, and Body Mass Index in Human Adults: A Systematic Review and Meta-analysis.' *Journal of the Academy of Nutrition and Dietetics*, *121*(5), 895–914. https://doi.org/10.1016/J.JAND.2020.12.002

13 Lohner S., Toews I., Meerpohl J. J. (2017). 'Health outcomes of non-nutritive

sweeteners: analysis of the research landscape.' *Nutrition Journal*, *16*(1). https://doi.org/10.1186/S12937-017-0278-X

14 Kim Y., Keogh J. B., Clifton P. M. (2019). 'Non-nutritive Sweeteners and Glycaemic Control.' *Current Atherosclerosis Reports*, *21*(12). https://doi.org/10.1007/S11883-019-0814-6

15 MV, B. and DM, S. (2015). 'Physiological mechanisms by which non-nutritive sweeteners may impact body weight and metabolism.' *Physiology & Behavior*, *152*(Pt B), 381–388. https://doi.org/10.1016/J.PHYSBEH.2015.05.036

16 Chen, X., Wu, Y. and Wang, L. (2013). 'Fat-resident Tregs: an emerging guard protecting from obesity-associated metabolic disorders.' *Obesity Reviews*, *14*(7), 568–578. https://doi.org/10.1111/OBR.12033

17 *Obesity and overweight* (n.d.). Retrieved 27 October 2021 from https://www.who.int/news-room/fact-sheets/detail/obesity-and-overweight

18 Spreckley, M., Seidell, J. and Halberstadt, J. (2021). 'Perspectives into the experience of successful, substantial long-term weight-loss maintenance: a systematic review.' *International Journal of Qualitative Studies on Health and Well-Being*, *16*(1). https://doi.org/10.1080/17482631.2020.1862481

19 *Overweight and obesity statistics | Cancer Research UK* (n.d.). Retrieved 27 October 2021 from https://www.cancerresearchuk.org/health-professional/cancer-statistics/risk/overweight-and-obesity#heading-Zero

20 Emmer C., Bosnjak M., Mata J. (2020). 'The association between weight stigma and mental health: A meta-analysis.' *Obesity Reviews: An Official Journal of the International Association for the Study of Obesity*, *21*(1). https://doi.org/10.1111/OBR.12935

21 Wansink, B. and Sobal, J. (2016). 'Mindless Eating: The 200 Daily Food Decisions We Overlook.' *Http://Dx.Doi.Org/10.1177/0013916506295573*, *39*(1), 106–123. https://doi.org/10.1177/0013916506295573

22 Perry, B. and Wang, Y. (2012). 'Appetite regulation and weight control: the role of gut hormones.' *Nutrition & Diabetes*, *2*(1), e26–e26. https://doi.org/10.1038/nutd.2011.21

23 Lee M. J., Kim E. H., Bae S. J., Choe J., Jung C. H., Lee W. J., Kim H. K. (2019). 'Protective role of skeletal muscle mass against progression from metabolically healthy to unhealthy phenotype.' *Clinical Endocrinology*, *90*(1), 102–113. https://doi.org/10.1111/CEN.13874

24 Westbury, L. D., Fuggle, N. R., Syddall, H. E., Duggal, N. A., Shaw, S. C., Maslin, K., Dennison, E. M., Lord, J. M. and Cooper, C. (2018). 'Relationships Between Markers of Inflammation and Muscle Mass, Strength and Function: Findings from the Hertfordshire Cohort Study.' *Calcified Tissue International*, *102*(3), 287. https://doi.org/10.1007/S00223-017-0354-4

25 Cruz-Jentoft, A. J., Bahat, G., Bauer, J., Boirie, Y., Bruyère, O., Cederholm, T., Cooper, C., Landi, F., Rolland, Y., Sayer, A. A., Schneider, S. M., Sieber, C. C., Topinkova, E., Vandewoude, M., Visser, M., Zamboni, M., (EWGSOP2), W. G. for the E. W. G. on S. in O. P. 2 and EWGSOP2, and the E. G. for EWGSOP2. (2019). 'Sarcopenia: revised European consensus on definition and diagnosis.' *Age and Ageing*, *48*(1), 16. https://doi.org/10.1093/AGEING/AFY169

CHAPTER 7

1 Calder, P. C., Carr, A. C., Gombart, A. F. and Eggersdorfer, M. (2020). 'Optimal Nutritional Status for a Well-Functioning Immune System Is an Important Factor to Protect against Viral Infections.' *Nutrients*, 12(4), 1181. https://doi.org/10.3390/NU12041181
2 Louca, P., Murray, B., Klaser, K., Graham, M. S., Mazidi, M., Leeming, E. R., Thompson, E., Bowyer, R., Drew, D. A., Nguyen, L. H., Merino, J., Gomez, M., Mompeo, O., Costeira, R., Sudre, C. H., Gibson, R., Steves, C. J., Wolf, J., Franks, P. W. . . . Menni, C. (2021). 'Modest effects of dietary supplements during the COVID-19 pandemic: insights from 445 850 users of the COVID-19 Symptom Study app.' *BMJ Nutrition, Prevention & Health*, 4(1), 250. https://doi.org/10.1136/BMJNPH-2021-000250
3 Kamangar, F. and Emadi, A. (2012). 'Vitamin and Mineral Supplements: Do We Really Need Them?' *International Journal of Preventive Medicine*, 3(3), 221. /pmc/articles/PMC3309636/
4 Siems W., Wiswedel I., Salerno C., Crifò C., Augustin W., Schild L., Langhans C. D., Sommerburg O. (2005). 'Beta-carotene breakdown products may impair mitochondrial functions—potential side effects of high-dose beta-carotene supplementation.' *Journal of Nutritional Biochemistry*, 16(7), 385–397. https://doi.org/10.1016/J.JNUTBIO.2005.01.009
5 Halliwell, B. (2013). 'The antioxidant paradox: less paradoxical now?' *British Journal of Clinical Pharmacology*, 75(3), 637. https://doi.org/10.1111/J.1365-2125.2012.04272.X
6 Franke, A. A., Cooney, R. V., Henning, S. M. and Custer, L. J. (2005). 'Bioavailability and antioxidant effects of orange juice components in humans.' *Journal of Agricultural and Food Chemistry*, 53(13), 5170. https://doi.org/10.1021/JF050054Y
7 Weiss, S. T. and Litonjua, A. A. (2015). 'Vitamin D dosing for infectious and immune disorders.' *Thorax*, 70(10), 919–920. https://doi.org/10.1136/THORAXJNL-2015-207334
8 Hosseini B., Berthon B. S., Saedisomeolia A., Starkey M. R., Collison A., Wark P. A. B., Wood L. G. (2018). 'Effects of fruit and vegetable consumption on inflammatory biomarkers and immune cell populations: a systematic literature review and meta-analysis.' *American Journal of Clinical Nutrition*, 108(1), 136–155. https://doi.org/10.1093/AJCN/NQY082
9 Saleh, H. A., Yousef, M. H. and Abdelnaser, A. (2021). 'The Anti-Inflammatory Properties of Phytochemicals and Their Effects on Epigenetic Mechanisms Involved in TLR4/NF-κB-Mediated Inflammation.' *Frontiers in Immunology*, 0, 919. https://doi.org/10.3389/FIMMU.2021.606069
10 Pandey, K. B. and Rizvi, S. I. (2009). 'Plant polyphenols as dietary antioxidants in human health and disease.' *Oxidative Medicine and Cellular Longevity*, 2(5), 270. https://doi.org/10.4161/OXIM.2.5.9498
11 Adusumilli, N. C., Zhang, D., Friedman, J. M. and Friedman, A. J. (2020). 'Harnessing nitric oxide for preventing, limiting and treating the severe pulmonary consequences of COVID-19.' *Nitric Oxide*, 103, 4–8. https://doi.org/10.1016/J.NIOX.2020.07.003
12 Milkowski A., Garg H. K., Coughlin J. R., Bryan N. S. (2010). 'Nutritional epidemiology in the context of nitric oxide biology: a risk-benefit evaluation for dietary nitrite and nitrate.' *Nitric Oxide: Biology and Chemistry*, 22(2), 110–119. https://doi.org/10.1016/J.NIOX.2009.08.004
13 Steinbrecher A., Linseisen J. (2009). 'Dietary intake of individual glucosinolates in participants of the EPIC-Heidelberg cohort study.' *Annals of Nutrition & Metabolism*, 54(2), 87–96. https://doi.org/10.1159/000209266

14 Wagner A.E., Boesch-Saadatmandi C., Dose J., Schultheiss G., Rimbach G. (2012). 'Anti-inflammatory potential of allyl-isothiocyanate—role of Nrf2, NF-(κ) B and microRNA-155.' *Journal of Cellular and Molecular Medicine*, 16(4), 836–843. https://doi.org/10.1111/J.1582-4934.2011.01367.X

15 Higdon J. V., Delage B., Williams D. E., Dashwood R. H. (2007). 'Cruciferous vegetables and human cancer risk: epidemiologic evidence and mechanistic basis.' *Pharmacological Research*, 55(3), 224–236. https://doi.org/10.1016/J.PHRS.2007.01.009

16 Bai Y., Wang X., Zhao S., Ma C., Cui J., Zheng Y. (2015). 'Sulforaphane Protects against Cardiovascular Disease via Nrf2 Activation.' *Oxidative Medicine and Cellular Longevity*, 2015. https://doi.org/10.1155/2015/407580

17 Ciecierska A., Drywień M. E., Hamulka J., Sadkowski T. (2019). 'Nutraceutical functions of beta-glucans in human nutrition.' *Roczniki Panstwowego Zakladu Higieny*, 70(4), 315–324. https://doi.org/10.32394/RPZH.2019.0082

18 Castro, E. D. M., Calder, P. C. and Roche, H. M. (2021). 'β-1,3/1,6-Glucans and Immunity: State of the Art and Future Directions.' *Molecular Nutrition & Food Research*, 65(1). https://doi.org/10.1002/MNFR.201901071

19 'Infection prevention in patients with severe multiple trauma with the immunomodulator beta 1-3 polyglucose (glucan).' *Cochrane Library* (n.d.). Retrieved 27 October 2021, from https://www.cochranelibrary.com/central/doi/10.1002/central/CN-00096453/full

20 Park, J. S., Chyun, J. H., Kim, Y. K., Line, L. L. and Chew, B. P. (2010). 'Astaxanthin decreased oxidative stress and inflammation and enhanced immune response in humans.' *Nutrition & Metabolism*, 7, 18. https://doi.org/10.1186/1743-7075-7-18

21 Scrimshaw N. S., SanGiovanni J. P. (1997). 'Synergism of nutrition, infection, and immunity: an overview.' *American Journal of Clinical Nutrition*, 66(2). https://doi.org/10.1093/AJCN/66.2.464S

22 Phillips, S. M. (2015). 'Nutritional Supplements in Support of Resistance Exercise to Counter Age-Related Sarcopenia.' *Advances in Nutrition*, 6(4), 452. https://doi.org/10.3945/AN.115.008367

23 Gutiérrez, S., Svahn, S. L. and Johansson, M. E. (2019). 'Effects of omega-3 fatty acids on immune cells.' *International Journal of Molecular Sciences*:, 20(20). https://doi.org/10.3390/ijms20205028

24 Ravaut, G., Légiot, A., Bergeron, K.-F. and Mounier, C. (2021). 'Monounsaturated Fatty Acids in Obesity-Related Inflammation.' *International Journal of Molecular Sciences*, 22(1), 1–22. https://doi.org/10.3390/IJMS22010330

25 Osborn, O., Sears, D. D. and Olefsky, J. M. (2010). 'Previews: Fat-Induced Inflammation Unchecked.' *Cell Metabolism*, 12, 553–554. https://doi.org/10.1016/j.cmet.2010.11.017

26 Pipoyan, D., Stepanyan, S., Stepanyan, S., Beglaryan, M., Costantini, L., Molinari, R. and Merendino, N. (2021). 'The Effect of Trans Fatty Acids on Human Health: Regulation and Consumption Patterns.' *Foods*, 10(10), 2452. https://doi.org/10.3390/FOODS10102452

27 Shan, Z., Rehm, C. D., Rogers, G., Ruan, M., Wang, D. D., Hu, F. B., Mozaffarian, D., Zhang, F. F. and Bhupathiraju, S. N. (2019). 'Trends in Dietary Carbohydrate, Protein, and Fat Intake and Diet Quality Among US Adults, 1999-2016.' *JAMA*, 322(12), 1178–1187. https://doi.org/10.1001/JAMA.2019.13771

28 Thorup, A. C., Kristensen, H. L., Kidmose, U., Lambert, M. N. T., Christensen, L. P., Fretté, X., Clausen, M. R., Hansen, S. M. and Jeppesen, P. B. (2021). 'Strong and Bitter Vegetables from Traditional Cultivars and Cropping Methods Improve the

Health Status of Type 2 Diabetics: A Randomized Control Trial.' *Nutrients, 13*(6), 1813. https://doi.org/10.3390/NU13061813

29 Patel, N. N., Workman, A. D. and Cohen, N. A. (2018). 'Role of Taste Receptors as Sentinels of Innate Immunity in the Upper Airway.' *Journal of Pathogens, 2018*, 1–8. https://doi.org/10.1155/2018/9541987

30 Di Bona, D., Malovini, A., Accardi, G., Aiello, A., Candore, G., Ferrario, A., Ligotti, M. E., Maciag, A., Puca, A. A. and Caruso, C. (2020). 'Taste receptor polymorphisms and longevity: a systematic review and meta-analysis.' *Aging Clinical and Experimental Research, 33*(9), 2369–2377. https://doi.org/10.1007/S40520-020-01745-3

31 Lee, R. J., Xiong, G., Kofonow, J. M., Chen, B., Lysenko, A., Jiang, P., Abraham, V., Doghramji, L., Adappa, N. D., Palmer, J. N., Kennedy, D. W., Beauchamp, G. K., Doulias, P.-T., Ischiropoulos, H., Kreindler, J. L., Reed, D. R. and Cohen, N. A. (2012). 'T2R38 taste receptor polymorphisms underlie susceptibility to upper respiratory infection.' *Journal of Clinical Investigation, 122*(11), 4145–4159. https://doi.org/10.1172/JCI64240

32 Maggs J. L., Staff J. (2017). 'No Benefit of Light to Moderate Drinking for Mortality From Coronary Heart Disease When Better Comparison Groups and Controls Included: A Commentary on Zhao et al.' *Journal of Studies on Alcohol and Drugs, 78*(3), 387–388. https://doi.org/10.15288/JSAD.2017.78.387

33 Hill, J. H. and Round, J. L. (2021). 'SnapShot: Microbiota effects on host physiology.' *Cell, 184*. https://doi.org/10.1016/j.cell.2021.04.026

34 Hooper L. V., Midtvedt T., Gordon J. I. (2002). 'How host-microbial interactions shape the nutrient environment of the mammalian intestine.' *Annual Review of Nutrition, 22*, 283–307. https://doi.org/10.1146/ANNUREV.NUTR.22.011602.092259

35 Zheng, D., Liwinski, T. and Elinav, E. (2020). 'Interaction between microbiota and immunity in health and disease.' *Cell Research, 30*(6), 492–506. https://doi.org/10.1038/s41422-020-0332-7

36 Pelton, R. (2020). 'Postbiotic Metabolites: How Probiotics Regulate Health.' *Integrative Medicine: A Clinician's Journal, 19*(1), 25. /pmc/articles/PMC7238912/

37 Li, M., van Esch, B. C. A. M., Henricks, P. A. J., Folkerts, G. and Garssen, J. (2018). 'The Anti-inflammatory Effects of Short Chain Fatty Acids on Lipopolysaccharide- or Tumor Necrosis Factor α-Stimulated Endothelial Cells via Activation of GPR41/43 and Inhibition of HDACs.' *Frontiers in Pharmacology, 0*(MAY), 533. https://doi.org/10.3389/FPHAR.2018.00533

38 Wells, J. M., Brummer, R. J., Derrien, M., MacDonald, T. T., Troost, F., Cani, P. D., Theodorou, V., Dekker, J., Méheust, A., Vos, W. M. de, Mercenier, A., Nauta, A. and Garcia-Rodenas, C. L. (2017). 'Homeostasis of the gut barrier and potential biomarkers.' *Https://Doi.Org/10.1152/Ajpgi.00048.2015, 312*, 171–193. https://doi.org/10.1152/AJPGI.00048.2015

39 Kamada, N., Chen, G. Y., Inohara, N. and Núñez, G. (2013). 'Control of Pathogens and Pathobionts by the Gut Microbiota.' *Nature Immunology, 14*(7), 685. https://doi.org/10.1038/NI.2608

40 Collins, S. L. and Patterson, A. D. (2020). 'The gut microbiome: an orchestrator of xenobiotic metabolism.' *Acta Pharmaceutica Sinica B, 10*(1), 19–32. https://doi.org/10.1016/J.APSB.2019.12.001

41 Furusawa Y., Obata Y., Fukuda S., Endo T. A., Nakato G., Takahashi D., Nakanishi Y., Uetake C., Kato K., Kato T., Takahashi M., Fukuda N. N., Murakami S., Miyauchi E., Hino S., Atarashi K., Onawa S., Fujimura Y., Lockett T., Clarke J. M., Topping D. L.,

Tomita M., Hori S., Ohara O., Morita T., Koseki H., Kikuchi J., Honda K., Hase K., Ohno H. (2013). 'Commensal microbe-derived butyrate induces the differentiation of colonic regulatory T cells.' *Nature*, 504(7480), 446–450. https://doi.org/10.1038/NATURE12721

42 Roediger, W. E. W. (1982). 'Utilization of Nutrients by Isolated Epithelial Cells of the Rat Colon.' *Gastroenterology*, 83(2). https://doi.org/10.1016/S0016-5085(82)80339-9

43 Heiman, M. L. and Greenway, F. L. (2016). 'A healthy gastrointestinal microbiome is dependent on dietary diversity.' *Molecular Metabolism*, 5(5), 317. https://doi.org/10.1016/J.MOLMET.2016.02.005

44 Hakansson, A. and Molin, G. (2011). 'Gut Microbiota and Inflammation.' *Nutrients*, 3(6), 637. https://doi.org/10.3390/NU3060637

45 DeGruttola, A. K., Low, D., Mizoguchi, A. and Mizoguchi, E. (2016). 'Current understanding of dysbiosis in disease in human and animal models.' *Inflammatory Bowel Diseases*, 22(5), 1137. https://doi.org/10.1097/MIB.0000000000000750

46 Campos-Rodríguez, R., Godínez-Victoria, M., Abarca-Rojano, E., Pacheco-Yépez, J., Reyna-Garfias, H., Barbosa-Cabrera, R. E. and Drago-Serrano, M. E. (2013). 'Stress modulates intestinal secretory immunoglobulin A.' *Frontiers in Integrative Neuroscience*, 7(DEC). https://doi.org/10.3389/FNINT.2013.00086

47 Qamar, N., Castano, D., Patt, C., Chu, T., Cottrell, J. and Chang, S. L. (2019). 'Meta-analysis of alcohol-induced gut dysbiosis and the resulting behavioral impact.' *Behavioural Brain Research*, 376, 112196. https://doi.org/10.1016/J.BBR.2019.112196

48 Li, J., Zhang, R., Ma, J., Tang, S., Li, Y., Li, Y. and Wan, J. (2021). 'Mucosa-Associated Microbial Profile Is Altered in Small Intestinal Bacterial Overgrowth.' *Frontiers in Microbiology*, 12, 710940. https://doi.org/10.3389/FMICB.2021.710940

49 Iliev, I. D. and Leonardi, I. (2017). 'Fungal dysbiosis: immunity and interactions at mucosal barriers.' *Nature Reviews. Immunology*, 17(10), 635. https://doi.org/10.1038/NRI.2017.55

50 Chakaroun, R. M., Massier, L. and Kovacs, P. (2020). 'Gut Microbiome, Intestinal Permeability, and Tissue Bacteria in Metabolic Disease: Perpetrators or Bystanders?' *Nutrients*, 12(4). https://doi.org/10.3390/NU12041082

51 Xie Y., Luo H., Duan J., Hong C., Ma P., Li G., Zhang T., Wu T., Ji G. (2014). 'Phytic acid enhances the oral absorption of isorhamnetin, quercetin, and kaempferol in total flavones of *Hippophae rhamnoides* L.' *Fitoterapia*, 93, 216–225. https://doi.org/10.1016/J.FITOTE.2014.01.013

52 Makki, K., Deehan, E. C., Walter, J. and Bäckhed, F. (2018). 'The Impact of Dietary Fiber on Gut Microbiota in Host Health and Disease.' *Cell Host & Microbe*, 23(6), 705–715. https://doi.org/10.1016/J.CHOM.2018.05.012

53 Heiman, M. L. and Greenway, F. L. (2016). 'A healthy gastrointestinal microbiome is dependent on dietary diversity.' *Molecular Metabolism*, 5(5), 317. https://doi.org/10.1016/J.MOLMET.2016.02.005

54 Gibson, G. R., Hutkins, R., Sanders, M. E., Prescott, S. L., Reimer, R. A., Salminen, S. J., Scott, K., Stanton, C., Swanson, K. S., Cani, P. D., Verbeke, K. and Reid, G. (2017). 'Expert consensus document: The International Scientific Association for Probiotics and Prebiotics (ISAPP) consensus statement on the definition and scope of prebiotics.' *Nature Reviews Gastroenterology & Hepatology*, 14(8), 491–502. https://doi.org/10.1038/nrgastro.2017.75

55 Naito, Y., Uchiyama, K. and Takagi, T. (2018). 'A next-generation beneficial microbe: *Akkermansia muciniphila*.' *Journal of Clinical Biochemistry and Nutrition*, 63(1), 33. https://doi.org/10.3164/JCBN.18-57

56 Hansson G. C. (2012). 'Role of mucus layers in gut infection and inflammation.' *Current Opinion in Microbiology*, 15(1), 57–62. https://doi.org/10.1016/J.MIB.2011.11.002
57 Zhou, K. (2017). 'Strategies to promote abundance of *Akkermansia muciniphila*, an emerging probiotic in the gut, evidence from dietary intervention studies.' *Journal of Functional Foods*, 33, 194. https://doi.org/10.1016/J.JFF.2017.03.045
58 Pierre J. F., Heneghan A. F., Feliciano R. P., Shanmuganayagam D., Roenneburg D. A., Krueger C. G., Reed J. D., Kudsk K. A. (2013). 'Cranberry proanthocyanidins improve the gut mucous layer morphology and function in mice receiving elemental enteral nutrition.' *Journal of Parenteral and Enteral Nutrition*, 37(3), 401–409. https://doi.org/10.1177/0148607112463076
59 Anhê, F. F., Nachbar, R. T., Varin, T. V., Vilela, V., Dudonné, S., Pilon, G., Fournier, M., Lecours, M. A., Desjardins, Y., Roy, D., Levy, E., & Marette, A. (2015). 'A polyphenol-rich cranberry extract protects from diet-induced obesity, insulin resistance and intestinal inflammation in association with increased Akkermansia spp. population in the gut microbiota of mice.' *Gut*, 64(6), 872–883. https://doi.org/10.1136/GUTJNL-2014-307142
60 Verhoog S., Taneri P. E., Roa Díaz Z. M., Marques-Vidal P., Troup J. P., Bally L., Franco O. H., Glisic M., Muka T. (2019). 'Dietary Factors and Modulation of Bacteria Strains of *Akkermansia muciniphila* and *Faecalibacterium prausnitzii*: A Systematic Review.' *Nutrients*, 11(7). https://doi.org/10.3390/NU11071565
61 Vlasova, A. N., Kandasamy, S., Chattha, K. S., Rajashekara, G. and Saif, L. J. (2016). 'Comparison of probiotic lactobacilli and bifidobacteria effects, immune responses and rotavirus vaccines and infection in different host species.' *Veterinary Immunology and Immunopathology*, 172, 72. https://doi.org/10.1016/J.VETIMM.2016.01.003
62 Kelesidis, T. and Pothoulakis, C. (2012). 'Efficacy and safety of the probiotic *Saccharomyces boulardii* for the prevention and therapy of gastrointestinal disorders.' *Therapeutic Advances in Gastroenterology*, 5(2), 111. https://doi.org/10.1177/1756283X11428502
63 Kwak M. K., Liu R., Kwon J. O., Kim M. K., Kim A. H., Kang S. O. (2013). 'Cyclic dipeptides from lactic acid bacteria inhibit proliferation of the influenza A virus.' *Journal of Microbiology (Seoul, Korea)*, 51(6), 836–843. https://doi.org/10.1007/S12275-013-3521-Y
64 Kwak, S.-H., Cho, Y.-M., Noh, G.-M. and Om, A.-S. (2014). 'Cancer Preventive Potential of Kimchi Lactic Acid Bacteria (*Weissella cibaria, Lactobacillus plantarum*).' *Journal of Cancer Prevention*, 19(4), 253. https://doi.org/10.15430/JCP.2014.19.4.253
65 Wastyk, H. C., Fragiadakis, G. K., Perelman, D., Dahan, D., Merrill, B. D., Yu, F. B., Topf, M., Gonzalez, C. G., Treuren, W. Van, Han, S., Robinson, J. L., Elias, J. E., Sonnenburg, E. D., Gardner, C. D. and Sonnenburg, J. L. (2021). 'Gut-microbiota-targeted diets modulate human immune status.' *Cell*, 0(0), 1–17. https://doi.org/10.1016/J.CELL.2021.06.019
66 David, L. A., Maurice, C. F., Carmody, R. N., Gootenberg, D. B., Button, J. E., Wolfe, B. E., Ling, A. V., Devlin, A. S., Varma, Y., Fischbach, M. A., Biddinger, S. B., Dutton, R. J. and Turnbaugh, P. J. (2014). 'Diet rapidly and reproducibly alters the human gut microbiome.' *Nature*, 505(7484), 559–563. https://doi.org/10.1038/nature12820
67 Aune, D., Giovannucci, E., Boffetta, P., Fadnes, L. T., Keum, N., Norat, T., Greenwood, D. C., Riboli, E., Vatten, L. J. and Tonstad, S. (2017). 'Fruit and vegetable intake and the risk of cardiovascular disease, total cancer and all-cause mortality – a systematic review and dose-response meta-analysis of prospective studies.' *International Journal of Epidemiology*, 46(3), 1029–1056. https://doi.org/10.1093/IJE/DYW319

68 Lam, M. C. L. and Adams, J. (2017). 'Association between home food preparation skills and behaviour, and consumption of ultra-processed foods: Cross-sectional analysis of the UK National Diet and nutrition survey (2008–2009).' *International Journal of Behavioral Nutrition and Physical Activity*, 14(1). https://doi.org/10.1186/S12966-017-0524-9
69 Wassermann, B., Müller, H. and Berg, G. (2019). 'An Apple a Day: Which Bacteria Do We Eat With Organic and Conventional Apples?' *Frontiers in Microbiology*, 10. https://doi.org/10.3389/fmicb.2019.01629
70 Doleman, J. F., Grisar, K., Liedekerke, L. Van, Saha, S., Roe, M., Tapp, H. S. and Mithen, R. F. (2017). 'The contribution of alliaceous and cruciferous vegetables to dietary sulphur intake.' *Food Chemistry*, 234, 38. https://doi.org/10.1016/J.FOODCHEM.2017.04.098
71 Mazarakis, N., Snibson, K., Licciardi, P. V. and Karagiannis, T. C. (2020).' The potential use of l-sulforaphane for the treatment of chronic inflammatory diseases: A review of the clinical evidence.' *Clinical Nutrition*, 39(3), 664–675. https://doi.org/10.1016/J.CLNU.2019.03.022
72 Fahey, J. W., Holtzclaw, W. D., Wehage, S. L., Wade, K. L., Stephenson, K. K. and Talalay, P. (2015). 'Sulforaphane Bioavailability from Glucoraphanin-Rich Broccoli: Control by Active Endogenous Myrosinase.' *PLOS ONE*, 10(11). https://doi.org/10.1371/JOURNAL.PONE.0140963

CHAPTER 8

1 Obermeier, B., Daneman, R. & Ransohoff, R. (2013). 'Development, maintenance and disruption of the blood-brain barrier.' *Nature Medicine*, 19(12), 1584–1596. https://doi.org/10.1038/NM.3407
2 Miller, A. H. and Raison, C. L. (2016). 'The role of inflammation in depression: from evolutionary imperative to modern treatment target.' *Nature Reviews. Immunology*, 16(1), 22. https://doi.org/10.1038/NRI.2015.5
3 Tracey, K. J. (2002). 'The inflammatory reflex.' *Nature*, 420(6917), 853–859. https://doi.org/10.1038/nature01321
4 Exton M. S., von Auer A. K., Buske-Kirschbaum A., Stockhorst U., Göbel U., Schedlowski M. (2000). 'Pavlovian conditioning of immune function: animal investigation and the challenge of human application.' *Behavioural Brain Research*, 110(1–2), 129–141. https://doi.org/10.1016/S0166-4328(99)00191-6
5 Papaioannou, V., Pneumatikos, I. and Maglaveras, N. (2013). 'Association of heart rate variability and inflammatory response in patients with cardiovascular diseases: current strengths and limitations.' *Frontiers in Physiology*, 4. https://doi.org/10.3389/FPHYS.2013.00174
6 Vedhara, K., Gill, S., Eldesouky, L., Campbell, B. K., Arevalo, J. M. G., Ma, J. and Cole, S. W. (2015). 'Personality and gene expression: Do individual differences exist in the leukocyte transcriptome?' *Psychoneuroendocrinology*, 52(1), 72–82. https://doi.org/10.1016/J.PSYNEUEN.2014.10.028
7 BioMed Centre Series blog (n.d.), *Quality of life and future risk of dying* – Retrieved 3 August 2021 from https://blogs.biomedcentral.com/bmcseriesblog/2020/11/06/quality-of-life-and-future-risk-of-dying/

8 Barak, Y. (2006). 'The immune system and happiness.' *Autoimmunity Reviews*, *5*(8), 523–527. https://doi.org/10.1016/J.AUTREV.2006.02.010
9 Cohen S., Doyle W. J., Turner R. B., Alper C. M., Skoner D. P. (2003). 'Emotional style and susceptibility to the common cold.' *Psychosomatic Medicine*, *65*(4), 652–657. https://doi.org/10.1097/01.PSY.0000077508.57784.DA
10 De Neve, J.-E., Diener, N. E., Tay, L. and Xuereb, C. (2013). 'The Objective Benefits of Subjective Well-Being Acknowledgements.' *World Happiness Report 2013*, Chapter 4: 'The objective benefits of subjective well-being.' Published by UN Sustainable Development Solutions Network.
11 Chatterjee, S. and Jethwani, D. J. (2020). 'A study of the Relationship between Mindful Self-Care and Subjective Well-Being among College Students and Working Professionals.' *International Journal of Innovative Research in Technology & Science*. 7(2), 417
12 Breines, J. G., Thoma, M. V., Gianferante, D., Hanlin, L., Chen, X. and Rohleder, N. (2014). 'Self-compassion as a predictor of interleukin-6 response to acute psychosocial stress.' *Brain, Behavior, and Immunity*, *37*, 109. https://doi.org/10.1016/J.BBI.2013.11.006
13 Terry, M. L. and Leary, M. R. (2011). 'Self and Identity: Self-compassion, self-regulation, and health.' https://doi.org/10.1080/15298868.2011.558404
14 Gilbert, P. and Procter, S. (2006). 'Compassionate Mind Training for People with High Shame and Self-Criticism: Overview and Pilot Study of a Group Therapy Approach.' *Clinical Psychology and Psychotherapy* 13, 353–379. https://doi.org/10.1002/cpp.507
15 Leary, M. R., Tate, E. B., Adams, C. E., Batts Allen, A. and Hancock, J. (2007). 'Self-Compassion and Reactions to Unpleasant Self-Relevant Events: The Implications of Treating Oneself Kindly.' https://doi.org/10.1037/0022-3514.92.5.887
16 Silverman, M. N. and Sternberg, E. M. (2012). 'Glucocorticoid regulation of inflammation and its functional correlates: from HPA axis to glucocorticoid receptor dysfunction.' *Annals of the New York Academy of Sciences*, *1261*(1), 55–63. https://doi.org/10.1111/J.1749-6632.2012.06633.X
17 Hall, J. M. F., Cruser, D., Podawiltz, A., Mummert, D. I., Jones, H. and Mummert, M. E. (2012). 'Psychological stress and the cutaneous immune response: Roles of the HPA Axis and the sympathetic nervous system in atopic dermatitis and psoriasis.' *Dermatology Research and Practice*. https://doi.org/10.1155/2012/403908
18 Slavich, G. M. (2020). 'Psychoneuroimmunology of Stress and Mental Health.' *The Oxford Handbook of Stress and Mental Health*, 518–546. https://doi.org/10.1093/OXFORDHB/9780190681777.013.24
19 Crum, A. J., Akinola, M., Martin, A. and Fath, S. (2017). 'The role of stress mindset in shaping cognitive, emotional, and physiological responses to challenging and threatening stress.' https://doi.org/10.1080/10615806.2016.1275585
20 Goyal, M., Singh, S., Sibinga, E. M. S., Gould, N. F., Rowland-Seymour, A., Sharma, R., Berger, Z., Sleicher, D., Maron, D. D., Shihab, H. M., Ranasinghe, P. D., Linn, S., Saha, S., Bass, E. B. and Haythornthwaite, J. A. (2014). 'Meditation Programs for Psychological Stress and Well-being: A Systematic Review and Meta-analysis.' *JAMA Internal Medicine*, 174(3), 357–368. https://doi.org/10.1001/JAMAINTERNMED.2013.13018
21 Marsland, A. L., Kuan, D. C.-H., Sheu, L. K., Krajina, K., Kraynak, T. E., Manuck, S. B. and Gianaros, P. J. (2017). 'Systemic Inflammation and Resting State Connectivity of the Default Mode Network.' *Brain, Behavior, and Immunity*, *62*, 162. https://doi.org/10.1016/J.BBI.2017.01.013

22 Zimmermann A., Bauer M. A., Kroemer G., Madeo F., Carmona-Gutierrez D. (2014). 'When less is more: hormesis against stress and disease.' *Microbial Cell (Graz, Austria)*, 1(5), 150–153. https://doi.org/10.15698/MIC2014.05.148

23 Mäkinen T. M., Mäntysaari M., Pääkkönen T., Jokelainen J., Palinkas L. A., Hassi J., Leppäluoto J., Tahvanainen K., Rintamäki H. (2008). 'Autonomic nervous function during whole-body cold exposure before and after cold acclimation.' *Aviation, Space, and Environmental Medicine*, 79(9), 875–882. https://doi.org/10.3357/ASEM.2235.2008

CHAPTER 9

1 Chastin S. F. M., Abaraogu U., Bourgois J. G., Dall P. M., Darnborough J., Duncan E., Dumortier J., Pavón D. J., McParland J., Roberts N. J., Hamer M. (2021). 'Effects of Regular Physical Activity on the Immune System, Vaccination and Risk of Community-Acquired Infectious Disease in the General Population: Systematic Review and Meta-Analysis.' *Sports Medicine (Auckland, N.Z.)*, 51(8). https://doi.org/10.1007/S40279-021-01466-1

2 Wen, C. P. and Wu, X. (2012). 'Stressing harms of physical inactivity to promote exercise.' *Lancet*, 380(9838), 192–193. https://doi.org/10.1016/S0140-6736(12)60954-4

3 Blair, S. N. (2009). 'Physical inactivity: the biggest public health problem of the 21st century.' *British Journal of Sports Medicine*, 43(1), 1–2. PMID: 19136507, https://pubmed.ncbi.nlm.nih.gov/19136507/

4 Duggal, N A., Pollock, R.D., Lazarus, N. R., Harridge, S. and Lord, J. M. (2018). 'Major features of immunesenescence, including reduced thymic output, are ameliorated by high levels of physical activity in adulthood,' *Aging Cell*, 17(2), e12750, https://doiord/10.1111/acel.12750

5 Ekkekakis, P., Parfitt, G. and Petruzzello, S. J. (2012). 'The Pleasure and DispleasurePeople Feel When They Exercise at Different Intensities.' *Sports Medicine*, 41(8), 641–671. https://doi.org/10.2165/11590680-000000000-00000

6 Koster A., Caserotti P., Patel K. V., Matthews C. E., Berrigan D., Van Domelen D. R., Brychta R. J., Chen K. Y., Harris T. B. (2012). 'Association of sedentary time with mortality independent of moderate to vigorous physical activity.' *PLOS ONE*, 7(6). https://doi.org/10.1371/JOURNAL.PONE.0037696

7 Chau, J. Y., Grunseit, A. C., Chey, T., Stamatakis, E., Brown, W. J., Matthews, C. E., Bauman, A. E. and Ploeg, H. P. van der. (2013). 'Daily Sitting Time and All-Cause Mortality: A Meta-Analysis.' *PLOS ONE*, 8(11), 80000. https://doi.org/10.1371/JOURNAL.PONE.0080000

8 Campbell, J. P. and Turner, J. E. (2018). 'Debunking the Myth of Exercise-Induced Immune Suppression: Redefining the Impact of Exercise on Immunological Health Across the Lifespan.' *Frontiers in Immunology*, 9, 648. https://doi.org/10.3389/fimmu.2018.00648

9 Law, T. D., Clark, L. A. and Clark, B. C. (2016). 'Resistance Exercise to Prevent and Manage Sarcopenia and Dynapenia.' *Annual Review of Gerontology & Geriatrics*, 36(1), 205. https://doi.org/10.1891/0198-8794.36.205

10 Nieman, D. C., Henson, D. A., Austin, M. D. and Sha, W. (2011). 'Upper respiratory tract infection is reduced in physically fit and active adults.' *British Journal of Sports Medicine*, 45(12), 987–992. https://doi.org/10.1136/BJSM.2010.077875

11 Bonilla, D. A., Pérez-Idárraga, A., Odriozola-Martínez, A. and Kreider, R. B. (2021). 'The 4R's Framework of Nutritional Strategies for Post-Exercise Recovery: A Review with Emphasis on New Generation of Carbohydrates.' *International Journal of Environmental Research and Public Health*, 18(1), 1–19. https://doi.org/10.3390/IJERPH18010103

12 Alemán-Mateo H., Carreón V. R., Macías L., Astiazaran-García H., Gallegos-Aguilar A. C., Enríquez J. R. (2014). 'Nutrient-rich dairy proteins improve appendicular skeletal muscle mass and physical performance, and attenuate the loss of muscle strength in older men and women subjects: a single-blind randomized clinical trial.' *Clinical Interventions in Aging*, 9, 1517–1525. https://doi.org/10.2147/CIA.S67449

13 Beaudart, C., Buckinx, F., Rabenda, V., Gillain, S., Cavalier, E., Slomian, J., Petermans, J., Reginster, J.-Y. and Bruyère, O. (2014). 'The Effects of Vitamin D on Skeletal Muscle Strength, Muscle Mass, and Muscle Power: A Systematic Review and Meta-Analysis of Randomized Controlled Trials.' *Journal of Clinical Endocrinology & Metabolism*, 99(11), 4336–4345. https://doi.org/10.1210/JC.2014-1742

14 Dupont, J., Dedeyne, L., Dalle, S., Koppo, K. and Gielen, E. (2019). 'The role of omega-3 in the prevention and treatment of sarcopenia.' *Aging Clinical and Experimental Research*, 31(6), 825. https://doi.org/10.1007/S40520-019-01146-1

15 Jenkins, E. M., Nairn, L. N., Skelly, L. E., Little, J. P. and Gibala, M. J. (2019). 'Do stair climbing exercise 'snacks' improve cardiorespiratory fitness?' *Applied Physiology, Nutrition and Metabolism*, 44(6), 681–684. https://doi.org/10.1139/APNM-2018-0675

16 Piercy K. L., Troiano R. P., Ballard R. M., Carlson S. A., Fulton J. E., Galuska D. A., George S. M., Olson R. D. (2018). 'The Physical Activity Guidelines for Americans.' *JAMA*, 320(19), 2020–2028. https://doi.org/10.1001/JAMA.2018.14854

17 Buckley, J. P., Hedge, A., Yates, T., Copeland, R. J., Loosemore, M., Hamer, M., Bradley, G. and Dunstan, D. W. (2015). 'The sedentary office: an expert statement on the growing case for change towards better health and productivity.' *British Journal of Sports Medicine*, 49(21), 1357–1362. https://doi.org/10.1136/BJSPORTS-2015-094618

CHAPTER 10

1 Besedovsky, L., Dimitrov, S., Born, J. and Lange, T. (2016). 'Nocturnal sleep uniformly reduces numbers of different T-cell subsets in the blood of healthy men.' *American Journal of Physiology – Regulatory, Integrative and Comparitive Physiology*, 311(4), R637–R642. https://doi.org/10.1152/AJPREGU.00149.2016

2 Scheiermann C., Kunisaki Y., Frenette P. S. (2013). 'Circadian control of the immune system.' *Nature Reviews. Immunology*, 13(3), 190–198. https://doi.org/10.1038/NRI3386

3 R, H. (2012). 'Neurobiology, pathophysiology, and treatment of melatonin deficiency and dysfunction.' *Scientific World Journal*, 2012. https://doi.org/10.1100/2012/640389

4 Galland-Decker C., Marques-Vidal P., Vollenweider P. (2019). 'Prevalence and factors associated with fatigue in the Lausanne middle-aged population: a population-based, cross-sectional survey.' *BMJ Open*, 9(8). https://doi.org/10.1136/BMJOPEN-2018-027070

5 Macfarlane, G. J., Kronisch, C., Atzeni, F., Häuser, W., Choy, E. H., Amris, K., Branco, J., Dincer, F., Leino-Arjas, P., Longley, K., McCarthy, G., Makri, S., Perrot, S., Puttini,

P. S., Taylor, A. and Jones, G. T. (2017). 'EULAR recommendations for management of fibromyalgia.' *Annals of the Rheumatic Diseases, 76*(12), e54–e54. https://doi.org/10.1136/ANNRHEUMDIS-2017-211587

CHAPTER 11

1 Gullone, E. (2000). 'The Biophilia Hypothesis and Life in the 21st Century: Increasing Mental Health or Increasing Pathology?' *Journal of Happiness Studies, 1*(3), 293–322. https://doi.org/10.1023/A:1010043827986
2 Ewert, A. and Chang, Y. (2018). 'Levels of Nature and Stress Response.' *Behavioral Sciences, 8*(5), 49. https://doi.org/10.3390/BS8050049
3 Danko, D., Bezdan, D., Afshin, E. E., Ahsanuddin, S., Bhattacharya, C., Butler, D. J., Chng, K. R., Donnellan, D., Hecht, J., Jackson, K., Kuchin, K., Karasikov, M., Lyons, A., Mak, L., Meleshko, D., Mustafa, H., Mutai, B., Neches, R. Y., Ng, A. . . . Zubenko, S. (2021). 'A global metagenomic map of urban microbiomes and antimicrobial resistance.' *Cell, 184*(13), 3376-3393.e17. https://doi.org/10.1016/J.CELL.2021.05.002
4 Roslund, M. I., Puhakka, R., Grönroos, M., Nurminen, N., Oikarinen, S., Gazali, A. M., Cinek, O., Kramná, L., Siter, N., Vari, H. K., Soininen, L., Parajuli, A., Rajaniemi, J., Kinnunen, T., Laitinen, O. H., Hyöty, H., Sinkkonen, A. and group A. research. (2020). 'Biodiversity intervention enhances immune regulation and health-associated commensal microbiota among daycare children.' *Science Advances, 6*(42), eaba2578. https://doi.org/10.1126/SCIADV.ABA2578
5 Saxbe, D. E. and Repetti, R. (2009). 'No Place Like Home: Home Tours Correlate with Daily Patterns of Mood and Cortisol.' http://Dx.Doi.Org/10.1177/0146167209352864, *36*(1), 71–81. https://doi.org/10.1177/0146167209352864
6 Thacher, P. V. and Reinheimer A. (2015). 'People at risk of hoarding disorder may have serious complaints about sleep.' *Sleep, 38,* Abstract Supplement.
7 Pandelaere, M. (2016). 'Materialism and well-being: The role of consumption.' *Current Opinion in Psychology, 10*, 33–38. https://doi.org/10.1016/J.COPSYC.2015.10.027
8 Lee, H.-H. M. (2017). 'In Pursuit of Happiness: Phenomenological Study of the Konmari Decluttering Method.' *ACR North American Advances, NA-45*, 2017. https://doi.org/10.1002/9781118989463.wbeccs201
9 Keith, N. R., Clark, D. O. and Miller, D. K. (2010). 'Environmental Correlates of Physical Activity in Middle-Aged, Urban-Dwelling African Americans.' *Medicine & Science in Sports & Exercise, 42*(5), 246–247. https://doi.org/10.1249/01.MSS.0000384314.31339.27
10 Vartanian, L., Kernan, K. and Wansink, B. (2016). 'Clutter, Chaos, and Overconsumption: The Role of Mind-Set in Stressful and Chaotic Food Environments.' *SSRN Electronic Journal*. https://doi.org/10.2139/SSRN.2711870
11 Rodin, J. and Langer, E. J. (1977). 'Long-term effects of a control-relevant intervention with the institutionalized aged.' *Journal of Personality and Social Psychology, 35*(12), 897–902. https://doi.org/10.1037/0022-3514.35.12.897
12 Lee, M., Lee, J., Park, B.-J. and Miyazaki, Y. (2015). 'Interaction with indoor plants may reduce psychological and physiological stress by suppressing autonomic nervous system activity in young adults: a randomized crossover study.' *Journal of Physiological Anthropology, 34*(1). https://doi.org/10.1186/S40101-015-0060-8

13 Nieuwenhuis, M., Knight, C., Postmes, T. and Haslam, S. A. (2014). 'The relative benefits of green versus lean office space: Three field experiments.' *Journal of Experimental Psychology: Applied*, 20(3), 199–214. https://doi.org/10.1037/XAP0000024

14 Park S. H., Mattson R. H. (2009). 'Ornamental indoor plants in hospital rooms enhanced health outcomes of patients recovering from surgery.' *Journal of Alternative and Complementary Medicine* (*New York, N.Y.*), 15(9), 975–980. https://doi.org/10.1089/ACM.2009.0075

15 Horoshenkov, K. V., Khan, A. and Benkreira, H. (2013). 'Acoustic properties of low growing plants.' *Journal of the Acoustical Society of America*, 133(5), 2554. https://doi.org/10.1121/1.4798671

16 Kreitinger, J. M., Beamer, C. A. and Shepherd, D. M. (2016). 'Environmental Immunology: Lessons Learned from Exposure to a Select Panel of Immunotoxicants.' *Journal of Immunology*, 196(8), 3217–3225. https://doi.org/10.4049/JIMMUNOL.1502149

17 DeWitt, J. C., Germolec, D. R., Luebke, R. W. and Johnson, V. J. (2016). 'Associating Changes in the Immune System with Clinical Diseases for Interpretation in Risk Assessment.' *Current Protocols in Toxicology*, 67(1), 1811. https://doi.org/10.1002/0471140856.TX1801S67

18 Smith, K. R., Corvalán, C. F. and Kjellström, T. (1999). 'How much global ill health is attributable to environmental factors?' *Epidemiology*, 10(5). https://doi.org/10.1097/00001648-199909000-00027

19 Mokdad A. H., Marks J. S., Stroup D. F., Gerberding J. L. (2005). 'Correction: actual causes of death in the United States, 2000.' *JAMA*, 293(3), 293–294. https://doi.org/10.1001/JAMA.293.3.293

20 Carvalho, A. M., Miranda, A. M., Santos, F. A., Loureiro, A. P. M., Fisberg, R. M. and Marchioni, D. M. (2015). 'High intake of heterocyclic amines from meat is associated with oxidative stress.' *British Journal of Nutrition*, 113(8), 1301–1307. https://doi.org/10.1017/S0007114515000628

21 Skorge, T. D., Villani, S., Jarvis, D., Zock, J. P. and Svanes, C.* (n.d.). 'Cleaning at home and at work in relation to lung function decline and airway obstruction.' *American Journal of Respiratory and Critical Car Medicine 2018, 197 (9), 1157–1164*, 3. Retrieved 28 October 2021, from www.atsjournals.org

22 Listing of POPs in the Stockholm Convention (n.d.). Retrieved 28 October 2021 from http://chm.pops.int/TheConvention/ThePOPs/ListingofPOPs/tabid/2509/Default.aspx

23 Hansen, J. F., Nielsen, C. H., Brorson, M. M., Frederiksen, H., Hartoft-Nielsen, M.-L., Rasmussen, Å. K., Bendtzen, K. and Feldt-Rasmussen, U. (2015). 'Influence of Phthalates on in-vitro Innate and Adaptive Immune Responses.' *PLOS ONE*, 10(6). https://doi.org/10.1371/JOURNAL.PONE.0131168

24 Yang Y. N., Yang Y. S. H., Lin I. H., Chen Y. Y., Lin H. Y., Wu C. Y., Su Y. T., Yang Y. J., Yang S. N., Suen J. L. (2019). 'Phthalate exposure alters gut microbiota composition and IgM vaccine response in human newborns.' *Food and Chemical Toxicology: An International Journal Published for the British Industrial Biological Research Association*, 132. https://doi.org/10.1016/J.FCT.2019.110700

25 Attina, T. M. and Trasande, L. (2015). 'Association of Exposure to Di-2-Ethylhexylphthalate Replacements With Increased Insulin Resistance in Adolescents From NHANES 2009–2012.' *Journal of Clinical Endocrinology and Metabolism*, 100(7), 2640. https://doi.org/10.1210/JC.2015-1686

26 Wang G., Chen Q., Tian P., Wang L., Li X., Lee Y. K., Zhao J., Zhang H., Chen W. (2020).

'Gut microbiota dysbiosis might be responsible to different toxicity caused by Di-(2-ethylhexyl) phthalate exposure in murine rodents.' *Environmental Pollution*, 1987, 261. Published by Elsevier, Barking, Essex. https://doi.org/10.1016/J.ENVPOL.2020.114164

27 Wolverton, B. C., Johnson, A. and Bounds, K. (1989). 'Interior Landscape Plants for Indoor Air Pollution Abatement.' Technical memorandum, NASA. https://ntrs.nasa.gov/citations/19930073077

28 Cummings, B. E. and Waring, M. S. (2019). 'Potted plants do not improve indoor air quality: a review and analysis of reported VOC removal efficiencies.' *Journal of Exposure Science & Environmental Epidemiology*, 30(2), 253–261. https://doi.org/10.1038/s41370-019-0175-9

CHAPTER 12

1 Yanuck, S., Pizzorno, J., Messier, H. and Fitzgerald, K. (2020). 'Evidence Supporting a Phased Immuno-physiological Approach to COVID-19 from Prevention Through Recovery.' *Integrative Medicine: A Clinician's Journal*, 19(Supplement. 1), 8. /pmc/articles/PMC7190003/

2 Pietrzik, K. (1985). 'Concept of borderline vitamin deficiencies.' *International Journal for Vitamin and Nutrition Research. Supplement = Internationale Zeitschrift für Vitamin- und Ernahrungsforschung. Supplement.*, 27.

3 I, Z., R, L., C, N. and A, T. (2020). 'COVID-19: The Inflammation Link and the Role of Nutrition in Potential Mitigation.' *Nutrients*, 12(5). https://doi.org/10.3390/NU12051466

4 Calder P. C., Carr A. C., Gombart A. F., Eggersdorfer M. (2020). 'Optimal Nutritional Status for a Well-Functioning Immune System Is an Important Factor to Protect against Viral Infections.' *Nutrients*, 12(4). https://doi.org/10.3390/NU12041181

5 Mora, J. R., Iwata, M. and von Andrian, U. H. (2008). 'Vitamin effects on the immune system: vitamins A and D take centre stage.' *Nature Reviews Immunology*, 8(9), 685–698. https://doi.org/10.1038/nri2378

6 Kluger, M. J. (2015). *Fever: Its Biology, Evolution, and Function*, 1–195. Published by Princeton University Press.

7 Kluger M. J., Kozak W., Conn C. A., Leon L. R., Soszynski D. (1996). 'The adaptive value of fever.' *Infectious Disease Clinics of North America*, 10(1), 1–20. https://doi.org/10.1016/S0891-5520(05)70282-8

8 Smith, A. P. (2012). 'Effects of the common cold on mood, psychomotor performance, the encoding of new information, speed of working memory and semantic processing.' *Brain, Behavior, and Immunity*, 26(7), 1072–1076. https://doi.org/10.1016/J.BBI.2012.06.012

9 Imeri, L. and Opp, M. R. (2009). 'How (and why) the immune system makes us sleep.' *Nature Reviews. Neuroscience*, 10(3), 199. https://doi.org/10.1038/NRN2576

10 Dimitrov, S., Lange, T., Gouttefangeas, C., Jensen, A. T. R., Szczepanski, M., Lehnnolz, J., Soekadar, S., Rammensee, H.-G., Born, J. and Besedovsky, L. (2019). 'Gαs-coupled receptor signaling and sleep regulate integrin activation of human antigen-specific T cells.' *Journal of Experimental Medicine*, 216(3), 517. https://doi.org/10.1084/JEM.20181169

11 Imeri and Opp, op. cit.

12 Mooventhan, A. and Nivethitha, L. (2014). 'Scientific Evidence-Based Effects of

Hydrotherapy on Various Systems of the Body.' *North American Journal of Medical Sciences, 6*(5), 199. https://doi.org/10.4103/1947-2714.132935
13 Popkin, B. M., D'Anci, K. E. and Rosenberg, I. H. (2010). 'Water, Hydration and Health.' *Nutrition Reviews, 68*(8), 439. https://doi.org/10.1111/J.1753-4887.2010.00304.X
14 Kurpad, A. V. (2006). 'The requirements of protein & amino acid during acute & chronic infections.' *Indian Journal of Medical Research*, 124(2), 129–48. PMID: 17015927. https://pubmed.ncbi.nlm.nih.gov/17015927/
15 Özkaya, I., Beyza, İ. and Üniversitesi, K. (2021). 'Effect of Protein Consumption Over the Immune System Responses Given During Covid-19.' *International Journal of Medical Science and Clinical Invention* 8(5), 5359–5363. https://doi.org/10.18535/ijmsci/v8i05.01
16 McRae, M. P. (2016). 'Therapeutic Benefits of l-Arginine: An Umbrella Review of Meta-analyses.' *Journal of Chiropractic Medicine*, 15(3), 184. https://doi.org/10.1016/J.JCM.2016.06.002
17 Cruzat, V., Rogero, M. M., Keane, K. N., Curi, R. and Newsholme, P. (2018). 'Glutamine: Metabolism and immune function, supplementation and clinical translation.' *Nutrients*, 10(11). MDPI AG. https://doi.org/10.3390/nu10111564
18 Hemilä, H. and Chalker, E. (2013). 'Vitamin C for preventing and treating the common cold.' *Cochrane Database of Systematic Reviews* 2013(1). Published by John Wiley & Sons Ltd. https://doi.org/10.1002/14651858.CD000980.pub4
19 Bai, X., Yang, P., Zhou, Q., Cai, B., Buist-Homan, M., Cheng, H., Jiang, J., Shen, D., Li, L., Luo, X., Faber, K. N., Moshage, H. and Shi, G. (2017). 'The protective effect of the natural compound hesperetin against fulminant hepatitis in vivo and in vitro.' *British Journal of Pharmacology*, 174(1), 41. https://doi.org/10.1111/BPH.13645
20 Parhiz H., Roohbakhsh A., Soltani F., Rezaee R., Iranshahi M. (2015). 'Antioxidant and anti-inflammatory properties of the citrus flavonoids hesperidin and hesperetin: an updated review of their molecular mechanisms and experimental models.' *Phytotherapy Research: PTR*, 29(3), 323–331. https://doi.org/10.1002/PTR.5256
21 Sharma S., Sheehy T., Kolonel L. N. (2013). 'Contribution of meat to vitamin B_{12}, iron and zinc intakes in five ethnic groups in the USA: implications for developing food-based dietary guidelines.' *Journal of Human Nutrition and Dietetics: The Official Journal of the British Dietetic Association*, 26(2), 156–68. https://doi.org/10.1111/JHN.12035
22 Wang M. X., Win S. S., Pang J. (2020). 'Zinc Supplementation Reduces Common Cold Duration among Healthy Adults: A Systematic Review of Randomized Controlled Trials with Micronutrients Supplementation.' *American Journal of Tropical Medicine and Hygiene*, 103(1), 86–99. https://doi.org/10.4269/AJTMH.19-0718
23 Beck M. A., Levander O. A., Handy J. (2003). 'Selenium deficiency and viral infection.' *Journal of Nutrition*, 133(50 Supplement 1. https://doi.org/10.1093/JN/133.5.1463S
24 Levy, E., Delvin, E., Marcil, V. and Spahis, S. (2020). 'Can phytotherapy with polyphenols serve as a powerful approach for the prevention and therapy tool of novel coronavirus disease 2019 (COVID-19)?' *American Journal of Physiology–Endocrinology and Metabolism*, 319(4), E689. https://doi.org/10.1152/AJPENDO.00298.2020
25 Research reveals levels of inappropriate prescriptions in England – GOV.UK (n.d.). Retrieved 3 August 2021 from https://www.gov.uk/government/news/research-reveals-levels-of-inappropriate-prescriptions-in-england
26 Nyquist A. C., Gonzales R., Steiner J. F., Sande M. A. (1998). 'Antibiotic prescribing for children with colds, upper respiratory tract infections, and bronchitis.' *JAMA*, 279(11), 875–877. https://doi.org/10.1001/JAMA.279.11.875

27 Coccimiglio, J., Alipour, M., Jiang, Z. H., Gottardo, C. and Suntres, Z. (2016). 'Antioxidant, antibacterial, and cytotoxic activities of the ethanolic *Origanum vulgare* extract and its major constituents.' *Oxidative Medicine and Cellular Longevity*, March 2016. https://doi.org/10.1155/2016/1404505

28 Sienkiewicz, M., Wasiela, M., Głowacka, A. (2012), *Aktywność przeciwbakteryjna olejku oreganowego (Origanum heracleoticum* L.) *wobec szczepów klinicznych Escherichia coli i Pseudomonas aeruginosa* ['The antibacterial activity of oregano essential oil (*Origanum heracleoticum* L.) against clinical strains of *Escherichia coli* and *Pseudomonas aeruginosa*']. *Med Dosw Mikrobiol*, 64(4), 297–307. Polish. PMID: 23484421.

29 Oduwole, O., Udoh, E. E., Oyo-Ita, A. and Meremikwu, M. M. (2018). 'Honey for acute cough in children.' *Cochrane Database of Systematic Reviews*, 2018(4). https://doi.org/10.1002/14651858.CD007094.PUB5

30 Carter, D. A., Blair, S. E., Cokcetin, N. N., Bouzo, D., Brooks, P., Schothauer, R. and Harry, E. J. (2016). 'Therapeutic Manuka Honey: No Longer So Alternative.' *Frontiers in Microbiology*, 7(Apr). https://doi.org/10.3389/FMICB.2016.00569

31 Bayan, L., Koulivand, P. H. and Gorji, A. (2014). 'Garlic: a review of potential therapeutic effects.' *Avicenna Journal of Phytomedicine*, 4(1), 1. /pmc/articles/PMC4103721/

32 Charron C. S., Dawson H. D., Albaugh G. P., Solverson P. M., Vinyard B. T., Solano-Aguilar G. I., Molokin A., Novotny J. A. (2015). 'A Single Meal Containing Raw, Crushed Garlic Influences Expression of Immunity- and Cancer-Related Genes in Whole Blood of Humans.' *Journal of Nutrition*, 145(11), 2448–2455. https://doi.org/10.3945/JN.115.215392

33 Borek C. (2001). 'Antioxidant health effects of aged garlic extract.' *Journal of Nutrition*, 131(3s). https://doi.org/10.1093/JN/131.3.1010S

34 Praditya, D., Kirchhoff, L., Brüning, J., Rachmawati, H., Steinmann, J. and Steinmann, E. (2019). 'Anti-infective Properties of the Golden Spice Curcumin.' *Frontiers in Microbiology*, 10(May). https://doi.org/10.3389/FMICB.2019.00912

35 Hewlings, S. J. and Kalman, D. S. (2017). 'Curcumin: A Review of Its Effects on Human Health.' *Foods*, 6(10). https://doi.org/10.3390/FOODS6100092

36 Daily, J. W., Yang, M. and Park, S. (2016). 'Efficacy of Turmeric Extracts and Curcumin for Alleviating the Symptoms of Joint Arthritis: A Systematic Review and Meta-Analysis of Randomized Clinical Trials.' *Journal of Medicinal Food*, 19(8), 717. https://doi.org/10.1089/JMF.2016.3705

37 De Flora S., Grassi C., Carati L. (1997). 'Attenuation of influenza-like symptomatology and improvement of cell-mediated immunity with long-term N-acetylcysteine treatment.' *European Respiratory Journal*, 10(7), 1535–1541. https://doi.org/10.1183/09031936.97.10071535

38 Liu, Q., Meng, X., Li, Y., Zhao, C.-N., Tang, G.-Y. and Li, H.-B. (2017). 'Antibacterial and Antifungal Activities of Spices.' *International Journal of Molecular Sciences*, 18(6). https://doi.org/10.3390/IJMS18061283

39 Langner, E. (1998). 'Ginger: History and use.' *Advances in Therapy*, 15(1). https://doi.org/10.1201/9781420040463

40 Rayati, F., Hajmanouchehri, F. and Najafi, E. (2017). 'Comparison of anti-inflammatory and analgesic effects of Ginger powder and Ibuprofen in postsurgical pain model: A randomized, double-blind, case-control clinical trial.' *Dental Research Journal*, 14(1), 1. /pmc/articles/PMC5356382/

41 Wakabayashi H., Oda H., Yamauchi K., Abe F. (2014). 'Lactoferrin for prevention of common viral infections.' *Journal of Infection and Chemotherapy: Official Journal of*

the Japan Society of Chemotherapy, 20(11), 666–671. https://doi.org/10.1016/J.JIAC.2014.08.003

42 Vitetta L., Coulson S., Beck S. L., Gramotnev H., Du S., Lewis S. (2013). 'The clinical efficacy of a bovine lactoferrin/whey protein Ig-rich fraction (Lf/IgF) for the common cold: a double-blind randomized study.' *Complementary Therapies in Medicine*, *21*(3), 164–171. https://doi.org/10.1016/J.CTIM.2012.12.006

43 Altarac, S. and Papeš, D. (2014). 'Use of d-mannose in prophylaxis of recurrent urinary tract infections (UTIs) in women.' *BJU International*, *113*(1), 9–10. https://doi.org/10.1111/BJU.12492

44 Porru, D., Parmigiani, A., Tinelli, C., Barletta, D., Choussos, D., Franco, C. Di, Bobbi, V., Bassi, S., Miller, O., Gardella, B., Nappi, R., Spinillo, A. and Rovereto, B. (2014). 'Oral D-mannose in recurrent urinary tract infections in women: a pilot study.' http://Dx.Doi.Org/10.1177/2051415813518332, 7(3), 208–213. https://doi.org/10.1177/2051415813518332

45 Sandhaus, S. and Swick, A. G. (2021). 'Specialized proresolving mediators in infection and lung injury.' *BioFactors*, *47*(1), 6–18. https://doi.org/10.1002/BIOF.1691

46 Rathnavelu, V., Alitheen, N. B., Sohila, S., Kanagesan, S. and Ramesh, R. (2016). 'Potential role of bromelain in clinical and therapeutic applications.' *Biomedical Reports*, *5*(3), 283. https://doi.org/10.3892/BR.2016.720

47 Malaguarnera, L. (2019). 'Influence of Resveratrol on the Immune Response.' *Nutrients*, *11*(5), 946. https://doi.org/10.3390/NU11050946

48 Mazarakis, N., Snibson, K., Licciardi, P. V. and Karagiannis, T. C. (2020). 'The potential use of l-sulforaphane for the treatment of chronic inflammatory diseases: A review of the clinical evidence.' *Clinical Nutrition*, *39*(3), 664–675. https://doi.org/10.1016/J.CLNU.2019.03.022

CHAPTER 13

1 Ortiz, R. A. and Barnes, K. C. (2015). 'Genetics of Allergic Diseases.' *Immunology and Allergy Clinics of North America*, *35*(1), 19. https://doi.org/10.1016/J.IAC.2014.09.014

2 Weidinger S., O'Sullivan M., Illig T., Baurecht H., Depner M., Rodriguez E., Ruether A., Klopp N., Vogelberg C., Weiland S. K., McLean W. H., von Mutius E., Irvine A. D., Kabesch M. (2008). 'Filaggrin mutations, atopic eczema, hay fever, and asthma in children.' *Journal of Allergy and Clinical Immunology*, *121*(5). https://doi.org/10.1016/J.JACI.2008.02.014

3 Yang L., Fu J., Zhou Y. (2020). 'Research Progress in Atopic March.' *Frontiers in Immunology*, *11*. https://doi.org/10.3389/FIMMU.2020.01907

4 Strachan, D. P. (1989). 'Hay fever, hygiene, and household size.' *British Medical Journal*, *299*(6710), 1259–1260. https://doi.org/10.1136/bmj.299.6710.1259

5 Guarner F., Bourdet-Sicard R., Brandtzaeg P., Gill H. S., McGuirk P., van Eden W., Versalovic J., Weinstock J. V., Rook G. A. (2006). 'Mechanisms of disease: the hygiene hypothesis revisited.' *Nature Clinical Practice. Gastroenterology & Hepatology*, *3*(5), 275–284. https://doi.org/10.1038/NCPGASTHEP0471

6 Moffatt M. F., Cookson W. O. (2017). 'The lung microbiome in health and disease.' *Clinical Medicine* (London, England), *17*(6), 525–529. https://doi.org/10.7861/CLINMEDICINE.17-6-525

7 Hanski I., von Hertzen L., Fyhrquist N., Koskinen K., Torppa K., Laatikainen T., Karisola P., Auvinen P., Paulin L., Mäkelä M. J., Vartiainen E., Kosunen T. U., Alenius H., Haahtela T. (2012). 'Environmental biodiversity, human microbiota, and allergy are interrelated.' *Proceedings of the National Academy of Sciences of the United States of America*, 109(21), 8334–8339. https://doi.org/10.1073/PNAS.1205624109

8 Polkowska-Pruszyńska B., Gerkowicz A., Krasowska D. (2020). 'The gut microbiome alterations in allergic and inflammatory skin diseases – an update.' *Journal of the European Academy of Dermatology and Venereology:* 34(3), 455–464. https://doi.org/10.1111/JDV.15951

9 Fyhrquist N., Ruokolainen L., Suomalainen A., Lehtimäki S., Veckman V., Vendelin J., Karisola P., Lehto M., Savinko T., Jarva H., Kosunen T. U., Corander J., Auvinen P., Paulin L., von Hertzen L., Laatikainen T., Mäkelä M., Haahtela T., Greco D., Hanski I., Alenius H. (2014). 'Acinetobacter species in the skin microbiota protect against allergic sensitization and inflammation.' *Journal of Allergy and Clinical Immunology*, 134(6), 1301–1309.e11. https://doi.org/10.1016/J.JACI.2014.07.059

10 Kantor R., Kim A., Thyssen J. P., Silverberg J. I. (2016). 'Association of atopic dermatitis with smoking: A systematic review and meta-analysis.' *Journal of the American Academy of Dermatology*, 75(6), 1119–1125.e1. https://doi.org/10.1016/J.JAAD.2016.07.017

11 Sedghy, F., Varasteh, A.-R., Sankian, M. and Moghadam, M. (2018). 'Interaction Between Air Pollutants and Pollen Grains: The Role on the Rising Trend in Allergy.' *Reports of Biochemistry & Molecular Biology*, 6(2), 219. /pmc/articles/PMC5941124/

12 Beck, I., Jochner, S., Gilles, S., McIntyre, M., Buters, J. T. M., Schmidt-Weber, C., Behrendt, H., Ring, J., Menzel, A. and Traidl-Hoffmann, C. (2013). 'High Environmental Ozone Levels Lead to Enhanced Allergenicity of Birch Pollen.' *PLOS ONE*, 8(11), e80147. https://doi.org/10.1371/JOURNAL.PONE.0080147

13 To, T., Zhu, J., Stieb, D., Gray, N., Fong, I., Pinault, L., Jerrett, M., Robichaud, A., Ménard, R., Donkelaar, A. van, Martin, R. V., Hystad, P., Brook, J. R. and Dell, S. (2020). 'Early life exposure to air pollution and incidence of childhood asthma, allergic rhinitis and eczema.' *European Respiratory Journal*, 55(2). https://doi.org/10.1183/13993003.00913-2019

14 Baumann, S. and Lorentz, A. (2013). 'Obesity – A Promoter of Allergy?' *International Archives of Allergy and Immunology*, 162(3), 205–213. https://doi.org/10.1159/000353972

15 Reznik, M. (2013). 'Fast Food Linked to Asthma and Allergies in Children.' *Science Translational Medicine*, 5(171), 171ec26-171ec26. https://doi.org/10.1126/SCITRANSLMED.3005803

16 A, Z. and JI, S. (2015). 'Association of atopic dermatitis with being overweight and obese: a systematic review and meta-analysis..' *Journal of the American Academy of Dermatology*, 72(4), 606-616.e4. https://doi.org/10.1016/J.JAAD.2014.12.013

17 P, C., AS, S., O, F. and A, L. (2018). 'The Circadian Clock Drives Mast Cell Functions in Allergic Reactions.' *Frontiers in Immunology*, 9(Jul). https://doi.org/10.3389/FIMMU.2018.01526

18 MH, S., B, L. and AE, R. (2007). 'Chronobiology and chronotherapy of allergic rhinitis and bronchial asthma.' *Advanced Drug Delivery Reviews*, 59(9–10), 852–882. https://doi.org/10.1016/J.ADDR.2007.08.016

19 Haahtela, T., Holgate, S., Pawankar, R., Akdis, C. A., Benjaponpitak, S., Caraballo, L., Demain, J., Portnoy, J. and von Hertzen, L. (2013). 'The biodiversity hypothesis and allergic disease: world allergy organization position statement.' *World Allergy Organization Journal*, 6(1), 3. https://doi.org/10.1186/1939-4551-6-3

20 Allergy UK | National Charity (n.d.). Retrieved 28 October 2021 from https://www.allergyuk.org/assets/000/001/287/Final_HayMax_Report_2016_Part_1_original.pdf?1502279669
21 Kurukulaaratchy, R. J., Karmaus, W., Raza, A., Matthews, S., Roberts, G. and Arshad, S. H. (2011). 'The influence of gender and atopy on the natural history of rhinitis in the first 18 years of life.' *Clinical & Experimental Allergy*, *41*(6), 851–859. https://doi.org/10.1111/J.1365-2222.2011.03765.X
22 Anderegg, W. R. L., Abatzoglou, J. T., Anderegg, L. D. L., Bielory, L., Kinney, P. L. and Ziska, L. (2021). 'Anthropogenic climate change is worsening North American pollen seasons.' *Proceedings of the National Academy of Sciences*, *118*(7). https://doi.org/10.1073/PNAS.2013284118
23 Ariano R., Canonica G. W., Passalacqua G. (2010). 'Possible role of climate changes in variations in pollen seasons and allergic sensitizations during 27 years.' *Annals of Allergy, Asthma & Immunology: Official Publication of the American College of Allergy, Asthma, & Immunology*, *104*(3), 215–222. https://doi.org/10.1016/J.ANAI.2009.12.005
24 Mukai, K., Tsai, M., Starkl, P., Marichal, T. and Galli, S. J. (2016). 'IgE and mast cells in host defense against parasites and venoms.' *Seminars in Immunopathology*, *38*(5), 581. https://doi.org/10.1007/S00281-016-0565-1
25 Sandilands, A., Sutherland, C., Irvine, A. D. and McLean, W. H. I. (2009). 'Filaggrin in the frontline: role in skin barrier function and disease.' *Journal of Cell Science*, *122*(9), 1285. https://doi.org/10.1242/JCS.033969
26 Tsakok, T., Marrs, T., Mohsin, M., Baron, S., Toit, G. du, Till, S. and Flohr, C. (2017). 'Does atopic dermatitis cause food allergy? A systematic review.' *The Lancet*, *389*, S95. https://doi.org/10.1016/S0140-6736(17)30491-9
27 Grewling, Ł., Bogawski, P. and Smith, M. (2016). 'Pollen nightmare: elevated airborne pollen levels at night.' *Aerobiologia*, *32*(4), 725. https://doi.org/10.1007/S10453-016-9441-7
28 Zhang, Y., Bielory, L., Mi, Z., Cai, T., Robock, A. and Georgopoulos, P. (2015). 'Allergenic pollen season variations in the past two decades under changing climate in the United States.' *Global Change Biology*, *21*(4), 1581. https://doi.org/10.1111/GCB.12755
29 Folkerts, J., Stadhouders, R., Redegeld, F. A., Tam, S.-Y., Hendriks, R. W., Galli, S. J. and Maurer, M. (2018). 'Effect of Dietary Fiber and Metabolites on Mast Cell Activation and Mast Cell-Associated Diseases.' *Frontiers in Immunology*, 0(May), 1067. https://doi.org/10.3389/FIMMU.2018.01067
30 Hagenlocher, Y. and Lorentz, A. (2015). 'Immunomodulation of mast cells by nutrients.' *Molecular Immunology*, *63*(1), 25–31. https://doi.org/10.1016/J.MOLIMM.2013.12.005
31 Mlcek, J., Jurikova, T., Skrovankova, S. and Sochor, J. (2016). 'Quercetin and Its Anti-Allergic Immune Response.' *Molecules* *21*(5), 623. https://doi.org/10.3390/MOLECULES21050623
32 Formica, J. V. and Regelson, W. (1995). 'Review of the biology of quercetin and related bioflavonoids.' *Food and Chemical Toxicology*, *33*(12), 1061–1080. https://doi.org/10.1016/0278-6915(95)00077-1
33 Li Y., Mattison C. P. (2018). 'Polyphenol-rich pomegranate juice reduces IgE binding to cashew nut allergens.' *Journal of the Science of Food and Agriculture*, *98*(4), 1632–1638. https://doi.org/10.1002/JSFA.8639
34 Mittman P. (1990). 'Randomized, double-blind study of freeze-dried *Urtica dioica* in

the treatment of allergic rhinitis.' *Planta Medica, 56*(1), 44–47. https://doi.org/10.1055/S-2006-960881

35 Thornhill S. M., Kelly A. M. (2000). 'Natural treatment of perennial allergic rhinitis.' *Alternative Medicine Review: A Journal of Clinical Therapeutic*, 5(5), 448–454. https://pubmed.ncbi.nlm.nih.gov/11056414/

36 Yuta A., Baraniuk J. N. (2005). 'Therapeutic approaches to mucus hypersecretion.' *Current Allergy and Asthma Reports*, 5(3), 243–251. https://doi.org/10.1007/S11882-005-0044-6

37 Wang X., Ma D. W., Kang J. X., Kulka M. (2015). 'n-3 Polyunsaturated fatty acids inhibit Fc ε receptor I-mediated mast cell activation.' *Journal of Nutritional Biochemistry, 26*(12), 1580–1588. https://doi.org/10.1016/J.JNUTBIO.2015.07.027

38 Barcelos R. C., de Mello-Sampayo C., Antoniazzi C. T., Segat H. J., Silva H., Veit J. C., Piccolo J., Emanuelli T., Bürger M. E., Silva-Lima B., Rodrigues L. M. (2015). 'Oral supplementation with fish oil reduces dryness and pruritus in the acetone-induced dry skin rat model.' *Journal of Dermatological Science, 79*(3), 298–304. https://doi.org/10.1016/J.JDERMSCI.2015.06.015

39 Kendall, A. C., Kiezel-Tsugunova, M., Brownbridge, L. C., Harwood, J. L. and Nicolaou, A. (2017). 'Lipid functions in skin: Differential effects of n-3 polyunsaturated fatty acids on cutaneous ceramides, in a human skin organ culture model.' *Biochimica et Biophysica Acta*, 1859(9 Part B), 1679. https://doi.org/10.1016/J.BBAMEM.2017.03.016

40 Schlichte, M. J., Vandersall, A. and Katta, R. (2016). 'Diet and eczema: a review of dietary supplements for the treatment of atopic dermatitis.' *Dermatology Practical & Conceptual, 6*(3): 23–29. https://doi:10.5826/dpc.0603a06

41 Hodges, R. E. and Minich, D. M. (2015). 'Modulation of Metabolic Detoxification Pathways Using Foods and Food-Derived Components: A Scientific Review with Clinical Application.' *Journal of Nutrition and Metabolism*. https://doi.org/10.1155/2015/760689

42 Rajan T. V., Tennen H., Lindquist R. L., Cohen L., Clive J. (2002). 'Effect of ingestion of honey on symptoms of rhinoconjunctivitis.' *Annals of Allergy, Asthma & Immunology: Official Publication of the American College of Allergy, Asthma, & Immunology*, 88(2), 198–203. https://doi.org/10.1016/S1081-1206(10)61996-5

43 Costa D. J., Marteau P., Amouyal M., Poulsen L. K., Hamelmann E., Cazaubiel M., Housez B., Leuillet S., Stavnsbjerg M., Molimard P., Courau S., Bousquet J. (2014). 'Efficacy and safety of the probiotic *Lactobacillus paracasei* LP-33 in allergic rhinitis: a double-blind, randomized, placebo-controlled trial (GA2LEN Study).' *European Journal of Clinical Nutrition, 68*(5), 602–607. https://doi.org/10.1038/EJCN.2014.13

44 Wickens K., Barthow C., Mitchell E. A., Kang J., van Zyl N., Purdie G., Stanley T., Fitzharris P., Murphy R., Crane J. (2018). 'Effects of *Lactobacillus rhamnosus* HN001 in early life on the cumulative prevalence of allergic disease to 11 years.' *Pediatric Allergy and Immunology: Official Publication of the European Society of Pediatric Allergy and Immunology*, 29(8), 808–814. https://doi.org/10.1111/PAI.12982

44 Ouwehand A. C., Nermes M., Collado M. C., Rautonen N., Salminen S., Isolauri E. (2009). 'Specific probiotics alleviate allergic rhinitis during the birch pollen season.' *World Journal of Gastroenterology*, 15(26), 3261–3268. https://doi.org/10.3748/WJG.15.3261

CHAPTER 14

1 Perricone, C. and Shoenfeld, Y. (2019). 'Mosaic of autoimmunity: The novel factors of autoimmune diseases.' *Mosaic of Autoimmunity: The Novel Factors of Autoimmune Diseases*, 1–728. https://doi.org/10.1016/C2017-0-01127-8
2 Mazzone, R., Zwergel, C., Artico, M., Taurone, S., Ralli, M., Greco, A. and Mai, A. (2019). 'The emerging role of epigenetics in human autoimmune disorders.' *Clinical Epigenetics* 11(1), 1–15. https://doi.org/10.1186/S13148-019-0632-2
3 Khan M.F., Wang G. (2018). 'Environmental Agents, Oxidative Stress and Autoimmunity.' *Current Opinion in Toxicology*, 7, 22–27. https://doi.org/10.1016/J.COTOX.2017.10.012
4 Shamriz O., Shoenfeld Y. (2018). 'Infections: a double-edge sword in autoimmunity.' *Current Opinion in Rheumatology*, 30(4), 365–372. https://doi.org/10.1097/BOR.000000000
0000490
5 Stojanovich L., Marisavljevich D. (2008). 'Stress as a trigger of autoimmune disease.' *Autoimmunity Reviews*, 7(3), 209–213. https://doi.org/10.1016/J.AUTREV.2007.11.007
6 Sharif, K., Watad, A., Coplan, L., Lichtbroun, B., Krosser, A., Lichtbroun, M., Bragazzi, N. L., Amital, H., Afek, A. and Shoenfeld, Y. (2018). 'The role of stress in the mosaic of autoimmunity: An overlooked association.' *Autoimmunity Reviews*, 17(10), 967–983. https://doi.org/10.1016/J.AUTREV.2018.04.005
7 Roberts, A. L., Malspeis, S., Kubzansky, L. D., Feldman, C. H., Chang, S.-C., Koenen, K. C. and Costenbader, K. H. (2017). 'Association of Trauma and Posttraumatic Stress Disorder with Incident Systemic Lupus Erythematosus in a Longitudinal Cohort of Women.' *Arthritis & Rheumatology*, 69(11), 2162–2169. https://doi.org/10.1002/art.40222
8 Dube, S. R., Fairweather, D., Pearson, W. S., Felitti, V. J., Anda, R. F. and Croft, J. B. (2009). 'Cumulative Childhood Stress and Autoimmune Diseases in Adults.' *Psychosomatic Medicine*, 71(2), 243. https://doi.org/10.1097/PSY.0B013E3181907888
9 Berube, L. T., Kiely, M., Yazici, Y. and Woolf, K. (2017). 'Diet quality of individuals with rheumatoid arthritis using the Healthy Eating Index (HEI)-2010.' http://Dx.Doi.Org/10.1177/0260106016688223, 23(1), 17–24. https://doi.org/10.1177/0260106016688223
10 Rondanelli, M., Perdoni, F., Peroni, G., Caporali, R., Gasparri, C., Riva, A., Petrangolini, G., Faliva, M. A., Infantino, V., Naso, M., Perna, S. and Rigon, C. (2021). 'Ideal food pyramid for patients with rheumatoid arthritis: A narrative review.' *Clinical Nutrition*, 40(3), 661–689. https://doi.org/10.1016/J.CLNU.2020.08.020
11 Philippou, E. and Nikiphorou, E. (2018). 'Are we really what we eat? Nutrition and its role in the onset of rheumatoid arthritis.' *Autoimmunity Reviews*, 17(11), 1074–1077. https://doi.org/10.1016/J.AUTREV.2018.05.009
12 Versini M., Jeandel P. Y., Rosenthal E., Shoenfeld Y. (2014). 'Obesity in autoimmune diseases: not a passive bystander.' *Autoimmunity Reviews*, 13(9), 981–1000. https://doi.org/10.1016/J.AUTREV.2014.07.001
13 SC, B. and YH, L. (2019). 'Causal association between body mass index and risk of rheumatoid arthritis: A Mendelian randomization study.' *European Journal of Clinical Investigation*, 49(4). https://doi.org/10.1111/ECI.13076
14 Xu, H., Liu, M., Cao, J., Li, X., Fan, D., Xia, Y., Lu, X., Li, J., Ju, D., Zhao, H. and Guan, Q. (2019). 'The Dynamic Interplay between the Gut Microbiota and Autoimmune Diseases.' *Journal of Immunology Research*, 2019. https://doi.org/10.1155/2019/7546047

15 Fasano A. (2012). 'Zonulin, regulation of tight junctions, and autoimmune diseases.' *Annals of the New York Academy of Sciences*, 1258(1), 25–33. https://doi.org/10.1111/J.1749-6632.2012.06538.X

16 Sturgeon C., Fasano A. (2016). 'Zonulin, a regulator of epithelial and endothelial barrier functions, and its involvement in chronic inflammatory diseases.' *Tissue Barriers*, 4(4). https://doi.org/10.1080/21688370.2016.1251384

17 Rondanelli, M., Perdoni, F., Peroni, G., Caporali, R., Gasparri, C., Riva, A., Petrangolini, G., Faliva, M. A., Infantino, V., Naso, M., Perna, S. and Rigon, C. (2021). 'Ideal food pyramid for patients with rheumatoid arthritis: A narrative review.' *Clinical Nutrition*, 40(3), 661–689. https://doi.org/10.1016/J.CLNU.2020.08.020

18 Xu, H., Liu, M., Cao, J., Li, X., Fan, D., Xia, Y., Lu, X., Li, J., Ju, D., Zhao, H. and Guan, Q. (2019). 'The Dynamic Interplay between the Gut Microbiota and Autoimmune Diseases.' *Journal of Immunology Research*, 2019. https://doi.org/10.1155/2019/7546047

19 Philippou, E. and Nikiphorou, E. (2018). 'Are we really what we eat? Nutrition and its role in the onset of rheumatoid arthritis.' *Autoimmunity Reviews*, 17(11), 1074–1077. https://doi.org/10.1016/J.AUTREV.2018.05.009

20 Khan H., Sureda A., Belwal T., Çetinkaya S., Süntar İ., Tejada S., Devkota H. P., Ullah H., Aschner M. (2019). 'Polyphenols in the treatment of autoimmune diseases.' *Autoimmunity Reviews*, 18(7), 647–657. https://doi.org/10.1016/J.AUTREV.2019.05.001

21 Ratnam D .V., Ankola D. D., Bhardwaj V., Sahana D. K., Kumar M. N. (2006). 'Role of antioxidants in prophylaxis and therapy: A pharmaceutical perspective.' *Journal of Controlled Release: Official Journal of the Controlled Release Society*, 113(3), 189–207. https://doi.org/10.1016/J.JCONREL.2006.04.015

22 Pae M., Wu D. (2013). 'Immunomodulating effects of epigallocatechin-3-gallate from green tea: mechanisms and applications.' *Food & Function*, 4(9), 1287–1303. https://doi.org/10.1039/C3FO60076A

23 Bright J. J. (2007). 'Curcumin and autoimmune disease.' *Advances in Experimental Medicine and Biology*, 595, 425–451. https://doi.org/10.1007/978-0-387-46401-5_19

24 Smallwood M. J., Nissim A., Knight A. R., Whiteman M., Haigh R., Winyard P. G. (2018). 'Oxidative stress in autoimmune rheumatic diseases.' *Free Radical Biology & Medicine*, 125, 3–14. https://doi.org/10.1016/J.FREERADBIOMED.2018.05.086

25 Aryaeian N., Shahram F., Mahmoudi M., Tavakoli H., Yousefi B., Arablou T., Jafari Karegar S. (2019). 'The effect of ginger supplementation on some immunity and inflammation intermediate genes expression in patients with active rheumatoid arthritis.' *Gene*, 698, 179–185. https://doi.org/10.1016/J.GENE.2019.01.048

26 Moosavian S. P., Paknahad Z., Habibagahi Z., Maracy M. (2020). The effects of garlic (*Allium sativum*) supplementation on inflammatory biomarkers, fatigue, and clinical symptoms in patients with active rheumatoid arthritis: A randomized, double-blind, placebo-controlled trial.' *Phytotherapy Research: PTR*, 34(11), 2953–2962. https://doi.org/10.1002/PTR.6723

27 Watad, A., Azrielant, S., Bragazzi, N. L., Sharif, K., David, P., Katz, I., Aljadeff, G., Quaresma, M., Tanay, G., Adawi, M., Amital, H. and Shoenfeld, Y. (2017). 'Seasonality and autoimmune diseases: The contribution of the four seasons to the mosaic of autoimmunity.' *Journal of Autoimmunity*, 82, 13–30. https://doi.org/10.1016/J.JAUT.2017.06.001

28 Rondanelli, M., Perdoni, F., Peroni, G., Caporali, R., Gasparri, C., Riva, A., Petrangolini, G., Faliva, M. A., Infantino, V., Naso, M., Perna, S. and Rigon, C. (2021). 'Ideal food

pyramid for patients with rheumatoid arthritis: A narrative review.' *Clinical Nutrition*, 40(3), 661–689. https://doi.org/10.1016/J.CLNU.2020.08.020

29 Gómez-Vaquero C., Nolla J. M., Fiter J., Ramon J. M., Concustell R., Valverde J., Roig-Escofet D.

30 Touger-Decker, R. (1988). 'Nutritional considerations in rheumatoid arthritis.' *Journal of American Dietetic Association*, 88(3) PMID: 3126221.

31 Singh, P., Arora, A., Strand, T. A., Leffler, D. A., Catassi, C., Green, P. H., Kelly, C. P., Ahuja, V. and Makharia, G. K. (2018). 'Global Prevalence of Celiac Disease: Systematic Review and Meta-analysis.' *Clinical Gastroenterology and Hepatology*, 16(6), 823-836.e2. https://doi.org/10.1016/J.CGH.2017.06.037

32 Clemente M. G., De Virgiliis S., Kang J. S., Macatagney R., Musu M. P., Di Pierro M. R., Drago S., Congia M., Fasano A. (2003). 'Early effects of gliadin on enterocyte intracellular signalling involved in intestinal barrier function.' *Gut*, 52(2), 218–223. https://doi.org/10.1136/GUT.52.2.218

33 Barbaro, M. R., Cremon, C., Stanghellini, V. and Barbara, G. (2018). 'Recent advances in understanding non-celiac gluten sensitivity.' *F1000Research*, 7, 1631. https://doi.org/10.12688/f1000research.15849.1

34 Carroccio, A., D'Alcamo, A., Cavataio, F., Soresi, M., Seidita, A., Sciumè, C., Geraci, G., Iacono, G. and Mansueto, P. (2015). 'High Proportions of People with Nonceliac Wheat Sensitivity Have Autoimmune Disease or Antinuclear Antibodies.' *Gastroenterology*, 149(3), 596-603.e1. https://doi.org/10.1053/J.GASTRO.2015.05.040

35 Igbinedion, S. O., Ansari, J., Vasikaran, A., Gavins, F. N., Jordan, P., Boktor, M. and Alexander, J. S. (2017). 'Non-celiac gluten sensitivity: All wheat attack is not celiac.' *Http://Www.Wjgnet.Com/*, 23(40), 7201–7210. https://doi.org/10.3748/WJG.V23.I40.7201

36 Nestel, P. J., Pally, S., MacIntosh, G. L., Greeve, M. A., Middleton, S., Jowett, J. and Meikle, P. J. (2012). 'Circulating inflammatory and atherogenic biomarkers are not increased following single meals of dairy foods.' *European Journal of Clinical Nutrition*, 66, 25–31.

37 Haase S., Wilck N., Kleinewietfeld M., Müller D. N., Linker R. A. (2019). 'Sodium chloride triggers Th17 mediated autoimmunity.' *Journal of Neuroimmunology*, 329, 9–13. https://doi.org/10.1016/J.JNEUROIM.2018.06.016

38 Zhang D., Jin W., Wu R., Li J., Park S. A., Tu E., Zanvit P., Xu J., Liu O., Cain A., Chen W. (2019). 'High Glucose Intake Exacerbates Autoimmunity through Reactive-Oxygen-Species-Mediated TGF-β Cytokine Activation.' *Immunity*, 51(4), 671-681.e5. https://doi.org/10.1016/J.IMMUNI.2019.08.001

39 Lanier, R. K., Gibson, K. D., Cohen, A. E. and Varga, M. (2013). 'Effects of Dietary Supplementation with the Solanaceae Plant Alkaloid Anatabine on Joint Pain and Stiffness: Results from an Internet-Based Survey Study.' *Clinical Medicine Insights. Arthritis and Musculoskeletal Disorders*, 6, 73. https://doi.org/10.4137/CMAMD.S13001

40 Konijeti G. G., Kim N., Lewis J. D., Groven S., Chandrasekaran A., Grandhe S., Diamant C., Singh E., Oliveira G., Wang X., Molparia B., Torkamani A. (2017). 'Efficacy of the Autoimmune Protocol Diet for Inflammatory Bowel Disease.' *Inflammatory Bowel Diseases*, 23(11), 2054–2060. https://doi.org/10.1097/MIB.0000000000001221

41 Chandrasekaran A., Groven S., Lewis J. D., Levy S. S., Diamant C., Singh E., Konijeti G. G. (2019). 'An Autoimmune Protocol Diet Improves Patient-Reported Quality of Life in Inflammatory Bowel Disease.' *Crohn's & Colitis 360*, 1(3). https://doi.org/10.1093/CROCOL/OTZ019

42 RD, A., A, S. and AG, A. (2019). 'Efficacy of the Autoimmune Protocol Diet as Part

of a Multi-disciplinary, Supported Lifestyle Intervention for Hashimoto's Thyroiditis.' *Cureus*, 11(4). https://doi.org/10.7759/CUREUS.4556

43 Choi, I. Y., Piccio, L., Childress, P., Bollman, B., Ghosh, A., Brandhorst, S., Suarez, J., Michalsen, A., Cross, A. H., Morgan, T. E., Wei, M., Paul, F., Bock, M. and Longo, V. D. (2016). 'A Diet Mimicking Fasting Promotes Regeneration and Reduces Autoimmunity and Multiple Sclerosis Symptoms.' *Cell Reports*, 15(10), 2136–2146. https://doi.org/10.1016/J.CELREP.2016.05.009

44 Liu, Y., Liu, S., Zheng, F., Cai, Y., Xie, K. and Zhang, W. (2016). 'Cardiovascular autonomic neuropathy in patients with type 2 diabetes.' *Journal of Diabetes Investigation*, 7(4), 615. https://doi.org/10.1111/JDI.12438

45 Liem, S. I. E., Meessen, J. M. T. A., Wolterbeek, R., Marsan, N. A., Ninaber, M. K., Vlieland, T. P. M. V. and Vries-Bouwstra, J. K. de. (2018). 'Physical activity in patients with systemic sclerosis.' *Rheumatology International*, 38(3), 443. https://doi.org/10.1007/S00296-017-3879-Y

46 An, H. J., Tizaoui, K., Terrazzino, S., Cargnin, S., Lee, K. H., Nam, S. W., Kim, J. S., Yang, J. W., Lee, J. Y., Smith, L., Koyanagi, A., Jacob, L., Li, H., Shin, J. I. and Kronbichler, A. (2020). 'Sarcopenia in Autoimmune and Rheumatic Diseases: A Comprehensive Review.' *International Journal of Molecular Sciences*, 21(16), 1–21. https://doi.org/10.3390/IJMS21165678

Index

acetate 127, 128, 136
acetic acid 94
acetylcholine (Ach) 194
acrylamides 258
adrenal glands 201, 202
adrenalin 201, 202
advanced glycaemic end products (AGEs) 91
ageing 17, 26, 84, 91, 92, 133
  effect of mitochondria on 87, 88
  immunological 27–9, 31, 83, 88, 325–6
aggregation of marginal gains 59
air quality 259, 262–3, 299
Akkermansia muciniphila 136
alcohol 124, 130, 133, 264, 317
alkaloids 343
allergic rhinitis *see* hay fever
allergies 23, 294–324
  allergic reactions 304–5
  biopsychosocial support 324
  diet, gut health and natural remedies 317–23
  increased frequency of 295–300
  sensitisation 303
  taking action against 314–17
  testing for 305–63
alliums 114–15
allostatic load 32, 39, 91
almonds: broccoli, garlic, almonds and preserved lemons 163–4
amino acids 118, 119, 228, 265–6, 284
antecedents, predisposing 36
anthocyanidins 112
anti-adhesins 289–90
antibiotics 130, 133, 286, 287, 332
antibodies 280, 281, 284, 325
antigens 16, 330, 353
antihistamines 304, 314, 316–17, 320
antimicrobials, nutritional 287–90
antioxidants 26, 104, 107, 109, 113, 117, 124, 229, 265, 286, 289, 318, 343
antipyretics 281–2
anxiety 37, 75, 252
appetite 75, 90, 100–1, 117, 193, 203, 284, 339
artichokes: artichoke tart 171–2
  watercress, pea and artichoke soup 161–2
astaxanthin 117, 118, 188
asthma 294, 295, 296, 299, 300, 304, 308, 315
ATP 86, 87
autoimmune diseases (AD) 23, 31, 88, 325–56
  anti-inflammatory eating for life 84, 85, 337–47
  autoimmune diet protocol (AIP) 345–6
  cause of 327–33
  definition 325–7
  elimination and restrictive diets 341–6, 347
  exercise and 348–51
  fasting 346–7
  flare ups 353–6
  leaky gut and 132, 332
  thriving with 333–7
autophagy 346

B cells 16, 17, 279–80, 303
β-glucans 116, 289
bacteria 126, 152, 273
balance 21–31
beans 118, 318
beef: cottage pie with a twist 178–9
  less-meat meatballs 184–5
beliefs 37, 65–6, 78–9
berries: cranachan 190–1
betacarotene 107, 161
Bifidobacterium 139, 290, 322, 340
biodiversity: improving your inner 133–6, 137, 141
  reduced biodiversity theory 297–8
bioflavonoids 135, 285, 319
biophilia hypothesis 246–7, 252
biotransformation 127
bitter taste 122–4
blood sugar 87, 88, 89–95, 101, 117, 119, 120, 202, 235, 331
body burden 254, 265, 329
body composition 96–102, 215, 226, 278
body mass index (BMI) 99, 331
bone marrow 30–1, 113
boundaries, healthy 336–7
the brain 192–214
  brain fog 87, 91, 341, 353
breath 206, 207, 292
broccoli 321
  broccoli, garlic, almonds and preserved lemons 163–4
broccoli sprouts 154–5, 163
brodo, feel-better 157–8
bromelain 293, 320
butyrate 127, 128–9

calories 80, 81, 97, 98, 104, 126
candida dysbiosis 131
capers, potato dischetti with anchovy 165–6
carbohydrates 93, 119–20, 122, 145, 126, 227
cardio exercise 223–5
cat-cow 220
chamomile 319
champit 167
chaos, reducing 248–50
chicken: feel-better brodo 157–8
chickpea (gram) flour: savoury crepes 182–3
chickpeas, roasted 186–7
chocolate 112
  granola florentines 189
chronic disease 2, 109, 271

flavonoids and 111
inflammation and 23, 151
and stress 203
chronic inflammation 23–4, 25, 27, 88, 102, 130–3, 151
cinnamon 94
circadian rhythms 75, 237, 238, 241, 244, 299–300, 310
citrus bioflavonoids 285
citrus flavanones 339
cleaning supplies 262
clutter 249–50, 261
co-morbidity 278, 331
coeliac disease 341–2
compassion, self- 76, 142, 143, 199–200, 210, 229–30, 310, 314, 348
consistency 57, 58–60, 61
control, taking 249–50
cooking 146, 151, 155
cortisol 201, 202, 205, 237–8, 247, 249
cottage pie with a twist 178–9
COVID-19 5, 23, 24, 57, 273, 274
antihistamines and 301
effect of nitric oxide on 114
future-proofing our fitness 217
importance of healthy immune system 27, 28, 104
lessons from a post-COVID world 67–9
mental-health crisis 193
spike proteins 274
spreading germs 277, 278
and suboptimal metabolic health 88–9
cranachan 190–1
cravings 75, 76, 91
crepes, savoury 182–3
curcumin 293, 339
curcuminoids 288
curries: curried vegetables 167–8
slow-cooker curry 176–7
cytokines 16, 28, 193, 199, 282, 283, 303, 339

dairy 342
damage-associated molecular patterns (DAMPs) 87
damp 262, 310
decluttering 249, 250–1
detoxification 263–6
DEXA (dual-energy X-ray absorptiometry) scans 99–100
dicarbonyls 91
diet 28–9, 37, 74–85
allergies and 317–23
anti-inflammatory eating for life 331, 337–47
diet patterns 83–5
dietary hazards 258–9
elimination and restrictive diets 341–6, 347
immune-nourishing nutrition 103–91
infections and 278, 292–3
metabolic health and 87, 89
nutrition, diet and gut-health assessment 44–6
your relationship with food 75–9
diversions, creating pleasant 251
dopamine 193–4, 198
downward dog 222
drugs, prescription 264, 271–2
dust 261
dust mites 294, 300, 310, 315
dysbiosis 130–1, 132, 135–6, 298, 332

eating 250
emotional 75–6
high-value eating 108–24
mindful 77, 133
overeating 75, 77, 104, 133, 151
ecotherapy 207–8
eczema (allergic dermatitis) 294, 295, 296, 299, 304, 306–13, 317, 321, 324
elimination diets 341–6, 347
endotoxins 132, 332
environment 87
allergies and 296–300
autoimmune diseases 328–33, 353
blueprint for 266–8
curating a healthy 245–68
environment assessment 52–3
environmental pollution 113
simplifying for better health 250–1
epigallocatechin-3-gallate (EGCG) 339
epigenetics 33–4, 111, 128–9, 154, 328
epinephrine 193–4
exercise 37, 133, 209, 215–35, 241, 250
and autoimmune diseases 348–51
and blood sugar levels 92, 94
exercise snacking 230, 235
fifteen-minute exercise 210–11
ten-minute morning mobility ritual 219–22
exposome 35, 82

fasting 346–7
fat, body 88, 90, 96–8, 99–100
fatigue 87, 203, 240, 291–2, 341, 348, 353, 355
fats 119–20, 133, 145, 347
fatty acids 97, 321
feel-better brodo 157–8
fermented foods 138, 140–1, 145, 155–6
fevers 87, 280–1
fibre 93, 118, 122, 126, 133, 134–5, 137, 141, 147, 188, 318, 342, 347
filaggrin 307–8, 321
fish 117, 118, 121, 144, 259, 293, 340
fresh anchovy fritto misto 169–70
potato dischetti with anchovy capers 165–6
flavanols 112
flavanones 112, 339
flavones 112
flavonoids 111–12, 189, 265, 318–19
flavonols 111, 161
flavour 145, 151–2
florentines, granola 189
folate 113, 126
food 74–85, 277
allergies 294, 295, 296, 308, 323
anti-inflammatory eating for life 331, 337–47
controversial foods 341–7
diet patterns 83–5
fermented foods 140–1, 155–6
food toxins 258–9
immune-nourishing nutrition 103–91
immunity-focused plates 145–8
seasonal 151–2
toxic food environment 79–83
your relationship with 75–9
food diaries 94, 142–4, 148
fragrance 261–2
free radicals 26, 27, 111, 113
fritto misto, fresh anchovy 169–70
fruit 109, 113, 145, 146, 147, 152

garlic 288, 339
broccoli, garlic, almonds and preserved lemons 163–4

Nonna's roasted tomato soup 159–60
genetics 16, 32
allergies and 295–6
autoimmune diseases 327, 328, 332
and body composition 100
epigenetics 33–4, 111, 128–9, 154, 328
immunodeficiency 275
predisposing antecedents 36
germs 276–81, 289
ghrelin 100–1
ginger 94, 339
glucose 89, 90, 93
glucosinolates 114, 154, 155, 266
gluten 341–2, 344
glycine 265–6
glycogen 224, 227
goals 40, 56–7, 59–60, 65, 66
achieving 69
food diaries and 143
identifying 60
limiting factors 150, 213
nutritional 347
setting 63–5, 148–50, 211–12, 232–3, 242–4, 267–8
SMART goals 64–5
granola florentines 189
gut health 125–41, 147
allergies and 297–8, 317–23
antibiotics 287
assessment of 44–6
and autoimmune diseases 331–2, 340
benefits of probiotics 138–41
and chronic inflammation 130–3
gut-immune axis 126–9
improving your inner biodiversity 133–6, 137, 141
organic produce and 152
sensitive guts 137
gut microbiota (GM) 125–41, 147, 318
allergies and 297–8
antibiotics 287
and autoimmune diseases 331–2, 340
and blood-sugar control 92
effect of the environment on 248
effect of NNS on 95
effect of UPFs on 81
fibre and 93, 122
reduced biodiversity theory 297–8

habits 60–3, 65, 66, 69, 143, 313
hayfever 294, 295, 296, 299, 300–6, 317, 318, 320, 324
health-related quality of life score (HRQOL) 85
heart rate variability (HRV) 195
hematopoietic stem cells 30–1
herbs 113, 145
heterocyclic amines 258
histamine 161, 296, 298, 301, 304–5, 318, 319, 322, 323
HLA (human leukocyte antigens) 16–17, 328
homeostasis 17, 292–3
honey 287–8, 321–2
hormetic stress tools 208–9
hormones 37, 75, 92, 97, 100–1, 120, 126, 193, 197, 264, 354
see also individual hormones
hunger 75, 76, 77, 100–1
hydration 124, 226, 266, 282, 283
hygiene 277, 278, 297
hypothalamic-pituitary-adrenal (HPA) axis 201, 202

identity 66
IgE antibodies 296, 303, 304, 306, 319, 324
immune cells: autoimmune diseases 325
bitter taste receptors 123
cytokine production 199
fat and 97
gut microbiota and 125, 126–7
infections and 274–5, 283
metabolic syndrome and 88
mitochondria in 86–7
phytonutrients and 110
production of 30, 54
protein and 117
immunobiography 32–53, 335
immunodeficiency 275
immunological ageing 27–9, 31, 83, 88, 325–6
immunometabolism 86–8
immunonutrition blueprint 141–50
immuno-plasticity 32
immunosenescent cells 28, 31
immunotoxicology 252–68
indoor spaces 246, 248–50
indoor hazards 259–62
infections 28, 273–93
autoimmune diseases 329–30
fighting 279–86
preventing 276–9
pro-resolution and the road back to health 291–3
probiotics for 290
protection 277–8

inflammation 17, 21, 87, 91
anti-inflammatory eating for life 85, 337–47
assessment 41–3
balancing 21–3, 25
and the brain 193–5
chronic 23–4, 25, 27, 88, 130–3, 151
effect of diet on 84, 97, 109
fever as sign of 280–1
flavonoids and 111
lowering baseline 54–5
oxidative stress and 26–7
signs of acute 21–2
switching off 194
vicious cycle of 24
innate immunity 16–17
insulin 90, 91, 92
interleukin 282, 303
intra-epithelial lymphocytes (IELs) 115
isoflavones 112
isothiocyanates 114–15, 154, 266

kefir 140, 141
kimchi 140, 141, 155
savoury crepes 182–3
kindness, self- 65–7, 201
kitchari 180–1

lactate 129
Lactobacillus 138, 139, 141, 152, 155, 290, 322, 340
lactoferrin 289
lactoperoxidase 289
leafy greens 113–14, 123, 145, 318
leaky gut 131–2, 332
leeks, jewelled 174–5
legumes 135, 137, 145
lentils: less-meat meatballs 184–5
slow-cooker curry 176–7
leptin 100, 101
letting go 336
leucine 118, 228
lifestyle: changes to 54–5, 68, 272
improving your gut microbiota 133
metabolic health and 87, 89
work-life balance 68
limiting factors 150, 213
liver 132, 253, 321
long-latency deficiency diseases 110, 111
lycopene 159, 343
lymphatic fluid 121, 124, 292

macronutrients 84, 119–20
see also carbohydrates; fats; protein

magnesium 113, 318
mast cells 296, 299–300, 303, 304, 305, 310, 319, 321
meals 76, 94
meatballs, less-meat 184–5
mediators 37–8
medication 271–2
meditation 206–7, 291
Mediterranean diet (MD) 84, 159–60, 338
melatonin 237, 238
mental health 46–8, 192–214, 326
metabolic health 86–102, 126, 215
metallic compounds 259
methylation 31, 34, 91, 113
microbiome *see* gut microbiota (GM)
microglia 193, 194
micronutrients 84, 118, 126, 229
 deficiencies in 278
 supplements 104–8
 see also individual micronutrients
mindfulness 200–1, 204, 206–7
 mindful eating 77, 133
mindset 241, 248
mitochondria 86–8, 102, 229
mobility 218–22
 ten-minute morning mobility ritual 219–22
momentum 223–5
monounsaturated fats 121, 145
motivation 57, 58, 59, 60–4, 66, 67, 144, 193–4, 213, 229, 234, 249
mould 310, 315
movement *see* exercise
mucus 135–6, 283, 286, 320
muscle mass 90, 101–2, 227
 and blood sugar levels 94
 breakdown of 284
 as indication of health 96
 sarcopenia 102
 strength training 222–3, 349–50
mushrooms 116, 289
myconutrients 115–16
myrosinase 154, 155

N-Acetylcysteine (NAC) 288–9, 320–1
nature 246–8, 291
nervous system 194, 195, 196–7, 206, 207, 225, 252
nettles 320
neuroinflammation 193–4
nightshades 343
nitric oxide (NO) 113–14
nitrosamines 258
noise pollution 251–2
non-exercise activity thermogenesis (NEAT) 217
non-nutritive sweeteners (NNS) 95
Nonna's roasted tomato soup 159–60
nutrition: anti-inflammatory eating for life 337–47
 fatigue and 241–2
 fuelling 119–24
 immune-nourishing 103–91
 and infections 278, 282, 284, 292–3
 nutrition assessment 44–6
 nutritional agnosticism 78–9, 85
 nutritional antimicrobials 287–90
 protective nutrition 109–17
 strengthening nutrition 117–19
 your immunonutrition blueprint 141–50

oatmeal: lemon oatmeal 173–5
 oatcakes 188
oats: cranachan 190–1
 granola florentines 189
obesity 96, 97–8, 99, 151, 299, 331
olive oil 121–2, 153, 159
omega-3 120–1, 144, 173, 188, 278, 293, 321, 339, 340
omega-6 120–1, 321
oral allergy symptoms (OAS) 302–3, 319
oregano oil 287
organic produce 152, 259
outdoor spaces 246–8
oxidative stress 26, 107, 111, 113, 292
autoimmune diseases 325–6, 354
 detoxification 265
 food toxins and 257, 258
 hormetic responses and 209
 intermittent fasting 346
 mitochondria 87, 88
 NAC and 320
 phytonutrients and 110
 senescent immune cells and 28
 sulforaphane and 154, 339

pathogens 152, 273, 276–9, 285, 328
peas: watercress, pea and artichoke soup 161–2
permaculture 19–20
persistent organic pollutants (POPs) 260
personality 196–7, 330
phthalates 260, 261
phytochemicals 108, 167, 338
phytoncides 247
phytonutrients 108, 110–12, 113, 132, 163, 176, 189, 209, 293, 321, 343
 and bitter taste 123
 glucosinolates 154, 155, 266
 herbal teas 124
 herbs 145
 rainbow colours 148
 and SCFA production 134
plants 146, 252, 262–3
plastics 258–9, 262
pollen 300–1, 302, 303, 305, 306, 310, 315, 321–2
pollution 87, 254
 air 259, 299
 environmental 113
 indoor 259–62
 noise 251–2
polycyclic aromatic hydrocarbons 258
polyphenols 121, 136, 265, 286, 318, 338
polyunsaturated fats 120–1, 145
pomegranate 319, 338
 jewelled leeks 174–5
postbiotics 127, 134, 165, 176
potatoes: cottage pie with a twist 178–9
 potato dischetti with anchovy capers 165–6
 summer salad 174
prebiotics 135, 137, 338
prefrontal cortex 61, 213
probiotics 138–41, 152, 155, 290, 322–3, 340
product labels 261, 309
propionate 127, 129
protein 93, 102, 117–19, 145, 147, 227, 278, 284
pulses 117–19, 135, 318
pyrexia 280–1

quercetin 111, 266, 285, 318–19, 320
quorum sensor inhibitors 289

recovery 226–8, 351
remedies, natural 317–23
resilience 25–7, 63, 210
rest 50–1, 69, 208, 229, 236–44, 283, 291
resting-squat sit 220–1
rice: kitchari 180–1

Saccharomyces boulardii 139
salads: baby turnip salad 168
 summer salad 174

salt 342, 347
salutogenesis 6–7
sarcopenia 102, 119, 350
satiety 77, 80, 100–1, 117, 119, 126
secretory IgA antibodies 127, 131, 206–7
sedentary behaviour 29, 68, 215–16, 217
  and blood sugar levels 94
  breaking up 234–5
  and gut dysbiosis 130
  sarcopenia and 102
seeds: granola florentines 189
  sprouting 154–5
selenium 285–6, 318
self-acceptance 271
self-advocacy 334–5
self-care 197–201, 282, 311–13, 351–2
self-compassion 76, 142, 143, 199–200, 210, 229–30, 310, 314, 348
self-efficacy 55–7, 59, 64
senescent immune cells 28, 31
sensitisation 303
serotonin 193, 198
short-chain fatty acids (SCFAs) 127, 128–9, 131, 134, 136, 138
short-latency-deficiency diseases 110
shoulder mobility 221–2
skin allergies 24, 306–13, 324
sleep 87, 193, 236–44, 356
  alcohol and 124
  allergies and 299, 310, 324
  effect on gut biodiversity 133
  and infection fighting 282–3
  and obesity 98
  restorative 292
  sleep disorders 326
  sleep and rest assessment 50–1
  and stress 203
small intestinal bacterial overgrown (SIBO) 81, 131
SMART goals 64–5, 148
smoking 29, 87, 130, 215, 260, 298–9, 329
snacking 133, 143
social pressure 75, 79
social support 149, 211, 232, 243
soups: feel-better brodo 157–8
  Nonna's roasted tomato soup 159–60
  watercress, pea and artichoke soup 161–2
spices 113, 145
Spiderman lunge to thoracic rotation 221
split yellow mung beans: kitchari 180–1
sprouting 154–5
stress 29, 37, 67, 201–9, 240, 249
  alcohol and 124
  allergies and 310, 324
  autoimmune diseases and 330, 352, 354
  and blood-sugar control 92
  eczema and 313
  effect on appetite 75, 76
  effect on gut health 130, 133
  environmental 245
  and exposure to nature 247
  infection risk 278
  long-term effects of 202–3
  managing 151, 203–9, 336–7, 252
  and obesity 98
  post-traumatic 192, 330
sugar 89–95, 331, 342, 347
sulforaphane 154, 155, 163, 293, 339
sulphur 114–15
summer salad 174
sunlight 237, 238, 244
supplements 104–8, 285–6, 289, 293
  allergies and 318–19
  auto-immune diseases 340
  probiotics 138, 139–40
  see also vitamins
sweat 253, 283
sweeteners 95

T cells 16, 17, 128, 274, 279–80, 281, 283, 296, 303, 334, 353–4
tart, artichoke 171–2
teas, herbal 124
technology 68
time management 241
tiredness 240–2
tomatoes: less-meat meatballs 184–5
  Nonna's roasted tomato soup 159–60
toxins 29, 245, 329
  biotransformation 127
  detoxification 263–6
  immunotoxicology 252–68
  levels of 255–6
  terminology 253–4
  top toxins 256–62
  toxic food environment 79–83
triggers 37, 62–3, 192
  for autoimmune diseases 328–33, 354, 355–6
  for eczema 309–10
  for emotional eating 75, 76
turmeric 176, 266, 288, 321
turnips 167

ultra-processed foods (UPFs) 79, 80–2, 83, 93, 98, 122, 146, 151, 342, 347
ultradian rhythms 241

vagus nerve 194, 207, 208–9
vegetables 109, 113, 135, 146, 152
  bitter taste 123–4
  cottage pie with a twist 178–9
  cruciferous 114–15, 154–5, 266, 321
  fermenting 155–6
  leafy greens 113–14
  recommended daily amount 145, 147
  root veggies four ways 167–8
  seasonal 152
  steaming 155
vinegar 94
visceral fat 98, 99
vitamins 105, 106, 107, 278
  vitamin A 113, 133, 161, 279
  vitamin B12 106, 118, 126
  vitamin C 110, 133, 159, 161, 285, 318, 319, 343
  vitamin D 106, 107–8, 116, 120, 133, 173, 279, 318, 339, 340, 354
  vitamin P 111–12, 145
volatile organic compounds (VOCs) 260, 261, 262, 263

walking 217, 224, 225, 228, 232, 247
watercress, pea and artichoke soup 161–2
weight 96, 97
wellbeing 8, 58, 192, 248
  autoimmune diseases 326
  future-proofing 67–9
  mental wellbeing assessment 46–8
  movement and 216
  subjective 197–8
white blood cells 16, 30
willpower 57, 62, 76, 144, 193, 230
work-life balance 68
xenobiotics 253, 254, 262, 263–4

yoghurt: cranachan 190–1

zinc 133, 285, 318
zoonutrients 117, 118

About the Author

Dr Jenna Macciochi specialises in understanding how nutrition and lifestyle interact with the immune system in health and disease. With over 20 years' experience she is on a mission to break down the science behind our health and share the secrets of how to be well, for good. Based in Brighton, Jenna is a lecturer at Sussex University, a qualified fitness instructor and health coach and author of *Immunity: The Science of Staying Well.* She is a mother of young twins and a keen home cook, creating recipes and rituals inspired by her farm-to-table Scottish roots and capturing her family's Italian heritage.